T0382683

Medication-Resistant Epilepsy

Fifty million people worldwide have epilepsy and yet up to 35% of patients experience seizures that are resistant to anti-epileptic drugs. Patients with medication-resistant epilepsy have increased risks of premature death, psychosocial dysfunction and a reduced quality of life. This key resource delivers guidance for all clinicians involved in caring for patients with medication-resistant epilepsy in order to reduce these risks.

Covering the epidemiology, biology, causes and potential treatments for medication-resistant epilepsy, this definitive and focused text reviews the clinical care needs of patients. Guidance is practical and includes treatment for specialized groups including paediatric patients and those with psychiatric comorbidities. Several promising non-pharmacologic interventions available for patients, such as surgery, neuromodulation diet therapy and botanical treatment, are explored in detail. Leading international figures from a range of disciplines bring their expertise together holistically in this essential manual.

John M. Stern is a Professor and Director of the Epilepsy Clinical Program in the Department of Neurology at the Geffen School of Medicine at UCLA, Los Angeles, USA.

Raman Sankar is Chief of Pediatric Neurology and Distinguished Professor in the Departments of Neurology and Pediatrics at the Geffen School of Medicine at UCLA, Los Angeles, USA.

Michael Sperling is Baldwin Keyes Professor of Neurology and Director of the Jefferson Comprehensive Epilepsy Center at the Sidney Kimmel Medical College at Thomas Jefferson University, Philadelphia, USA.

Medication-Resistant Epilepsy

Diagnosis and Treatment

Edited by

John M. Stern
Department of Neurology, Geffen School of Medicine at UCLA, Los Angeles, CA

Raman Sankar
Departments of Neurology and Pediatrics, Geffen School of Medicine at UCLA, Los Angeles, CA

Michael Sperling, Associate Editor
Jefferson Hospital for Neurosciences, Philadelphia, PA

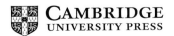

CAMBRIDGE
UNIVERSITY PRESS

CAMBRIDGE
UNIVERSITY PRESS

University Printing House, Cambridge CB2 8BS, United Kingdom

One Liberty Plaza, 20th Floor, New York, NY 10006, USA

477 Williamstown Road, Port Melbourne, VIC 3207, Australia

314–321, 3rd Floor, Plot 3, Splendor Forum, Jasola District Centre, New Delhi – 110025, India

79 Anson Road, #06–04/06, Singapore 079906

Cambridge University Press is part of the University of Cambridge.

It furthers the University's mission by disseminating knowledge in the pursuit of education, learning, and research at the highest international levels of excellence.

www.cambridge.org
Information on this title: www.cambridge.org/9781107139886
DOI: 10.1017/9781316492376

First published 2020

Printed in the United Kingdom by TJ International Ltd, Padstow Cornwall

A catalogue record for this publication is available from the British Library.

ISBN 978-1-107-13988-6 Hardback

Contents

Contents

Contributors

Kofi-Buaku Atsina MD
Clinical neuroradiology fellow at Penn Health System, Univeristy of Pennsylvania, PA, USA

Pauls Auce PhD
Walton Centre, NHS Foundation Trust, Liverpool, UK

Charles E. Begley PhD
School of Public Health, The University of Texas Health Science Center, Houston, TX, USA

Felix Benninger MD
Rabin Medical Center, Campus Beilinson, Sackler Faculty of Medicine, Tel Aviv University, Israel

Jeffrey W. Britton MD
Department of Neurology, Mayo Clinic, Rochester, MN, USA

Martin J. Brodie PhD
Epilepsy Unit, West Glasgow ACH-Yorkhill, Glasgow, Scotland, UK

Krzyszof A. Bujarski MD
Dartmouth-Hitchcock Epilepsy Center, Geisel School of Medicine at Dartmouth, NH, USA

Russell J. Buono PhD
Cooper Medical School of Rowan University, NJ, USA

Fahmida Amin Chowdhury MBChB, MRCP, PhD
Department of Clinical Neurophysiology, National Hospital for Neurology and Neurosurgery, Queen Square, London, UK

Amy Crepeau MD
Department of Neurology, Mayo Clinic, Scottsdale, AZ, USA

Beate Diehl MD, PhD, FRCP
Department of Clinical and Experimental Epilepsy, University College London Institute of Neurology, and Department of Clinical Neurophysiology,

National Hospital for Neurology and Neurosurgery, Queen Square, London, UK

Jerome Engel Jr MD, PhD
Departments of Neurology, Neurobiology and Psychiatry and Biobehavioral Sciences and the Brain Research Institute, David Geffen School of Medicine at UCLA, Los Angeles, CA, USA

Amr Ewida MD
Department of Neurology, Upstate Medical University, Syracuse, NY, USA

Thomas N. Ferraro PhD
Cooper Medical School of Rowan University, NJ, USA

Anteneh M. Feyissa MD, MSc
Department of Neurology, Mayo Clinic, Jacksonville, FL, USA

Bradford D. Fischer PhD
Cooper Medical School of Rowan University, NJ, USA

Cynthia Harden MD
Department of Neurology, Icahn School of Medicine at Mount Sinai, New York, NY, USA

Christianne Heck MD
Department of Neurology, University of Southern California, CA, USA

Christian Hoelscher MD
Sidney Kimmel Medical College, Thomas Jefferson University, PA, USA

Martin Holtkamp MD
Epilepsy-Center Berlin-Brandenburg, Department of Neurology, Charité – Universitätsmedizin Berlin, Berlin, Germany

Shin Jeong PhD
School of Public Health, The University of Texas Health Science Center, Houston, TX, USA

Barbara C. Jobst MD, PhD
Dartmouth-Hitchcock Epilepsy Center,
Geisel School of Medicine at Dartmouth, NH,
USA

Colin B. Josephson MD, MSc
Department of Clinical Neurosciences, Cumming
School of Medicine, University of Calgary, Calgary,
AB, Canada

Andres M. Kanner MD
Comprehensive Epilepsy Center and Epilepsy
Division, Department of Neurology, University of
Miami, Miller School of Medicine, FL, USA

Ritu Kapur PhD
NeuroPace, Inc., Mountain View, CA, USA

Sung-Eun Kim MD, PhD
Department of Neurology, Inje University School of
Medicine, Haeundae Paik Hospital, Korea

Eric H. Kossoff MD
Johns Hopkins Hospital, Baltimore, MD, USA

Mohamad Z. Koubeissi MD
Epilepsy Center, The GW Medical Faculty Associates,
Washington, DC, USA

Ruben Kuzniecky MD
Northwell Health Epilepsy Program, Department of
Neurology, Zucker-Hofstra School of Medicine,
New York, NY, USA

Nuria Lacuey MD
Clinical Fellow in Epilepsy, University Hospitals Case
Medical Center, Cleveland, OH, USA

Samden D. Lhatoo MD, FRCP (Lon)
Center, University Hospitals Case Medical Center,
Cleveland, OH, USA

Byungin Lee MD
Epilepsy Center, Inje University School of Medicine,
Haeundae Paik Hospital, Korea

Daniel B. Lowenstein MD
Johns Hopkins Hospital, Baltimore, MD, USA

Anthony G. Marson MD, FRCP
The University of Liverpool, The Walton Centre for
Neurology and Neurosurgery, UK

Martha J. Morrell MD
Neurology & Neurological Sciences, Stanford
University, NeuroPace, Inc., Mountain View, CA,
USA

George Nune MD
Department of Neurology, University of Southern
California, CA, USA

Elia M. Pestana Knight MD
Epilepsy Center, Cleveland Clinic, Cleveland, OH,
USA

Graham A. Powell PhD, MRCP
The University of Liverpool, The Walton Centre for
Neurology and Neurosurgery, UK

Raman Sankar MD, PhD
Departments of Neurology and Pediatrics, Geffen
School of Medicine at UCLA and UCLA Children's
Discovery and Innovation Institute, Los Angeles, CA,
USA

Steven C. Schachter MD
Consortia for Improving Medicine with Innovation
and Technology, Departments of Neurology, Beth
Israel Deaconess Medical Center, Massachusetts
General Hospital, and Harvard Medical School,
Boston, MA, USA

Lara M. Schrader MD
Department of Neurology, Geffen School of Medicine
at UCLA, Los Angeles, CA, USA

Ashwini Sharan MD
Division of Epilepsy and Neuromodulation
Neurosurgery, Department of Neurosurgery, Thomas
Jefferson University Hospital Philadelphia, PA, USA

Joseph I. Sirven MD
Department of Neurology, Mayo Clinic, Scottsdale,
AZ, USA

John M. Stern MD
Department of Neurology, Geffen School of
Medicine at UCLA, Los Angeles, CA, USA

Maria Thom BSc, MBBS, FRCPath, MD
Department of Clinical and Experimental Epilepsy,
University College London Institute of Neurology,
London, UK

Samuel Wiebe MD, MSc
Department of Clinical Neurosciences, Cumming School of Medicine, University of Calgary, Calgary, AB, Canada

Chengyuan Wu MD MSBmE
Division of Epilepsy and Neuromodulation Neurosurgery, Department of Neurosurgery, Thomas Jefferson University Hospital Philadelphia, PA, USA

Elaine Wyllie MD
Epilepsy Center, Cleveland Clinic, Cleveland, OH, USA

Jiyeoun Yoo MD
Department of Neurology, Icahn School of Medicine at Mount Sinai, New York, NY, USA

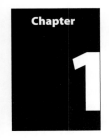

The Natural History of Epilepsy

Byungin Lee and Sung-Eun Kim

Natural History of Untreated Epilepsy

Understanding the natural course of epilepsy influences the advice given to patients, the treatment strategies and the timing of referral for surgery-based treatments. As such, it is integral to clinical care. The natural course of epilepsy at population level also has important implications for understanding the underlying neurobiology and for developing means for epilepsy prevention, new treatments and allocation of healthcare resources.

However, an understanding of the natural history or course of epilepsy depends upon knowing the clinical manifestations of epilepsy without treatment or other intervention from the time of onset until disease resolution or death, and such studies are unethical when treatment is available and requested by patients. One approach to such studies uses epidemiological studies in developing countries where patients with epilepsy are not offered any treatment throughout their illness. However, differences in aetiology, diagnostic accuracy and environmental factors need to be considered before generalization of the results.

A household survey in northern Ecuador identified 1029 patients with epilepsy and found a high rate of disease inactivity; 44% of all patients were seizure-free during the preceding 12 months, despite 70% never receiving anti-seizure medication (ASM) [1]. In this study, the lifetime prevalence (19.5/1000) and incidence (190/100 000/year) of epilepsy were much higher than other nations, but the prevalence of active epilepsy (8/1000) was comparable. A WHO-commissioned household survey in a rural region of China identified an epilepsy prevalence rate of 7/1000, which is comparable to developed countries, and 63% of 257 patients with active epilepsy were not receiving treatment, whereas 41% of the 130 patients with inactive epilepsy had never been treated [2]. A longitudinal study of 103 patients who were diagnosed with active epilepsy but not treated with an ASM was conducted in Bolivia [3]. After 10 years of follow-up, 31 of the 71 patients (44%) with seizure occurrence information were seizure-free for longer than five years. If the study included all 103 patients of the original cohort in the denominator, the spontaneous remission rate would be 30%, if all who were lost to follow-up continued to experience seizures.

The prevalence of epilepsy is dependent on both epilepsy incidence and duration. Based on a prevalence of 5 per 1000 and incidence of 50 per 100 000 per year, the expected average duration of active epilepsy should be around 10 years [4], which implies that a significant proportion of patients eventually achieve spontaneous remission. However, this average duration would be impacted by the already recognized self-limited epilepsies of childhood and mortality in older adults from other causes. The incidence of epilepsy is generally higher in developing countries, while prevalence of active epilepsy is approximately equal throughout the world. Although there has been a speculation about higher premature mortality in developing countries, a high spontaneous remission rate of epilepsy (30–40%) among incident cases seems to be an important contribution to the higher incidence and comparable prevalence, assuming diagnostic accuracy is comparable to developed countries [5].

Natural History of Treated Epilepsy

ASM treatment is usually started at the time of diagnosis in the developed world, and outcome studies carried out in these countries mostly reflect the prognosis of treated epilepsy. Accurate assessment of treated epilepsy is best achieved by prospective follow-up of newly diagnosed patients at the point of treatment initiation. In a Rochester, Minnesota study, five-year remission (5-YR) rates were 65% at 10 years and 76% at 20 years after diagnosis [6]; 70% of patients achieved five-year terminal remission (5-YTR) with 50% being off ASMs (Figure 1.1). Favourable predictors were idiopathic/cryptogenic aetiology,

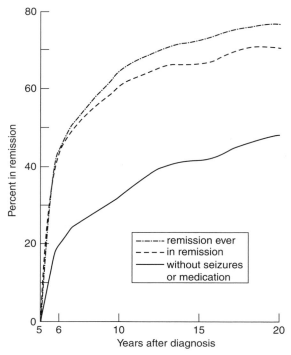

Figure 1.1 Time-dependent five-year remission rates among 457 patients with newly diagnosed epilepsy in Rochester study (with permission from [6])

Remission ever: percentage of patients who achieved five-year remission status.

In remission: percentage who have been seizure-free during the last five years or more.

Without seizures or medication: percentage of patients who were seizure-free off medication during the last five years

generalized tonic-clonic seizures (GTCS), and age of onset before age 10 years. In comparison, a community-based study in Kenya of ASM treatment on the natural course of epilepsy showed that either carbamazepine or phenobarbital therapy in patients with chronic epilepsies resulted in 53% seizure freedom at 12 months of treatment [7]. As such, a similar outcome was observed in a developing country, which supports comparability between developing and developed countries. In the Kenya study, there was no association between the remission rate and either the duration of epilepsy or the total number of lifetime seizures before treatment, suggesting that the impact of current ASM treatment on the natural course of epilepsy is probably not significant.

The National General Practice Study of Epilepsy (NGPSE) from the United Kingdom is a prospective community-based study of 564 patients with definite

epileptic seizures [8]. Chances of achieving 3-YR and 5-YR at nine years of follow-up were 86% and 68%, respectively. After 25 years of follow-up, 82% of 327 patients with definite epilepsy achieved 5-YTR [9]. Analysis of seizure patterns showed that 27% had early seizure remission continuing to 5-YTR, while 8% had continuous seizure recurrences without having any 1-YR. Late terminal remission was achieved in 22% of patients and the remaining patients had complex patterns of alternating 'remission and relapse'.

Response to sequential ASM trials on the clinical course in adults with newly diagnosed epilepsy were investigated in a hospital-based cohort [10–13]. Among 1098 newly diagnosed patients, 68% achieved at least 1-YTR by 7.5 years of follow-up. Successful response to the first drug regimen was achieved in 49.5%, 36.7% to the second drug, and 12% to 24% in response to the third or subsequent drugs [13]. The clinical courses of newly diagnosed people with epilepsy (PWE) were classified into four patterns: 'early and sustained seizure freedom' was achieved in 37%, 'delayed but sustained seizure freedom' in 22%, alternating periods of 'remission and relapse' in 16% and no achievement of 1–YR ever in 25%.

Several long-term paediatric cohort studies provided further insights into the natural course of childhood-onset epilepsy. A Finnish paediatric cohort included 245 patients (150 incident and 95 prevalent cases) under the age of 16 years in 1964 [14]. At 37 years of follow-up for 144 incident cases, 67% of patients were in 5-YTR on or off ASMs. Early remission, starting within the first year of treatment, was seen in 45 (32%) patients and 23 (16%) of them maintained remission until the end of follow-up without any relapse. Late remission with a mean delay of nine years was achieved by 72 (50%), and 46 (32%) achieved 5-YTR without any relapse. Following a relapse after early or late remission, 28 (19%) patients achieved 5-YTR, indicating a 'remission-relapse' pattern and 20 (14%) patients did not re-enter remission, indicating a worsening course of epilepsy. Twenty-seven (19%) patients failed to achieve any 5-YR throughout the follow-up, while 7% of patients failed to achieve 1-YR ever. Thus, half of the patients eventually entered 5-YTR without relapse and a fifth after relapse. A later study on the outcome at 45 years of follow-up reported that 66% of 133 patients were in 10-YTR and 50% were in 10-YTR without ASM over the preceding five years [15]. 10-YR did not guarantee lasting seizure freedom because seizure relapse occurred in 29% of patients

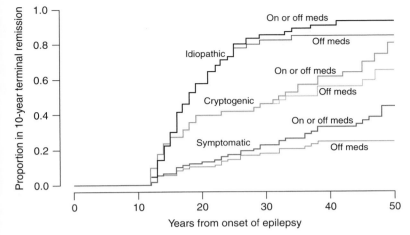

Figure 1.2 10-year terminal remission rate in relation to aetiology of seizures in 50 years of follow-up of the Finnish Childhood Onset Epilepsy(TACOE) cohort (with permission from [15])

Thick lines indicate 10-YTR on anti-seizure medications and thin lines indicate 10-YTR off medications during the last five years of follow-up.

All 245 cases in the cohort, including those who subsequently died, were lost or withdrew, are included to the analysis.

who had achieved at least one 10-YR. The outcome was strongly influenced by aetiology. Most idiopathic cases attained resolved epilepsy state (10-YR without ASM for at least five years) and did so within 30 years. Cryptogenic cases took longer to do so, and achieved remission by 45 to 50 years to an extent that approached that of idiopathic cases. The remission rate in symptomatic cases remained relatively low even after 45 years, but its slope was still up-going (Figure 1.2).

A Connecticut paediatric cohort consisted of a prospective community-based registry of children with newly diagnosed epilepsy [16]. Among 516 patients who had follow-up for at least 10 years, 95% experienced 1-YR and 257 (52%) relapsed after the initial remission with more than half regaining remission. Complete remission (CR: seizure-free and ASM-free for at least five years) was achieved by 328 (63.6%), but 23 of these patients (7%) had subsequent relapses. In summary, 60% of patients achieved CR, while 5% failed to achieve any 1-YR during the course; 35% of patients were between CR and medication-resistant epilepsy (MRE) with chronic epilepsy that had not resolved.

A Dutch hospital-based paediatric cohort study included children aged 1 month to 16 years with newly diagnosed epilepsy [17]. Among 413 patients who were followed-up for 15 years, 293 (71%) of patients had 5-YTR and 62% were receiving ASMs. Epilepsy was still active (one or more seizures during the past five years) in 120 (29%) subjects and 35 (8.5%) subjects were intractable in the final year of follow-up. Comparison of seizure outcome at 2, 5 and 15 years suggested that 48.4% had a favourable course (no

seizures throughout) and 29% had an improving course with seizures in the second year, but with remission in the fifth year or later. Clinical courses in remaining patients were categorized into poor course (9.9%), deteriorating course (6.1%) and varying course (6.5%).

These paediatric cohorts provided relatively comparable long-term courses consisting of about 67% of the study population achieving prolonged remission and 50–60% of patients discontinuing ASMs. Another 33% of patients showed dynamic courses characterized by alternating periods of 'remission and relapse' and a minority (5–10%) did not achieve any 1-YR (Table 1.1). However, individual patients have unique paths, and this is not easily summarized by the remission status at the end of an arbitrary follow-up period.

Natural History of Medication-Resistant Epilepsy

The long-term outcome of newly diagnosed epilepsy is generally expected to be favourable for most patients; however, a substantial minority continue to experience seizures in spite of a range of ASMs at typically therapeutic doses in either monotherapy or polytherapy. Those patients with MRE are characterized by higher mortality and morbidity, risk of medication adverse effects, higher stigma and social handicap, higher somatic and emotional comorbidities, and compromised quality of life. The natural course of patients with MRE is an essential research area to establish effective strategies for the relief of epilepsy burden.

Table 1.1 Patients with clinical courses of newly diagnosed epilepsy in selected studies

Studies	Number of patients	Duration of follow-up (years)	Clinical courses					Relapse
			Terminal Remission			Remission		
			Early	Late	Total	Ever	None	
Annegers et al., 1979 [7] – Population based – Children and adults	457	20	–	–	70%	76%	24%	16%
Brodie et al., 2012 [13][a] – Hospital Based – Adults	1098	7.5	37%	22%	58%	–	25%	15%
Bell et al., 2016 [9] – Population based – Children and adults	354	23.6	27%	22%	82%	–	8%	42%
Sillanpää and Schmidt, 2006 [15] – Population based – Children	144	37	16%	32%	67%	81%	27% (7%[b])	27%
Berg and Rychlik, 2015 [16] – Population based – Children	516	17	33%	10%	72%	81%	5% [b]	16% (52%)[c]

Remission indicates five-year remission except Brodie et al. [13].

[a] Remission indicates longer than one-year terminal remission.

[b] Proportion of patients who failed to achieve one-year remission.

[c] Proportion of patients who did relapse after achievement of one year or more remission.

Definition

The conceptual definition of medication resistance is 'failure to control seizures despite trials of all available ASMs in both monotherapy and combination therapy', but this is not applicable in clinical practice because of the interval of time needed to determine response to treatment and the multiplicity of ASM combinations. The historical lack of consensus on the practical definition of MRE has generated significant confusion in research and communication. Berg et al. applied several previously published definitions to their own paediatric cohort to compare the sensitivities and predictive values of individual definitions [18]. The proportion of subjects meeting the criteria for individual definitions in the cohort varied from 9% to 24%, with considerable differences in predictive values for later outcome, which raised concerns about the lack of consensus on the definition of MRE. In 2010, an ILAE Task Force proposed an operating definition of MRE, which defined drug resistant-epilepsy (DRE) as the failure of adequate trials of two tolerated, appropriately chosen and used ASM schedules to achieve sustained seizure freedom for either longer than one year or at least three times the longest inter-seizure interval, whichever is longer [19]. Use of the failure of the first two ASM treatments as the criterion was based on the observation that if two appropriate ASMs have failed to produce seizure freedom, the probability of success with subsequent ASM treatments is low [13]. The Task Force also recognized that the classification of a patient's epilepsy as medication resistant at a given point in time is valid only at the time of the assessment and does not necessarily imply that the patient will never become seizure-free on further manipulation of ASM therapy. Therefore, the ILAE definition is considered not to be the final confirmative diagnosis of medical 'intractability', but rather 'resistance', and a useful guideline for practicing neurologists in referring patients to dedicated epilepsy centres. The ILAE definition is discussed in detail in Chapter 3.

Epidemiology

Picot et al. conducted an epidemiological study in a medium-sized city in France to find 360 patients older than the age of 15 years with active epilepsy [20]. The age-adjusted prevalence rate was 5.4 per 1000 and the percentage with uncontrolled epilepsy (one or more seizure/year) was 22.5%, corresponding to a prevalence of 1.36 per 1000. Among those with uncontrolled epilepsy, 57.1% had tried two first-line drugs, 23.8% had tried three and 16.7% had tried four or more treatments. The seizure frequencies varied across these patients, with 32% having more than one a week, 43% having between one a week and one a month and 25% having fewer than one a month. Thus, patients with one or more seizures a month constituted 15.6% of patients with active epilepsy, corresponding to a prevalence of 0.84 per 1000. Among patients with MRE, localization-related epilepsy comprised 75.3%, idiopathic generalized epilepsy 6.2% and cryptogenic or symptomatic generalized epilepsy 6.2%.

A Connecticut paediatric cohort study showed that 14% of 603 patients met the stringent criteria of intractability (one or more seizures per month for 18 months) and 23% met the criteria of two ASM failures, which was in agreement with the French adult-prevalence study [20,21]. In the Dutch paediatric cohort, at least 12% of patients had a period of intractability (not seizure-free for longer than 3 months during the previous 12 months) during a 15-year follow-up, and 8.5% were intractable in the final year, suggesting a gradual reduction of patients with MRE over long-term follow-up [22]. In a hospital-based cohort of adults with newly diagnosed epilepsy, 35.4% of 780 patients did not achieve 1-YTR and an additional 42 (5.4%) patients failed to achieve 1-YTR after relapse following initial remission at a follow-up of 79 months [12]. Thus, about 40% of patients were considered to have MRE, which was somewhat higher than paediatric cohorts.

Timing of MRE Diagnosis

The assumption that MRE will be apparent at the time of epilepsy onset has not been fully supported by either retrospective or prospective studies [10,12]. A large US multi-centre study found that the average time from onset of epilepsy to the diagnosis of MRE was 9.1 years [23]; 26% of patients with MRE had a history of 1-YR remission at some point during the course of their disorder and a prior 5-YR remission was reported by 8.5% of study participants. Onset before the age of five years was strongly associated with longer latency time to the diagnosis of MRE and higher probability of past remission. In the Connecticut paediatric cohort study, temporal patterns of MRE were dependent

on the epilepsy context; when accompanied by developmental delay, 52% of 67 children met the criteria of MRE, but only 14% of children showed delayed diagnosis of MRE [21]. Among 203 children with genetic epilepsy syndromes without developmental delay, only 8 (4%) were diagnosed as MRE and 3 of them had a delayed MRE diagnosis. Of 294 children with focal epilepsy, 39 (13%) were diagnosed with MRE during the follow-up periods and 18 (46%) had a delayed appearance of MRE, with 13 having at least 1-YR before the diagnosis of MRE (Figure 1.3). Among focal epilepsies, temporal lobe epilepsy (TLE) had the highest probability of MRE (24%), as compared to other lobar epilepsies (11%)

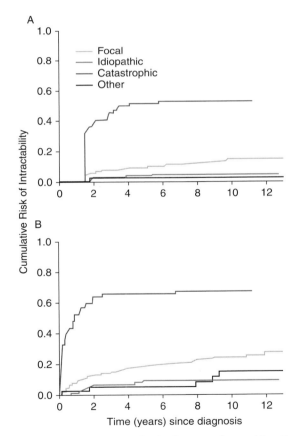

Figure 1.3 Cumulative risk for development of intractable epilepsy by syndrome groups(with permission from [21])
Red lines indicate focal epilepsy; green lines for idiopathic epilepsy; blue lines for catastrophic epilepsies; and black lines for others. (A) The stringent criteria for intractable epilepsy: ≥1 seizure/month for 18 months after the failure of two anti-seizure medications. (B) The criteria for the ILAE practical definition: failure of two anti-seizure medications and not seizure-free for one year or three times the longest inter-seizure interval, whichever is greater.

or unlocalized epilepsies (7%); however, the temporal patterns of developing MRE did not differ significantly.

In the Dutch paediatric cohort, 15 (3.3%) of 453 patients were medication resistant only during the first five years, 19 (4.2%) were medication resistant during both the first five years and the last year (15th year) of follow-up, and 16 (3.5%) had a late onset (more than five years after onset) of medication resistance, sometimes after long periods of remission [22]. Therefore, many patients had a changing MRE diagnosis during their illness, which indicates a highly dynamic epilepsy course. No significant predictive characteristics were found across these three groups.

The dynamic course of MREs was also reported in adult hospital-based cohorts. Schiller reported that 40% of 256 patients who achieved remission for one year or more had a seizure relapse at five years after entering remission, with 16% of them ultimately developing MRE [24]. In another study, a hospital cohort of 290 patients with MRE, Neligan et al. found that 70% of patients had a continuous pattern of seizures (no remissions after the onset of epilepsy) and the remaining 30% had an intermittent pattern [25].

These observations imply that the presentation of MRE is not straightforward and early identification of MRE may be elusive in a significant proportion of patients.

Predictive Factors for MRE

Identification of patients with MRE at an early stage of treatment is important in determining whether to consider alternative therapies, referral to epilepsy centres, parental counselling and individual support. Previous studies have proposed a long list of predictive factors for future development of MRE, which are divided into epilepsy-related, patient-related and treatment-related (Table 1.2) [21,26,27]. Many variables are directly or indirectly inter-related. For example, a symptomatic aetiology may include MRI lesions, focal neurological deficits and cognitive deficits. Younger age of onset may also relate to symptomatic or cryptogenic generalized epilepsies, which are common during infancy and early childhood. As such, caution is recommended when considering proposed predictive factors from different studies.

Among the long list of predictors of MRE, 'aetiology and epilepsy syndromes' was the most consistent factor, followed by high numbers of seizures or

Table 1.2 Predictive factors for MRE proposed from previous investigations

Disease-related factors	Symptomatic aetiology, including MRI lesions, partial seizures, multiple types of seizure, symptomatic generalized epilepsy High seizure frequency before treatment High seizure density before or during early treatment, seizure clustering during drug treatment Duration of epilepsy Electroencephalogram (EEG) abnormality Status epilepticus
Patient-related factors	Neurological deficits, mental retardation, developmental delay Early childhood age of onset Psychiatric comorbidities Non-adherence to ASMs, poor lifestyle, use of alcohol and recreational drugs Family history of epilepsy History of febrile convulsion or neonatal seizures
Treatment-related factors	Early response to drug treatment Delayed time to remission after treatment start

From: [6,12,21,22,26–33]

seizure density prior to initial treatment. The presence of an MRI lesion has been proposed as an important predictor; however, hippocampal sclerosis, cortical malformation and traumatic brain lesions were specific MRI lesions predicting worse outcome while other lesions were not predictive in a large-scale hospital-based study [28]. Most other predictors were either inconsistent or conflicting across studies. Even among patients with a symptomatic aetiology of epilepsy, up to 60% of children were able to enter long-term remission with prolonged treatment, which indicates a lack of any reliable way to identify medication resistance at presentation [29].

Other investigators proposed failure of the first ASM as a reliable predictor for MRE [10,12,34]. Kwan and Brodie reported that patients whose first ASM failed due to inefficacy have only an 11% chance of seizure freedom in subsequent ASM trials [10]. Dlugos et al. reported that failure of first ASM was the only variable predicting MRE in children with TLE, which was associated with high positive and negative predictive values [34]. However, Camfield et al. reported a case series of 72 children whose first ASM failed and found that 42% of them later achieved seizure freedom and only 29% had MRE at the end of eight years of follow-up [35]. A follow-up analysis of the SANAD trial found that 70% of patients whose first ASM failed later achieved 1-YR at five-year follow-up, which occurred in 65% of patients whose ASM failed due to inefficacy and 80% of those whose ASM failed due to adverse effects [36]. Therefore, the significance of failure of first ASM seems to be more reliable for childhood TLE and requires a further confirmation by other studies.

Trajectory of Medication-Resistant Epilepsy

The long-term outcomes of patients with MRE were considered pessimistic; however, several follow-up studies from tertiary epilepsy centres have reported that 20% to 30% of patients with highly refractory epilepsy have achieved late, prolonged remission with long-term follow-up. Luciano and Shorvon reported that systematic add-on ASM trials in 155 patients with chronic and highly refractory epilepsy resulted in 1-YR in 28% of patients [37]. Callaghan et al. and Choi et al. reported remission rates of 4–5% per year in their cohorts of refractory patients [38,39]. About two-thirds of them relapsed again after remission, but often with significant improvement in seizure frequency. This is a more optimistic outlook for MRE than previously believed and has kindled research interest in the long-term trajectory of patients who satisfy the ILAE criteria for MRE.

Berg et al. reported a long-term outcome (median 10.1 years) for 128 patients for whom two first-line ASMs had failed [40]; 57% of them achieved 1-YR, but 68% of these had relapses. At the last clinic visit, 1-YTR and 3-YTR were achieved in 38% and 23%, respectively. In multi-variate analysis, 'symptomatic aetiology' was the only negative predictor for 3-YTR. Among 69 patients with idiopathic or cryptogenic aetiologies, 22 (32%) patients achieved 3-YTR, while only 6 (10%) of 59 patients with symptomatic epilepsy did so. Wirrell et al. reported the long-term outcome of 75 patients who met the ILAE criteria of MRE during the first two years of treatment [41]. At follow-up of 11.5 years, 45% of them remained medically intractable, but another 45% were seizure-free on and off ASMs. Neuroimaging was the single most important predictor, with only 9% of patients with abnormal neuroimaging achieving seizure remission, compared to 60% of patients with normal neuroimaging. Both paediatric cohort studies strongly indicated that patients with ILAE-criteria MRE still have a good chance of achieving prolonged remission when the epilepsy is idiopathic or cryptogenic.

Recently, Choi et al. reported the trajectory of adult patients starting a third ASM after failure of two ASMs at a tertiary medical centre. Over the mean follow-up period of 65 months, 212 (53%) of 403 patients did not achieve a 1-YR, 63 (16%) had a complex trajectory of 'remission and relapse', 62 (15%) achieved seizure freedom after one year of treatment (delayed TR) and 66 (16%) had an early TR (within one year of treatment) [42]. Independent predictors associated with more favourable outcomes were epilepsy type and length of follow-up. TLE and generalized epilepsy were predictors of poor outcome. Remission rate was higher in patients with cryptogenic epilepsy than in symptomatic aetiology (37% vs. 25%), but the difference was not significant. The longer the follow-up, the more likely the patients were to experience a better trajectory, which was in agreement with the outcome of lifelong follow-up of patients with chronic MRE showing increasing rates of spontaneous remission in patients surviving to older age [43].

Mortality

PWE have increased premature mortality compared to the general population: almost twice as high in cryptogenic epilepsy, three to four times in symptomatic epilepsy, but not elevated in idiopathic epilepsy [44]. Mortality is highest in childhood epilepsies due to congenital or developmental causes (Table 1.3). The highest standard mortality ratio (SMR: the ratio of the observed deaths in the study population to the expected deaths in the population from which it came) is found in children, primarily due to the low mortality in the reference population and the high mortality in children with epilepsy and neurological deficits. However, the highest excess mortality was found in the elderly, which was 47/1000 person-years, or eight times higher than mortality in children with epilepsy (6/1000 person-years) [45].

The increase in mortality is most pronounced during the first years following diagnosis. In an NGPSE study, the SMR was 6.5 in the first year, decreased to 2.4 in the second year, stayed between 1 and 2 during years 5–10, and then gradually increased to >2 up to 25 years (Figure 1.4) [46]. A similar temporal pattern was also found in other population-based cohorts [45]. The reasons for a continuously high SMR persisting throughout the illness or a late increase of SMR in these cohorts are not clear, although adverse effects of chronic ASM treatment, increasing incidence of comorbidities among patients

Table 1.3 Pooled relative excess mortality risk in epilepsy by clinical characteristics across all age groups, including population-based and representative hospital-based cohorts (modified from [44])

	Incidence cases		All cases (including prevalent)	
	Pooled RR	95% CI	Pooled RR	95%CI
Aetiology				
Idiopathic/cryptogenic	1.56	1.36–1.79	1.61	1.42–1.82
Idiopathic	1.29	0.75–2.20	1.05	0.55–2.01
Cryptogenic	1.75	1.20–2.54	1.75	1.20–2.54
Symptomatic	4.73	3.27–6.83	4.48	3.24–6.21
Congenital or developmental causes	10.27	4.03–26.17	10.27	4.03–26.17
Seizures				
Seizure-free or five-year terminal remission	0.97	0.73–1.30	1.56	1.14–2.13
Highest seizure frequency category	4.69	1.41–15.60	4.65	2.70–8.01

Abbreviations: CI = confidence interval; pooled RR = pooled relative risk of death in epilepsy in a random-effects model.

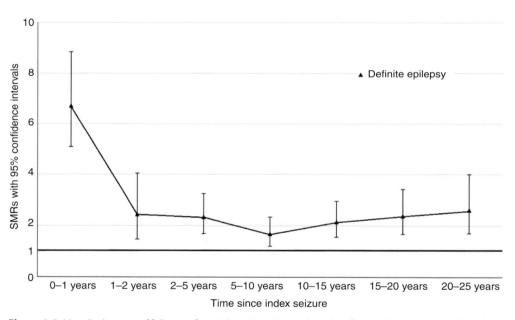

Figure 1.4 Mortality by years of follow-up from index seizure in people with definite epilepsy in UK-NGPSE study (modified with permission from [46]). Mortality is highest during the first year and rapidly decreases to an SMR level between 1 and 2 at 5–10 years after index seizure. Thereafter, SMR gradually increases and remains above 2.0 at 25 years of follow-up.

with chronic epilepsy and potential genetic influences have been proposed as potential explanations.

Cause of Death

Causes of death (COD) in PWE, which are classified into seizure-related and aetiology-related, are diverse, with significant differences among individual studies (Table 1.4).

Proportionate mortality ratio (PMR; ratio of the number of deaths for a particular cause in a study population to the total number of deaths in the same period) in population-based studies was 12–17% for cerebrovascular diseases, 12–37% for ischaemic heart diseases, 18–40% for neoplasia (including brain tumours), 8–18% for pneumonia, 0–7% for suicides, 0–12% for accidents, 0–4% for SUDEP, 0–10% for seizure-related causes (including status epilepticus) and 5–30% for other causes [47]. Seizure-related causes play a minor role in increased mortality in population-based incident studies, whereas they are found more

Table 1.4 Classification of causes of death in patients with epilepsy

Seizure-related causes	SUDEP (definite, probable, possible) Status epilepticus Complication of seizures: includes any deaths that resulted from documented complications of a seizure (e.g. aspiration pneumonia due to seizure) or iatrogenic complications as the result of treating seizures
Natural causes	Directly related to epilepsy aetiology: death attributable to any acute or chronic neurological conditions responsible for the development of epilepsy Not related to epilepsy aetiology: death attributable to any acute or chronic medical or neurological conditions not responsible for the development of epilepsy
Non-natural causes (external causes)	Suicide Accidents: Vehicle Non-vehicle: falls, burns, drowning, drug poisoning, or other unspecified Assault
Unknown	Inadequate information available to make an attribution of the specific cause of death or to group it into the scheme above

Modified from [48–50,52]

frequently in studies of prevalent cases having chronic epilepsies. In particular, the incidence of SUDEP is 0–0.35/1000 patient-years in population-based cohorts, whereas it increases to 1–5/1000 patient-years in epilepsy clinic populations, and to 6–10/1000 patient-years in patients who are considering epilepsy surgery [47]. In a recent NGPSE study [48], the three most common underlying causes of deaths were non-cerebral neoplasm, and cardiovascular and cerebrovascular disease, accounting for 59% of deaths, while external causes (e.g. suicide, accidents) and seizure-related causes (e.g. SUDEP) accounted for 4.2% and 3% of deaths, respectively [48]. Underlying COD was directly related to epilepsy aetiology in 23%, which was significantly more likely if death occurred within two years of the index seizure. At follow-up of 15 years and more, death in patients with idiopathic/cryptogenic cases becomes a major proportion with minor contributions from epilepsy aetiology and seizure-related causes (Figure 1.5).

Pneumonia was the most common immediate COD, accounting for 31%, followed by cancer-related conditions. Most of the patients who died had a significant number of comorbid conditions, among which neoplasm, neurologic diseases and substance abuse were independently associated with increased mortality risk. The substantial contribution of psychiatric comorbidities was also found in a Swedish national patient registry by Fazel et al., who found that external causes (suicide, accidents

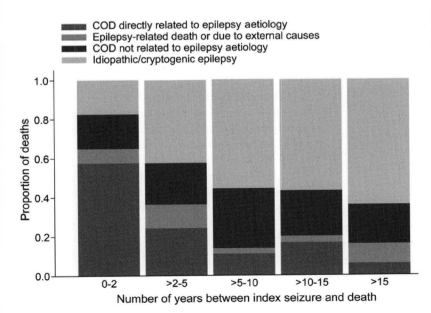

Figure 1.5 Relationship between epilepsy aetiology and underlying cause of death (COD) (with permission from [49]). During the first two years after diagnosis, epilepsy aetiology is the major COD, which declines to a minority on long-term follow-up. Mortality among patients with non-symptomatic epilepsy gradually increases to comprise more than 50% of death after five years of follow-up. Epilepsy-related deaths and external causes comprise a small proportion of mortality throughout the follow-up but their contribution increases after 15 years of follow-up.

COD directly related to epilepsy aetiology
Epilepsy-related death or due to external causes
COD not related to epilepsy aetiology
Idiopathic/cryptogenic epilepsy

and assaults) accounted for 15.8% of mortality in PWE, with 75% of them carrying a lifetime psychiatric diagnosis, especially a history of substance misuse and depression [49].

The Finnish paediatric cohort had the longest follow-up to provide details of premature mortality in childhood-onset epilepsy [51]. Among 245 patients, 60 (24%) died during 40 years of follow-up, which was 6.9/1000 person-years. Mortality was much higher in the remote symptomatic group and 85% of patients who died were not in 5-YR at the time of death. Death during childhood primarily occurred in the remote symptomatic group and was mostly related to the underlying disease, whereas deaths due to seizure-related causes occurred later, primarily in adolescence and adulthood. Of 60 deaths, 33 (55%) were seizure-related, including SUDEP in 18 subjects (30%), definite or probable seizures in 9 (15%) and accidental drowning in 6 (10%). The cumulative risk of SUDEP was 7% at 40 years overall and the median age of death was 25 years with the 'absence of 5-YTR' being a significant risk factor. However, the mortality outcome of the Finnish cohort was not confirmed by other subsequent studies. In a pooled analysis of four large paediatric cohorts, which included 2239 subjects with follow-up of more than 30000 person-years, 69 died, with an overall death rate of 228/100000 person-years [52]. Mortality rate was high only in complicated epilepsy, not in uncomplicated (idiopathic/cryptogenic) epilepsy. Seizure-related death occurred in 13 subjects (10 SUDEP and 3 others), accounting for 19% of all deaths. The SUDEP rate was similar to that for sudden infant death rates in the general population. Different outcomes between paediatric cohorts may be related to the exclusion of lethal metabolic conditions in the combined cohort study, as well as a higher proportion of remote symptomatic patients, combined incident and prevalent cases, and a longer follow-up period in the Finnish cohort [53]. In summary, COD linked to epilepsy aetiology is the major player in the earlier phase of premature mortality, whereas comorbidities unrelated to epilepsy aetiology provide a major contribution during the later phase. Seizure-related COD plays a relatively minor role throughout the course, although its contribution slowly increases during the later phase. It is likely that seizure-related COD, especially SUDEP, is more important in patients with chronic MRE.

Mortality in patients with MRE

Mortality in patients with MRE is that of prevalent cases, which is different from that of newly diagnosed epilepsy (incident cases). Premature mortality in incident cases is highest during the first two years of diagnosis, largely related to death from the underlying aetiology of epilepsy. Because the high mortality rate during the initial two years rapidly declines to a level near to that of the general population, the mortality of prevalent cases is generally expected to be lower than that of incident cases. However, in a hospital-based cohort of 2689 patients who did not respond to ASM treatment, 316 patients died during a follow-up period of 108 months, giving a crude death rate of 11.8% and an SMR of 2.04 [53]. There were 55 cases of probable SUDEP, resulting in an incidence of 2.46/1000 person-years, which was higher than the newly diagnosed epilepsy cohort (1.08/1000 person-years). Nevalainen et al. reported comparable outcomes from a hospital-based study of 1383 PWE, in which the hazard ratio of premature death was 2.66 [54]. Mortality was a product of interactions of aetiology and seizure frequencies; the SMR was 2.9 in patients with symptomatic epilepsy and seizure-free, whereas those with more than one seizure per month had a 6.3-fold higher mortality.

Callaghan et al. [55] identified 433 prevalent patients with MRE defined as failure of more than two ASMs and one or more seizures a month. Median duration of illness was 25 years and median age at the index date was 40 years. More than 80% of the population had focal epilepsy and 50% had symptomatic epilepsy; 33 patients died during the follow-up period of six years giving a case fatality of 7.6%. COD included seizure-related in 10 patients (SUDEP in 5, status epilepticus in 3, 1 accident and 1 suicide), underlying aetiology of epilepsy in 7 patients and causes unrelated to epilepsy aetiology in 16. Therefore, the contribution of seizure-related death to the increased mortality in patients with MRE was only modest, but largely related to diverse causes or comorbidities unrelated to epilepsy aetiology. However, there is accumulating evidence indicating the importance of seizure control for its preventive effects on mortality. In the study of patients with chronic MRE, SUDEP was responsible for 18% of death and high seizure frequency was a significant independent predictor of premature death, as well as SUDEP [43]. The reduction in years of life for those who had more than four seizures a month compared with those who had less than one seizure a month was 13 years. In a recent long-term outcome study of epilepsy surgery, the mortality rate of surgically treated patients was only one-third that of non-surgically treated patients and the SMR of patients who became seizure-free after surgery was no different from that of the general population, which reflects the preventive effects of seizure control on premature mortality in patients with MRE [56]. How seizure recurrences affect premature mortality in patients with MRE is certainly a prime target for future research.

Key Points

- Studies from developing countries indicate that about 30–40% of patients with untreated epilepsy achieve spontaneous remission, whereas in developed countries, about 67% of patients with newly diagnosed epilepsy achieve prolonged terminal remission (five years or more) and 50% of patients are able to discontinue anti-seizure medications (ASM) in a long-term follow-up.
- The clinical courses of newly diagnosed epilepsy are classified into four patterns: 'early and sustained seizure freedom', 'delayed but sustained seizure freedom', alternating periods of 'remission and relapse' and 'no prolonged seizure remission (≥1-YR)'. Approximately one-third of patients have fluctuating courses of 'remission and relapse', thus the outcome for an individual patient is not easily judged by the remission status at the end of an arbitrary follow-up period.
- The long-term outcomes for patients with medication-resistant epilepsy (MRE) were considered pessimistic; however, several follow-up studies from tertiary epilepsy centres have reported that 20–30% of patients with highly refractory epilepsy have achieved late, prolonged remission.
- PWE have increased premature mortality compared to the general population: almost twice as high in cryptogenic epilepsy, three to four times in symptomatic epilepsy, but not elevated in idiopathic epilepsy.
- Premature mortality in PWE is affected by interactions of aetiology and frequency of recurrent seizures, thus achieving seizure remission by either medical or surgical treatment may be important for reducing the higher mortality in patients with MRE.

References

1. Placencia M, Sander JWAS, Roman M, et al. The characteristics of epilepsy in a largely untreated population in rural Ecuador. *J Neurol Neurosurg Psychiatry* 1994:320–325

2. Wang WZ, Wu JZ, Wang DS, et al. The prevalence and treatment gap in epilepsy in China: an ILAE/IBE/WHO study. *Neurology* 2003;**60**:1544–1545

3. Nicoletti A, Sofia V, Vitale G, et al. Natural history and mortality of chronic epilepsy in an untreated population of rural Bolivia: a follow-up after 10 years. *Epilepsia* 2009;**50**:2199–2206

4. Beghi E, Giussani G, Sander JW. The natural history and prognosis of epilepsy. *Epileptic Disord* 2015;**17**:245–253

5. Beghi E, Hesdorffer D. Prevalence of epilepsy- an unknown quantity. *Epilepsia* 2014;**55**:963–967

6. Annegers JF, Hauser WA, Elverback LR. Remission of seizures and relapse in patients with epilepsy. *Epilepsia* 1979;**20**:729–737

7. Feksi AT, Kaamugisha J, Sander JWAS, Gatiti S, Shorvon SD. Comprehensive primary health care antiepileptic drug treatment programme in rural and semi-urban Kenya. ICBERG (International Community-based Epilepsy Research Group). *Lancet* 1991;**337**:406–409

8. Cockerell OC, Johnson AL, Sander JW, Shorvon SD. Prognosis of epilepsy: a review and further analysis of the first nine years of the British National General Practice Study of Epilepsy, a prospective population-based study. *Epilpesia* 1997;**38**:31–46

9. Bell GS, Neligan A, Giavasi C, et al. Outcome of seizures in the general population after 25 years: a prospective follow-up, observational cohort study. *J Neurol Neurosurg Psychiatry* 2016;**87**(8):843–850

10. Kwan P, Brodie MJ. Early identification of refractory epilepsy. *N Engl J Med* 2000;**342**:314–319

11. Chen Z, Brodie MJ, Liew D, Kwan P. Treatment outcomes in patients with newly diagnosed epilepsy treated with established and new antiepileptic drugs: a 30-year longitudinal cohort study. *JAMA Neurol* 2018;**75**:279–286

12. Mohanraj R, Brodie MJ. Diagnosing refractory epilepsy: response to sequential treatment schedules. *Eur J Neurol* 2006;**13**:277–282

13. Brodie MJ, Barry SJE, Bamagous G, Norrie JD, Kwan P. Patterns of treatment response in newly diagnosed epilepsy. *Neurology* 2012;**78**:1548–1554

14. Sillanpää M, Schmidt D. Natural history of treated childhood-onset epilepsy: prospective, long-term population-based study. *Brain* 2006;**129**:617–624

15. Sillanpää M, Anttinen A, Rinne JO, et al. Childhood-onset epilepsy five decades later. A prospective population-based cohort study. *Epilepsia* 2015;**56**:1774–1783

16. Berg AT, Rychlik K. The course of childhood-onset epilepsy over the first two decades: a prospective, longitudinal study. *Epilepsia* 2015;**56**:40–48

17. Geerts A, Arts WF, Stroink H, et al. Course and outcome of childhood epilepsy: a 15-year follow-up of the Dutch Study of Epilepsy in Childhood. *Epilepsia* 2010;**51**:1189–1197

18. Berg AT, Kelly MM. Defining intractability: comparisons among published definitions. *Epilepsia* 2006;**47**:431–436

19. Kwan P, Arzimanoglou A, Berg AT, et al. Definition of drug resistant epilepsy: consensus proposal by the ad hoc Task Force of the ILAE Commission on Therapeutic Strategies. *Epilepsia* 2010;**51**:1069–1077

20. Picot MC, Baldy-Moulinier M, Daures JP, Dujols P, Crespel A. The prevalence of epilepsy and pharmacoresistant epilepsy in adults: a population-based study in a Western European country. *Epilepsia* 2008;**49**:1230–1238

21. Berg AT, Vickrey BG, Testa FM, et al. How long does it take for epilepsy to become intractable?: a prospective investigation. *Ann Neurol* 2006;**60**:73–79

22. Geerts A, Brouwer O, Stoink H, et al. Onset of intractability and its course over time: the Dutch study of epilepsy in childhood. *Epilepsia* 2012;**53**:741–751

23. Berg AT, Langfitt J, Shinnar S, et al. How long does it take for partial epilepsy to become intractable? *Neurology* 2003;**60**:186–190

24. Schiller Y. Seizure relapse and development of drug resistance following long-term seizure remission. *Arch Neurol* 2009;**66**:1233–1239

25. Neligan A, Bell GS, Sander JW, Shorvon SD. How refractory is refractory epilepsy?: patterns of relapse and remission in people with refractory epilepsy. *Epilepsy Res* 2011;**96**:225–230

26. Hitiris N, Mohanraj R, Norrie J, Sills GJ, Brodie MJ. Predictors of pharmacoresistant epilepsy. *Epilepsy Res* 2007;**75**:192–196

27. Wirrell EC. Predicting pharmacoresistance in pediatric epilepsy. *Epilepsia* 2013;**54**(suppl. S2):19–22

28. Semah F, Picot MC, Adam C, et al. Is the underlying cause of epilepsy a major prognostic factor for recurrence? *Neurology* 1998;**51**:1256–1262

29. Sillanpää M, Schmidt D. Predicting antiepileptic drug response in children with epilepsy. *Expert Rev Neurother* 2011;**11**:877–886

30. Brorson LO, Wranne L. Long term prognosis in childhood epilepsy: survival and seizure prognosis. *Epilepsia* 1987;**28**:324–330

31. Kanner AM. Is depression associated with an increased risk of treatment-resistant epilepsy?: research strategies to investigate this question. *Epilepsy Behav* 2014;**38**:3–7

32. MacDonald BK, Johnson AL, Goodridge DM, et al. Factors predicting prognosis of epilepsy after presentation with seizures. *Ann Neurol* 2000;**48**:833–841

33. Mohanraj R, Brodie MJ. Early predictors of outcome in newly diagnosed epilepsy. *Seizure* 2013;**22**:333–344

34. Dlugos DJ, Sammel MD, Strom BL, Farrar JT. Response to first drug trial predicts outcome in childhood temporal lobe epilepsy. *Neurology* 2001;**57**:2259–2264

35. Camfield PR, Camfield CS, Gordon K, Dooley JM. If a first antiepileptic drug fails to control a child's epilepsy, what are the chances of success with the next drug? *J Pediatr* 1997;**131**:821–824

36. Bonnett LJ, Smith CT, Donegan S, Marson AG. Treatment outcome after failure of a first antiepileptic drug. *Neurology* 2014;**83**:552–560

37. Luciano AL, Shorvon SD. Results of treatment changes in patients with apparently drug-resistant chronic epilepsy. *Ann Neurol* 2007;**62**: 375–381

38. Callaghan B, Schlesinger M, Rodemer W, et al. Remission and relapse in a drug-resistant epilepsy population followed prospectively. *Epilepsia* 2011;**93**:115–119

39. Choi H, Heiman GA, Munger CH, et al. Seizure remission in adults with long-standing intractable epilepsy: an extended follow-up. *Epilepsy Res* 2011;**93**:115–119

40. Berg AT, Levy SR, Testa FM, D'Souza R. Remission of epilepsy after two drug failures in children: a prospective study. *Ann Neurol* 2009;**65**:510–597

41. Wirrell, EC, Song-Kisiel LCL, Mandrekar J, Nickels KC. What predicts enduring intractability in children who appear medically intractable in the first 2 years after diagnosis? *Epilepsia* 2013;**54**:1056–1064

42. Choi H, Hayat MJ, Zhang R, et al. Drug-resistant epilepsy in adults: outcome trajectories after failure of two medications. *Epilepsia* 2016;**57**(7):1152–1160

43. Novy J, Belluzzo M, Caboclo LO, et al. The lifelong course of chronic epilepsy: the Chalfont experience. *Brain* 2013;**136**:3187–3199

44. Nevalainen O, Ansakorpi H, Simola M, et al. Epilepsy-related clinical characteristics and mortality: a systematic review and meta-analysis. *Neurology* 2014;**83**:1–10

45. Forsgren L, Hauser WA, Olafsson E, et al. Mortality of epilepsy in developed countries: a review. *Epilepsia* 2005;**46**(suppl. 11):18–27

46. Neligan A, Bell GS, Johnson AL, et al. The long-term risk of premature mortality in people with epilepsy. *Brain* 2011;**134**:388–395

47. Hitiris N, Mohanraj R, Norrie J, Brodie MJ. Mortality in epilepsy. *Epilepsy Behav* 2007;**10**:363–376

48. Keezer MR, Bell GS, Neligan A, Novy J, Sander JW. Cause of death and predictors of mortality in a community-based cohort of people with epilepsy. *Neurology* 2016;**86**:1–9

49. Fazel S, Wolf A, Langstrom N, Newton CR, Lichtenstein P. Premature mortality in epilepsy and the role of psychiatric comorbidity: a total population study. *Lancet* 2013;**382** (9905):1646–1654

50. Devinsky O, Spruill T, Thurman D, Friedman D. Recognizing and preventing epilepsy-related mortality: a call for action. *Neurology* 2016;**86**:779–786

51. Sillanpää M, Shinnar S. Long-term mortality in childhood-onset epilepsy. *N Engl J Med* 2010;**363**:2522–2529

52. Berg AT, Nickels K, Wirrell C, et al. Mortality risks in new-onset childhood epilepsy. *Pediatrics* 2013;**132**:124–131

53. Mohanraj R, Norrie J, Stephen L, et al. Mortality in adults with newly diagnosed and chronic epilepsy: a retrospective comparative study. *Lancet Neurol* 2006;**5**:481–487

54. Nevalainen O, Auvinen A, Ansakorpi H, et al. Mortality by clinical characteristics in a tertiary care cohort of adult patients with chronic epilepsy. *Epilepsia* 2012;**53**:e212–e214

55. Callagahn B, Choi H, Schesigner M, et al. Increased mortality persists in an adult drug-resistant epilepsy prevalent cohort. *J Neurol Neurosurg Psychiatry* 2014;**85**:1084–1090

56. Sperling MR, Barshow S, Nei M, Asadi-Pooya AA. A reappraisal of mortality after epilepsy surgery. *Neurology* 2016;**86**:1938–1944

Challenges in Identifying Medication-Resistant Epilepsy

Martin J. Brodie and Pauls Auce

Introduction

This chapter will focus on the challenges in identifying medication-resistant epilepsy for the common focal and generalized epilepsies in children, adolescents and adults. The encephalopathies of infancy and seizures secondary to single gene mutations have been excluded from consideration, because many of these patients will never attain seizure freedom. Over the years, variations surrounding definitions and strategies across a range of studies in children and adults have complicated the picture and resulted in artificial differences in outcomes across different patient populations studied in various parts of the world using different methodologies. Many of these analyses have been undertaken retrospectively in patients with chronic epilepsy. There has been an increasing awareness of the necessity to follow prospectively only patients with newly diagnosed epilepsy. In 2010, a task force of the International League against Epilepsy (ILAE) published a definition of medication-resistant epilepsy, which has brought some clarity and cohesion to this complex issue [1]. This definition has reduced variation among subsequent studies, helping to clarify questions surrounding population selection, sample size, seizure classification and terminology, and characterization of intractability [2].

Definition

Medication-resistant epilepsy has been defined by the ILAE as a 'failure of adequate trials of two tolerated, appropriately chosen and used anti-seizure medication (ASM) schedules (whether as monotherapy or in combination) to achieve sustained seizure freedom' [3]. An 'adequate trial' requires failure of treatment at potentially therapeutic dosing due to lack of efficacy of an ASM appropriate for the seizure type(s). Thus, poor tolerability with an ASM at low dosage and withdrawal due to an idiosyncratic reaction do not constitute an adequate trial. Continuing seizure activity in patients with intermittent adherence to their drug schedule for whatever reason also does not conform to the ILAE definition. In the latest published data following outcomes of newly diagnosed epilepsy in adolescents and adults undertaken at the Epilepsy Unit in the Western Infirmary in Glasgow over 25 years, around 68% of the 1098 patients were in remission at the time of analysis [4]. However, only 44% of the patients remaining uncontrolled fulfilled the ILAE definition of medication-resistant epilepsy [5]. In a similar analysis undertaken in 194 patients with chronic 'refractory' epilepsy in Hong Kong, only 59% of the population could be defined as having medication-resistant epilepsy. Thus, many patients with continuing seizures arguably could have been made seizure-free with appropriate treatment and a much smaller cohort than highlighted in many publications has truly medication-resistant epilepsy, i.e. uncontrolled does not necessarily mean uncontrollable!

Similar data are available for children with uncontrolled seizures in a number of settings. In the Dutch study of epilepsy in childhood, involving 453 patients, more than 12% of the cohort had a period of intractability during the 15-year follow-up [6]. The mean time to onset of intractability during the first five years of follow-up was 1.6 years. This was more likely to occur in patients with focal than generalized epilepsies. Five-year terminal remission was reached by 71% of the cohort in an earlier analysis of 413 children [7]. In a prospective longitudinal study of 516 children in the United States, an initial one-, two-, three- and five-year remission occurred, respectively, in 95%, 92%, 89% and 81% of the population, with relapses following in 52%, 41%, 29% and 15% [8]. In another retrospective US cohort of 351 children, 19.7% demonstrating early medical intractability had abnormal neurologic examination and/or neuroimaging, supporting early surgery as an option for some of these [9]. The higher number of seizure-free children vs. adults with similar epilepsies occurring across a range of studies is likely to be, in part at least, due to better adherence with medication and simpler supervized lifestyles.

Patterns of Response

The only appropriate way to understand the natural history of treated epilepsy is to follow up newly diagnosed patients prospectively after the introduction of their first ASM [10]. In the Glasgow cohort, four different patterns of response have been recently identified [4]. In the first group (n = 408; 37%) seizure freedom was obtained immediately or within six months of starting treatment and continued throughout follow-up, often with a modest or moderate dose of any suitable ASM. A smaller group (n = 246; 22%) demonstrated a delayed response, but these patients also eventually attained remission. In some, this occurred when treatment was begun with a well-tolerated ASM after failure of a number of other drug choices due to side effects. Other patients took some time to accept the diagnosis and to regularize their lifestyle and become fully adherent with their treatment regimen. A further 172 patients (16%) demonstrated a fluctuating course with periods of seizure freedom followed by relapses or vice versa. After attaining a seizure-free period of at least a year either early (within six months, n = 116) or following a modest delay (after six months, n = 56), some of these patients reported up to five periods of poor control intercalated with episodes of seizure freedom lasting more than one year. Around 45% of this population remained uncontrolled at the time of analysis. The final group of patients (25%) never became seizure-free for any 12-month period, although seizure numbers and severity often will have been reduced. Over the years of follow-up the percentage of seizure-free patients fell from 68% at two years to just 52%

after 10 years [4]. Table 2.1 summarizes outcomes in the Glasgow newly diagnosed population over the past 15 years studied in four separate analyses supporting the proposition that the overall prognosis has not materially changed despite the introduction of many new ASMs during this period.

One major problem in the pharmacological management of epilepsy is that all ASMs, no matter their mechanism of action, were developed as a consequence of their anti-seizure rather than their anti-epilepsy properties in animal models [11]. Thus, epilepsy in some patients will remit, sometimes permanently, while in others it will relapse, resulting in refractory epilepsy with many patients having a period of good control at some point in their trajectory [12–14]. The scenario for children is similar [8]. Accordingly, a surprisingly large cohort of around 21% of patients turned down for epilepsy surgery in the United States subsequently had an extended period of seizure freedom [15]. There is a large, unpredictable variation in the time of onset, causation and duration of optimal seizure control in childhood epilepsy with a higher chance of final intractability after a poor course during the first five years of follow-up [6].

Thus, although two-thirds of all patients follow a stable pattern, that is to become seizure-free early and remain seizure-free or have refractory epilepsy lifelong, up to 33% demonstrate an unstable course [16]. These patients will either enter remission after many years of seizures or will relapse after many years of seizure freedom despite continued treatment with a range of ASMs. A number of studies have supported the reliability and validity of the ILAE criteria for the diagnosis of medication-resistant epilepsy [2,17,18]. The effect of ASM treatment, however, on the eventual outcome seemed to be minimal for both children and adults, i.e. ASM treatment does not materially influence the natural history of the epilepsy [19].

Table 2.1 Remission rates (%) in an expanding cohort of patients with newly diagnosed epilepsy followed for up to 34 years

Recruitment	Analysis	N	One drug	Multiple drugs	Total
1982–1997[1]	1999	470	61	3.0	64.0
1982–2001[1]	2003	780	59	5.4	64.4
1982–2006[1]	2008	1098	62	6.4	68.4
1982–2014[2]	2015	1805	55	9.0	64.0

Data from: [10], [41].

Predictors of Medication-Resistant Epilepsy

In a recent analysis of 11 cohort studies, younger age at seizure onset, symptomatic aetiology, high initial seizure frequency, epileptic electroencephalographic abnormalities and failure of treatment with at least two previous ASMs were all documented as independent prognostic factors of intractability in at least two studies [20,21]. Overall, poor response to the first few ASMs, underlying symptomatic aetiology and high seizure counts prior to diagnosis were consistent predictors of subsequent medication resistance [21]. In our database, high seizure density within the three to six months before starting treatment was the best predictor of subsequent uncontrolled epilepsy, arguably indicating more severe underlying processes [22]. Lesions on brain magnetic resonance imaging predicted poor seizure outcome in children with temporal lobe epilepsy [23], whereas EEG changes were not useful biomarkers of medication-resistant epilepsy [24]. There is a consistency across different studies in picking out high number of pre-treatment seizures, prior neurologic insult and abnormal brain imaging, and failure of response due to lack of efficacy of the first well-tolerated ASM in predicting poorer outcomes [25]. In a recent cohort study in patients with generalized epilepsy, predictors of medication resistance were epilepsy diagnosis below 12 years of age, prior history of status epilepticus, developmental delay and cryptogenic aetiology [26].

One of the major problems in identifying predictability of medication-resistant epilepsy was the influence of definition and design across the individual studies [27]. The publication of the ILAE definition of medication-resistant epilepsy has helped investigators to narrow down these anomalies [2]. In addition, all future studies should be undertaken prospectively in patients with newly diagnosed epilepsy. This approach should be linked, whenever possible, to an objective measurement of seizures, since subjective counts in children and adults significantly underestimate seizure numbers, sometimes by as much as 50% [28,29]. Most patients (85.5%) are unable to report seizures at night [28], whereas the majority can recognize them during the day [30].

Responses to consecutive drug regimens in our cohort of newly diagnosed epilepsy are outlined in Table 2.2. Only 1.8% of these patients subsequently became seizure-free after failing the first three ASM schedules for any reason. However, some of these patients did not actually receive further drug regimens. Overall, 16.2%, 12.5%, 12.5% and 22.2% of patients treated with a fourth, fifth, sixth or seventh schedule, respectively, became seizure-free, highlighting again the difference between uncontrolled and uncontrollable epilepsy. Thus, many of these patients were not actually medication resistant. This observation was supported by data from an earlier study, in which adding previously unused ASMs to the treatment regimen in patients with apparently uncontrollable epilepsy resulted in short-term seizure freedom in 28% of the population [31].

Table 2.2 Seizure-free rates with successive anti-seizure medication regimens in newly diagnosed epilepsy

Drug regimens	No. of patients	Seizure-free on monotherapy	Seizure-free on combination	Total number seizure-free	Seizure-free overall (%)	Seizure-free on each regimen (%)
First	1098	543	0	543	49.5	49.5
Second	398	101	45	146	13.3	36.7
Third	168	26	15	41	3.7	24.4
Fourth	68	6	5	11	1.0	16.2
Fifth	32	1	3	4	0.4	12.5
Sixth	16	1	1	2	0.2	12.5
Seventh	9	1	1	2	0.2	22.2
Eighth	3	0	0	0	0.0	0.0
Ninth	2	0	0	0	0.0	0.0

Data from [4].

Table 2.3 Predictors of refractoriness in 780 patients with newly diagnosed epilepsy

	Odds ratio	95% CI	p value
Family history	1.89	1.15–3.00	0.011
Febrile seizures	3.36	1.58–7.18	0.002
Traumatic brain injury	3.26	1.59–4.69	<0.001
Psychiatric comorbidity	2.17	1.33–3.55	0.002
Recreational drug use	4.26	2.03–8.94	<0.001
10 or more seizures	2.77	1.98–3.89	<0.001

Data from [32]
CI, confidence interval

In an earlier analysis of 780 patients, a number of other predictive factors for 'refractoriness' were identified (Table 2.3), including family history of epilepsy, traumatic brain injury and the presence of psychiatric comorbidities [32]. These psychiatric symptoms may facilitate the development and/or exacerbation in the severity of the epilepsy and can be regarded as possible biomarkers for medication resistance [33]. This observation suggests that some of the pathogenic mechanisms operant in psychiatric comorbidities may play a role in epileptogenesis.

MicroRNAs (miRNA) are small non-coding RNAs that regulate gene expression at post-transcriptional level [34]. In a preliminary study evaluating 77 patients with medication-resistant epilepsy, 81 patients with medication responsiveness and 85 healthy controls, 5 MiRNAs were de-regulated in the patients with medication resistance compared to the other groups [35]. Overall miR-301a-3p provided the best diagnostic value for medication resistance. It has also been linked to inflammatory response [35], and inflammatory cytokines have been linked to psychiatric comorbidities in rodent models [36,37]. This is an exciting and potentially important area for future research. However, there are no clinically applicable biomarkers either of epileptogenesis or treatment response [38].

Conclusions

The challenge in diagnosing medication-resistant epilepsy has become more complicated with time, partly as a consequence of a range of issues surrounding the classification of the epilepsies, many of which have still to be fully resolved [39]. The many types of epilepsy and substrates responsible for seizure generation, together with the paucity of data on the underlying pathophysiology in the individual patient make a cohesive understanding of this topic problematic. There is increasing awareness that outcomes have not markedly improved over the last 30 years, despite the global introduction of more than 15 new ASMs, many with unique mechanisms of action, for the common epilepsies [40]. This is a likely consequence of the symptomatic anti-seizure effects of these agents, which cosmetically reduce seizure numbers without affecting the processes generating them and making the epilepsy medication resistant. Thus, more patients benefit in the short term from these new agents, but some are more likely to relapse in the longer term, maintaining the status quo of a good outcome in just under two-thirds of the population [41]. A new approach to ASM development is necessary if this disappointing situation is to be improved.

Identifying medication-resistant epilepsy early is possible for some patients and perhaps this will provide a way forward to identifying anti-epilepsy rather than anti-seizure therapy. This requires to be accomplished by following patients with newly diagnosed epilepsy using accurate objective seizure detection systems [30]. Although in some patients medication resistance can be recognized within a year or two of diagnosis, an increasing number of children and adults demonstrate a relapsing and remitting pattern, for which no biomarkers currently provide the necessary predictive power to allow useful scientific exploration and management of this phenomenon [38]. Medication-resistant epilepsy must be regarded as a dynamic process and not a static concept if we are to improve the lives of the many people who do not currently respond to the expanding ASM armamentarium.

Key Points

- Some children and adults with the common epilepsies will do well de novo while others do badly from the outset with an increasing number now recognized as demonstrating a relapsing/ remitting pattern.
- Predictors of poor prognosis include high pre-treatment seizure density, symptomatic aetiology, with or without abnormal brain imaging, psychiatric comorbidities and suboptimal response to the first two well-tolerated anti-seizure medications (ASMs).

- Publication of the International League against Epilepsy's definition of 'drug-resistant' epilepsy in 2010 has brought some cohesion to the design of subsequent outcome studies.
- Despite the introduction of around 15 new ASMs, many with apparently unique mechanisms of action, over the past 20 years outcomes for patients with the common epilepsies have not substantially improved.

References

1. Kwan P, Brodie MJ. Definition of refractory epilepsy: defining the indefinable? *Lancet Neurol* 2010;**9**:27–29

2. Tellez-Zenteno JF, Hernandez-Ronquillo L, Buckley S, et al. A validation of the new definitions of drug resistant epilepsy by the International League against Epilepsy. *Epilepsia* 2014;**55**:829–834

3. Kwan P, Arzimanoglou A, Berg AT, et al. Definition of drug resistant epilepsy: consensus proposal by the ad hoc Task Force of the ILAE Commission on Therapeutic Strategies. *Epilepsia* 2010;**51**:1069–1077

4. Brodie MJ, Barry SJE, Bamagous GA, et al. Patterns of treatment response in newly diagnosed epilepsy. *Neurology* 2012;**78**:1548–1554

5. Hao X, Goldberg D, Kelly K, et al. Uncontrolled epilepsy is not necessarily the same as drug resistant epilepsy. Differences between populations with newly diagnosed and chronic epilepsy. *Epilepsy Behav* 2013;**29**:4–6

6. Geerts A, Brouwer O, Stroink H, et al. Onset of intractability and its course over time: The Dutch study of epilepsy in childhood. *Epilepsia* 2012;**53**:741–751

7. Geerts A, Arts WF, Stroink H, et al. Course and outcome of childhood epilepsy: a 15-year follow-up of the Dutch Study of Epilepsy in Childhood. *Epilepsia* 2010;**51**:1189–1197

8. Berg AT, Rychlik K. The course of childhood-onset epilepsy over the first two decades: a prospective longitudinal study. *Epilepsia* 2015;**56**:40–48

9. Wirrell EC, Wong-Kisiel LC, Mandrek AR, Nickels KC. What predicts enduring intractability in children who appear medically intractable in the first 2 years after diagnosis? *Epilepsia* 2013;**54**:1056–1064

10. Brodie MJ. Road to refractory epilepsy: the Glasgow story. *Epilepsia* 2013;**54**:(suppl 2):5–8

11. Brodie MJ, Covanis A, Lerche H, et al. Antiepileptic drug therapy: does mechanism of action matter? *Epilepsy Behav* 2011;**21**:331–341

12. Neligan A, Bell GS, Sander JW, Shorvon SD. How refractory is refractory epilepsy?: patterns of relapse and remission in people with refractory epilepsy. *Epilepsy Res* 2011;**96**:225–230

13. Callaghan B, Schlesinger M, Rodemer W, et al. Remission and relapse in a drug resistant epilepsy population followed prospectively. *Epilepsia* 2011;**52**:619–626

14. Choi H, Heiman GA, Munger CH, et al. Seizure remission in adults with long-standing intractable epilepsy: an extended follow-up. *Epilepsy Res* 2011;**93**:115–119

15. Selwa LM, Schmidt SL, Malow BA, Beydoun A. Long-term outcome of non-surgical candidates with medically refractory localization-related epilepsy. *Epilepsia* 2003;**44**:1568–1572

16. Schmidt D, Sillanpaa M. Evidence-based review on the natural history of the epilepsies. *Curr Opin Neurol* 2012;**25**:159–163

17. Ramos-Lizana J, Aguilegra-Lopez P, Aguirre-Rodriguez J, Cassinello-Garcia EA. A study of drug-resistant childhood epilepsy testing the new ILAE criteria. *Seizure* 2012;**21**:266–272

18. Kong ST, Ho CS, Ho PC, Lim SH. Prevalence of drug resistant epilepsy in adults with epilepsy attending a neurology clinic of a tertiary referral hospital in Singapore. *Epilepsy Res* 2014;**108**:1253–1262

19. Löscher W, Schmidt D. Modern antiepileptic drug development has failed to deliver: ways out of the current dilemma. *Epilepsia* 2011;**52**:657–678

20. Wassenaar M, Leijten FSS, Egberts TCG, et al. Prognostic factors for medically intractable epilepsy: a systematic review. *Epilepsy Res* 2013;**108**:301–310

21. Mohanraj R, Brodie MJ. Early predictors of outcome in newly diagnosed epilepsy. *Seizure* 2013;**22**:333–344

22. Mohanraj R, Brodie MJ. Diagnosing refractory epilepsy: response to sequential treatment schedules. *Eur J Neurol* 2006;**13**:277–282

23. Spooner CG, Berkovic SF, Mitchell LA, et al. New onset temporal lobe epilepsy in children-lesions on MRI predict poor seizure outcome. *Neurology* 2006;**67**:2147–2153

24. Selvitelli MF, Walker LM, Schomer DL, Chang BS. The relationship of interictal epileptiform discharges to clinical epilepsy severity: a study of routine electroencephalograms and review of the literature. *Clin Neurophysiol* 2010;**27**:87–92

25. Bonnett LJ, Smith CT, Donegan S, Marson AG. Treatment outcome after failure of a first antiepileptic drug. *Neurology* 2014;**83**:552–560

26. Voll A, Hernandez-Ronquillo L, Buckley S, Tellez-Zenteno JF. Predicting drug resistance in adult patients with generalised epilepsy: a case controlled study. *Epilepsy Behav* 2015;**53**:126–130

27. Abimbola S, Martinivic ALC, Hackett ML, Anderson CS. The influence of design and definition in

the population of general epilepsy cohorts with remission and intractability. *Neuroepidemiology* 2011;**36**:204–212

28. Hoppe C, Poepel A, Elger CE. Accuracy of patient seizure counts. *Arch Neurol* 2007;**64**:1595–1599

29. Akman CI, Montenegro MA, Jacob S, et al. Seizure frequency in children with epilepsy: factors influencing accuracy and parental awareness. *Seizure* 2009;**18**:524–529

30. Bidwell J, Khuwatsamrit T, Askew B, et al. Seizure reporting technologies for epilepsy treatment: a review of clinical information needed and supporting technologies. *Seizure* 2015;**32**:109–117

31. Luciano AL, Shorvon SD. Results of treatment changes in patients with apparently drug-resistant chronic epilepsy. *Ann Neurol* 2007;**62**:375–381

32. Hitiris N, Mohanraj R, Norrie J, et al. Predictors of pharmacoresistant epilepsy. *Epilepsy Res* 2007;**75**:192–196

33. Kanner AM, Mazarati A, Koepp M. Biomarkers of epileptogenesis: psychiatric comorbidities? *Neurotherapeutics* 2014;**11**:358–372

34. Barter DP. MicroRNAs: genomics, biogenesis, mechanism and function. *Cell* 2004;**116**:281–297

35. Wang J, Tan L, Tan L. Circulating microRNAs are promising novel biomarkers for drug resistant epilepsy. *Sci Rep* 2015;**5**:10201

36. Mazarati AM, Pineda E, Shin D, et al. Comorbidity between epilepsy and depression: role of hippocampal interleukin 1β. *Neurobiol Dis* 2010;**37**(2):461–467

37. Pineda EA, Hensler JG, Sankar R, et al. Interleukin-1β causes fluoxetine resistance in an animal model of epilepsy-associated depression. *Neurotherapeutics* 2012;**9**(2):477–485

38. Pitkänen A, Löscher W, Vezzani A, et al. Advances in the development of biomarkers for epilepsy. *Lancet Neurology* 2016;**15**:843–856

39. Berg AT, Berkovic SF, Brodie MJ, et al. Revised terminology and concepts for organisation of the epilepsies: report of the ILAE Commission on Classification and Terminology. *Epilepsia* 2010;**51**:676–685

40. Löscher W, Klitgaard H, Twyman RE, Schmidt D. New avenues for antiepileptic drug discovery and development. *Nature Revs* 2013;**12**:757–776

41. Chen Z, Brodie MJ, Liew D, Kwan P. Long-term outcome of 1,805 people with newly diagnosed epilepsy. Presented at the 31st International Epilepsy Congress, Istanbul, Turkey 5–9 September 2015

International League Against Epilepsy's Definition of Medication-Resistant Epilepsy

Colin B. Josephson and Samuel Wiebe

Medication-Resistant Epilepsy

Scope of the Problem

Epilepsy is a common condition affecting people of all ages, sex and socioeconomic status. Many patients with epilepsy, once diagnosed, can be successfully managed with anti-seizure medication (ASMs) [1]. However, up to 30–40% of patients will continue to have seizures despite optimal medical management [1]. Thus, the World Health Organization (WHO) estimates that 15 million people (of 50 million worldwide with epilepsy) will not achieve complete seizure freedom despite appropriate ASM therapy [2]. These patients consume more healthcare resources than those with well-controlled epilepsy, as the 15% who are most refractory account for ≥50% of the total costs of the disease [3].

Patients with medication-resistant epilepsy are at increased risk of worse health outcomes. They suffer more somatic, cognitive and psychiatric comorbidities than people whose epilepsy is well controlled. Furthermore, they are at greater risk of epilepsy-related morbidity and mortality. This includes seizure-related injuries, social stigmatization and lower rates of employment. These patients have a 4.69-fold increase in risk of death and their estimated risk of sudden unexpected death in epilepsy is between 1.5 and 2.2 per 1000 person-years (95% CI 1.3–3.6) [4].

Pseudo-Resistance

Anti-seizure medications used in the context of paroxysmal conditions mimicking seizures are therapeutically ineffective. Thus, a patient with presumed drug resistance may not in fact be treatment refractory but, rather, may have another condition masquerading as epilepsy. Alternatively, a patient with true epilepsy may be treated with an inappropriate or an insufficient amount of an ASM. Hence, they spuriously appear 'medication resistant'. This issue of

'pseudo-resistance' must be addressed in all patients prior to declaring them resistant to medical management.

Up to 26% of patients presenting to a tertiary care epilepsy clinic may be misdiagnosed with epilepsy prior to the referral. Unlike some other medical conditions, no standardized criteria or laboratory tests exist that can confirm or refute the diagnosis of epilepsy. Rather, detailed histories and physical examinations, in conjunction with clinical expertise, are required to distinguish it from common conditions mimicking epilepsy that include syncope, cardiac arrhythmias, psychogenic non-epileptic attacks and paroxysmal or brief disorders such as migraines or transient ischaemic attacks.

Inadequate dosing or use of inappropriate ASMs may be a particular problem leading to pseudo-resistance. Insufficient dosing or using an ASM in the presence of an enzyme-inducing medication may result in subtherapeutic serum levels. Furthermore, certain ASMs, such as phenytoin, carbamazepine or lamotrigine may worsen absence or myoclonic seizures. Hence, careful attention must be paid to the selection and dosing of ASMs prior to labelling a patient's epilepsy as medication resistant (Table 3.1).

The Need for a Consensus Definition of Medication Resistance

Why an Empirical, Evidence-Based Definition is Required

The promotion of evidence-based, precision medicine is critical in today's world, where judicious allocation of finite resources is becoming increasingly relevant. This can only be achieved through systematic, methodical approaches to the study of medication resistance. Towards this end, the International League Against Epilepsy (ILAE) aimed to develop a widely accepted operational definition of medication-resistant epilepsy. Operational case definitions are predicated on practical,

Table 3.1 Anti-seizure medication efficacy for specific seizure and epilepsy types

Anti-seizure medication	Focal onset	Generalized onset	Absence	Myoclonic	LGS*
Brivaracetam	X				X
Cannabidiol	X				X
Carbamazepine	X	X			
Clobazam	X	X		X	X
Clonazepam	X	X	X	X	X
Ethosuximide			X	X	
Felbamate	X	X	X	X	X
Gabapentin	X	X			
Lacosamide	X	X			
Lamotrigine	X	X	X	X	X
Levetiracetam	X	X	X	X	X
Oxcarbazepine	X	X			
Perampanel	X	X			
Phenobarbital	X	X		X	X
Phenytoin	X	X			
Pregabalin	X	X			
Primidone	X	X		X	X
Rufinamide	X	X	X	X	X
Stiripentol		X		X	
Tiagabine	X	X			
Topiramate	X	X	X	X	X
Valproic acid	X	X	X	X	X
Vigabatrin	X	X			
Zonisamide	X	X	X	X	X

* Lennox–Gastaut syndrome

quantifiable statements that can be used to guide clinicians, researchers and policy-makers in the effort to improve the lives of those with epilepsy. Drawing upon carefully defined, concrete measures, these definitions permit a uniform application of the definition to patients with epilepsy in clinical practice. An empirical, universally accepted definition for medication-resistant epilepsy permits clinicians to accurately identify patients who will benefit from pre-surgical evaluations. Furthermore, it promotes multi-centre research collaborations by encouraging the consistent application of key definitions, thus promoting amalgamation of data, increasing statistical power, and enhancing internal and external validity. According to the ILAE, epilepsy is considered to be medication resistant when there is demonstrated 'failure of adequate trials of two tolerated and appropriately chosen and used ASM schedules (whether used as monotherapies or in combination) to achieve sustained seizure freedom' [6]. We will expand on the rationale and specific aspects of the definition.

Barriers to a Consensus Definition

Prior to 2009, the literature was rife with discrepant definitions of medication resistance [6], a phenomenon that is likely related to the fact that the question of drug resistance is more complex than it superficially appears. The natural history of epilepsy is such that there are inherent periods of relapse and remission. Thus, any putative 'response' to an ASM may alternatively be explained by the natural history of the disease process. Additionally, patients' seizures improve at differing ASM doses. Thus, close attention must be paid to the WHO's defined daily dose (DDD) for each ASM (Table 3.2), as attempts should be made to meet or exceed this level before declaring a drug ineffective,

Table 3.2 Defined daily doses for anti-seizure medication as determined by the World Health Organization

Anti-seizure medication	DDD (mg)
Brivaracetam	100
Carbamazepine	1000
Clobazam	20
Clonazepam	8
Felbamate	2400
Gabapentin	1800
Lacosamide	300
Lamotrigine	300
Levetiracetam	1500
Oxcarbazepine	1000
Perampanel	8
Phenobarbital	100
Phenytoin	300
Pregabalin	300
Primidone	1250
Rufinamide	1400
Stiripentol	1000
Tiagabine	30
Topiramate	300
Valproic acid	1500
Vigabatrin	2000
Zonisamide	200

barring the occurrence of intolerable side effects, which may require slow titration of the medication to avoid adverse effects. Finally, the issue of what constitutes 'failure' must be carefully considered. The disability conveyed by seizures varies according to their frequency and type (e.g. focal, focal with impaired awareness and generalized seizures), and to the personal perspective of the patient. Some patients may tolerate brief, focal seizures without altered awareness, whilst others may demand complete seizure freedom. Therefore, what one patient may consider a success another may consider a failure.

Derivation of an Empirical, Evidence-Based Definition

With these caveats in mind, the onus becomes identifying clinical criteria that accurately predict future unresponsiveness to any adequately chosen ASM. Such a definition requires a comprehensive assessment involving:

1. The appropriateness of the chosen ASM
2. The dose of the ASM
3. Defining what constitutes an adequate response to ASMs
4. Defining why an ASM failed (did not achieve an adequate response)
5. Establishing how many ASMs should be tried before deciding that further attempts at medical therapy will be unlikely to produce seizure freedom.

Steps 1 and 2 (establishing whether an appropriate ASM and dosages were used) require addressing pseudo-resistance through careful evaluation of the patient's putative diagnosis. Once the diagnosis is confirmed, subsequent attention must be paid to the ASMs and their dose. As an example, medications with efficacy for focal seizures, such as lamotrigine, carbamazepine and levetiracetam should be tried [7,8], medications with efficacy for generalized-onset tonic–clonic seizures, such as valproic acid, lamotrigine and levetiracetam, should be tried [8,9] and medications with efficacy for absence seizures, such as ethosuximide and valproic acid, should be tried [10]. In contrast, medications that may exacerbate absence or myoclonic seizures, such as carbamazepine, phenytoin and, in some situations, lamotrigine, should be avoided in relevant patients. The prevailing notion is that DDDs should be reached prior to deciding that an agent lacks efficacy. However, there is recent evidence that failure of an ASM at 50% or more of the DDD increases the likelihood of another ASM failing [11]. In other words, seizure control achieved at lower dosages of an ASM predicts a good response to future ASMs and a lower likelihood of drug resistance. This raises the question of whether response at lower doses should be incorporated into the determination of medication resistance in individual patients.

Step 3, determining what constitutes an adequate response to an ASM, necessitates intensive investigation into the minimum time required to confidently assert that a patient has achieved seizure freedom with a specific ASM, i.e. better than chance occurrence. To this end, high-quality, epidemiological evaluations of patient outcomes with sufficient follow-up that can account for the natural history of the patient's own disease are crucial. For instance, a patient whose seizures occur only once per year would be at high risk of being inadvertently labelled seizure-free if the study follow-up was restricted to six months or even one year. Here, it is appropriate to employ the statistical 'rule of 3' as it applies to zero event scenarios [12]. Essentially, the upper 95% confidence limit of the probability of observing an event that has not yet occurred can be estimated by dividing the number 3 by the ratio of events over the inverse of the longest inter-seizure interval the patient has ever experienced (n). The resultant upper 95% confidence limit will be 3/(1/n), which equates to three times the longest inter-seizure interval. In other words, to be 95% certain that an ASM is controlling seizures adequately, the patient should be seizure-free for a period equal to three times the previous longest seizure-free period.

In contrast, 12-months of seizure freedom is typically considered clinically significant. Many physicians would be reluctant to alter medications in patients who have seizures at a frequency of less than one per year. Additionally, complete seizure freedom, at one year, is associated with improved measures of quality of life [13] and is sufficient to drive in most jurisdictions, leading to higher rates of employment. Thus, a reasonable definition is one that takes both approaches into consideration. On this basis, the ILAE proposes that a patient may be considered seizure-free (i.e. responsive to ASMs) if they either achieve seizure freedom for a minimum of three times the longest pre-intervention inter-seizure interval, or if they reach 12 months of seizure freedom, whichever is longer. If patients do not achieve either of these parameters, they are considered resistant to the ASMs they are receiving, provided that the type and dose are appropriate, as described in steps 1 and 2 above.

Step 4 entails determining why the ASM failed. Specifically, in the ILAE definition of drug resistance, cessation of an ASM due to adverse effects does not constitute failure. All ASMs have unique adverse effect profiles that include both non-specific and idiosyncratic phenomena. Thus, attributing specific symptoms to medications can be difficult. Despite this challenge, it has been estimated that up to 40–50% of patients with epilepsy may experience adverse effects during monotherapy [14]. However, the propensity to report adverse events is directly related to the methods used to ascertain their presence [15]. Furthermore, the threshold for reporting such symptoms varies by patient tolerance. Although standardized means of identifying symptoms and attributing their causality to ASMs exist, simple ascertainment through clinician interviews should

suffice for the purposes of establishing medication resistance. Should an adverse effect become intolerable, a compelling case can then be made for discontinuation of the ASM. Unfortunately, most adverse effects that fall under this rubric are dose-dependent, thus impeding attempts to reach therapeutic drug concentrations. In this situation, the medication cannot be considered to lack efficacy.

Step 5 involves establishing how many ASMs should be tried before determining that a patient is drug resistant. There are currently over 20 ASMs available, so cycling through each one in monotherapy and subsequently through all permutations of polytherapy is not only impractical but is logistically impossible. Unnecessary polytherapy leaves the patient susceptible to medication toxicity, may detract from adherence and burdens them with higher costs. However, more critically, this approach will defer surgical evaluations, thus delaying potentially more effective interventions. This is exacerbated by the fact that medication-resistant patients may achieve periods of seizure freedom that are frequently short-lived [16]. Fallaciously believing these periods to represent bona fide seizure freedom will further delay referral for surgical evaluation. Already, patients typically wait an average of 22 years prior to referral for epilepsy surgery, thus relegating them to extended periods of increased risk for significant morbidity and mortality due to uncontrolled seizures [17].

Although features exist that are consistently linked to medication resistance, these are not 100% sensitive or specific (Table 3.3) [18]. Thus, current attention is exclusively paid to the patient's response to ASMs. The number of ASMs trialled before a patient is determined to be medication resistant should ideally be established through rigorous population-based studies that employ clear inception dates and extensive follow-up. Although there is a paucity of studies that meet these criteria, the best evidence accrued to date suggests that the likelihood of becoming seizure-free diminishes significantly following the failure of two ASMs. A landmark study addressing this issue enrolled 525 consecutive patients of all ages at a single tertiary care centre in Glasgow, Scotland, over a 13-year period [19]. Patients with all-cause epilepsy were included and the outcome indices included one-year seizure freedom. Of 470 (90%) patients never exposed to ASM therapy, 222 (47%) achieved one-year seizure freedom following prescription of their first medication. Of those failing to achieve seizure freedom on their first medication, 61 (13%) responded to monotherapy with a second ASM, while only 18 (4%) met this outcome after receiving monotherapy with a third ASM or ASM polytherapy [19]. An extension of this study later refined these estimates to a seizure-free percentage of 50.4% following monotherapy with a first-ever ASM, 10.7% following monotherapy with a second-ever ASM and 2.7% following monotherapy with a third-ever ASM or polytherapy [20] (Figure 3.1). A study limited to paediatric populations has corroborated these results, thus further emphasizing the generalizability of the importance of two ASM efficacy failures [21]. Finally, the response to future ASMs appears to be exquisitely linked to the patient's prior experience with medications, as the corresponding response curve for seizure freedom appears to have a half-decay constant of 1.5 to 2 ASMs [22]. In other words, the probability of seizures being controlled in an individual patient decreases by 50% for every 1.5 ASM that was ineffective in the past.

Based on data from these cohort studies, the ILAE task force assembling the definition of drug-resistant epilepsy concluded that the precipitous decline in the chances of achieving seizure freedom to single-digit numbers following failure of a second-ever ASM was significant enough to deem this an appropriate threshold for defining drug resistance. Although seizure freedom is still theoretically possible after failure of a second ASM, the probability is low and unpredictable, the time to achieving such remissions is usually several years and the remissions are typically self-limited [21]. Thus, obstinate pursuance of medical therapy following failure of two ASMs is not expected to yield a good outcome in the vast majority of patients, and rather is more likely to delay time to potentially curative surgery, should the patient be a candidate.

Table 3.3 Features consistently (>90% of studies) associated with medication-resistant epilepsy

Demographics and history
- Age of onset <1 year or >12 years
- Neonatal seizures
- Focal or multiple seizure types
- High initial seizure frequency

Epilepsy syndrome
- Structural, metabolic, autoimmune epilepsies
- Lennox–Gastaut syndrome
- Early myoclonic encephalopathy

Physical examination and imaging findings
- Development delay
- Neurological deficits
- Malformations of cortical development
- Hippocampal sclerosis (in temporal lobe epilepsy)
- Dual pathology

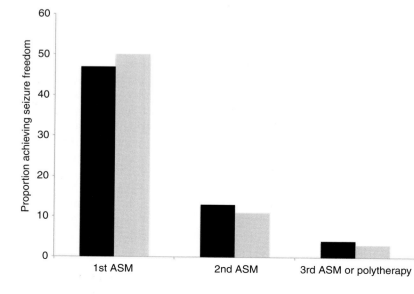

Figure 3.1 Proportion of patients achieving seizure freedom following a first-ever ASM in monotherapy, second-ever ASM in monotherapy and a third-ever ASM in monotherapy or polytherapy. The black bars are from the initial trial by Kwan and Brodie (2000)[19] and the yellow bars are from an expansion of this study with additional follow-up [20]. ASM = anti-seizure medication

Applications of the Definition

The validity and applicability of the definition has now been appraised by a number of studies. The inter-rater reliability is high (kappa = 0.77 to 0.91) [23,24], thus instilling confidence in the consistency of use of the definition between practitioners. A comparative study has further revealed that the inter-rater reliability of the ILAE definition outperforms prior attempts to define to drug resistance both in paediatric and adult populations [24].

However, despite the robust inter-rater reliability, the uptake of the definition amongst physicians referring patients for surgical evaluations remains subpar [25]. Furthermore, there remains controversy as one single-centre study found that up to 27% of patients could still become seizure-free after two adequately chosen trials of ASMs [25]. Under these circumstances, ongoing review and periodic critical re-evaluation of the definition and the means of disseminating it to relevant parties is crucial to ensure that it continues to remain both germane and valid as the therapeutic landscape in epilepsy continues to evolve.

Despite this, the clinical applications of the definition remain manifold in nature. The potential exists whereby it may be used to monitor patients consistently across centres for the purposes of determining candidacy for surgical evaluations. It may also be used as a quality indicator by which centres can evaluate referral rates, time to referral and time to operation for those who are surgical candidates. Incorporating this definition as a quality indicator could potentially have a major clinical impact by improving quality of care, increasing uptake rates of surgery and reducing healthcare costs by minimizing the burden conveyed by medication-resistant epilepsy.

Aside from direct clinical utility, the new definition also has clear implications for research. Prior epidemiological and outcomes studies have used varied definitions of drug resistance. This has led to discrepancies in reported incidence, prevalence and overall outcomes in the literature. This also complicates attempts to amalgamate data for meta-analytical purposes. Use of a consistent definition with high inter-rater reliability will permit inter-study consistency and facilitate future multi-centre efforts to firmly establish the scope and impact of medication-resistant epilepsy with a high degree of precision and validity. These studies are imperative as much of the research conducted to date has suffered from low statistical power and the lack of a consensus definition frequently restricts external validity.

Summary

The new ILAE definition constitutes a major accomplishment that has direct clinical and research applications. As aforementioned, the definition has immediate implications for epilepsy surgery. The risk–benefit profile attendant to surgery is considered favourable only for patients with medication-resistant epilepsy. This definition is therefore critical to avoid inadvertently exposing medically remediable patients to unnecessary risk. From a research perspective, harmonizing the definition of medication-resistant epilepsy will facilitate future attempts to elucidate the pathophysiological underpinnings and epidemiological expression of the disease. Uniform patient populations can be studied and amalgamation of multi-centre data, both through collaborative trials and through individual patient data meta-analyses, will now be feasible as a result of this consensus definition. As new data emerge, continued re-evaluation and refinement of the definition will ensure that it remains a central component of clinical care and research endeavours dedicated to improving outcomes for this uniquely vulnerable patient population.

Key Points

- Medication-resistant epilepsy is defined as failure of adequate trials of two tolerated, appropriately chosen and used ASM schedules (whether as monotherapy or in combination) to achieve sustained seizure freedom [6].

- Medication-resistant epilepsy is an important clinical entity to recognize as these patients are at increased risk of worse health outcomes. They suffer more somatic, cognitive and psychiatric comorbidities than the people whose epilepsy is well controlled and have a greater risk of epilepsy-related morbidity and mortality.

- A consensus driven, universally accepted definition of medication-resistant epilepsy is critical to consistently identify this patient population across clinical centres. To this end, a task force of the International League Against Epilepsy was convened in 2010 to generate an operational definition that incorporates the number, dose and appropriateness of medications, clear time frames over which seizure freedom should be evaluated and precise explanations of what constitutes medication failure.

- This definition has direct clinical applications in that it is intuitive, easy to use and unambiguously identifies patients who warrant surgical evaluations.

- The definition may also have a role as a quality indicator, as all geographically dispersed centres can use a universal definition to monitor the rate and time to referral for surgical evaluations and time from assessment to operation.

- The definition also has research implications in that it improves consistency across studies, minimizes heterogeneity, enhances external validity and facilitates future multi-centre and meta-analytic studies.

References

1. Kwan P, Brodie MJ. Early identification of refractory epilepsy. *N Engl J Med* 2000;**342**:314–319

2. Banerjee PN, Filippi D, Allen Hauser W. The descriptive epidemiology of epilepsy – a review. *Epilepsy Res* 2009;**85**:31–45

3. Begley CE, Annegers JF, Lairson DR, et al. Cost of epilepsy in the United States: a model based on incidence and prognosis. *Epilepsia* 1994;**35**:1230–1243

4. Derby LE, Tennis P, Jick H. Sudden unexplained death among subjects with refractory epilepsy. *Epilepsia* 1996;**37**:931–935

5. Siddiqui A, Kerb R, Weale ME, et al. Association of multidrug resistance in epilepsy with a polymorphism in the drug-transporter gene ABCB1. *N Engl J Med* 2003;**348**:1442–1448

6. Kwan P, Arzimanoglou A, Berg AT, et al. Definition of drug resistant epilepsy: consensus proposal by the ad hoc Task Force of the ILAE Commission on Therapeutic Strategies. *Epilepsia* 2010;**51**:1069–1077

7. Marson AG, Al-Kharusi AM, Alwaidh M, et al. The SANAD study of effectiveness of carbamazepine, gabapentin, lamotrigine, oxcarbazepine, or topiramate for treatment of partial epilepsy: an unblinded randomised controlled trial. *Lancet* 2007;**369**:1000–1015

8. Schmidt D, Schachter SC. Drug treatment of epilepsy in adults. *BMJ* 2014;**348**:g254

9. Marson AG, Al-Kharusi AM, Alwaidh M, et al. The SANAD study of effectiveness of valproate, lamotrigine, or topiramate for generalised and unclassifiable epilepsy: an unblinded randomised controlled trial. *Lancet* 2007;**369**:1016–1026

10. Glauser TA, Cnaan A, Shinnar S, et al. Ethosuximide, valproic acid, and lamotrigine in childhood absence epilepsy. *N Engl J Med* 2010;**362**:790–799

11. Brodie MJ, Barry SJ, Bamagous GA, et al. Effect of dosage failed of first antiepileptic drug on subsequent outcome. *Epilepsia* 2013;**54**:194–198

12. Hanley JA, Lippman-Hand A. If nothing goes wrong, is everything all right?: interpreting zero numerators. *JAMA* 1983;**249**:1743–1745

13. Jacoby A, Gamble C, Doughty J, et al. Quality of life outcomes of immediate or delayed treatment of early epilepsy and single seizures. *Neurology* 2007;**68**:1188–1196

14. Baker GA, Jacoby A, Buck D, et al. Quality of life of people with epilepsy: a European study. *Epilepsia* 1997;**38**:353–362

15. Carreno M, Gil-Nagel A, Sanchez JC, et al. Strategies to detect adverse effects of antiepileptic drugs in clinical practice. *Epilepsy Behav* 2008;**13**:178–183

16. Callaghan B, Schlesinger M, Rodemer W, et al. Remission and relapse in a drug-resistant epilepsy population followed prospectively. *Epilepsia* 2011;**52**:619–626

17. Berg AT, Langfitt J, Shinnar S, et al. How long does it take for partial epilepsy to become intractable? *Neurology* 2003;**60**:186–190

18. Wiebe S, Jette N. Pharmacoresistance and the role of surgery in difficult to treat epilepsy. *Nat Rev Neurol* 2012;**8**:669–677

19. Kwan P, Brodie MJ. Early identification of refractory epilepsy. *N Engl J Med* 2000;**342**:314–319

20. Mohanraj R, Brodie MJ. Diagnosing refractory epilepsy: response to sequential treatment schedules. *Eur J Neurol* 2006;**13**:277–282

21. Berg AT, Levy SR, Testa FM, et al. Remission of epilepsy after two drug failures in children: a prospective study. *Ann Neurol* 2009;**65**:510–519

22. Schiller Y, Najjar Y. Quantifying the response to antiepileptic drugs: effect of past treatment history. *Neurology* 2008;**70**:54–65

23. Hao XT, Wong IS, Kwan P. Interrater reliability of the international consensus definition of drug-resistant epilepsy: a pilot study. *Epilepsy Behav* 2011;**22**:388–390

24. Tellez-Zenteno JF, Hernandez-Ronquillo L, Buckley S, et al. A validation of the new definition of drug-resistant epilepsy by the International League Against Epilepsy. *Epilepsia* 2014;**55**:829–834

25. Ramos-Lizana J, Rodriguez-Lucenilla MI, Aguilera-Lopez P, et al. A study of drug-resistant childhood epilepsy testing the new ILAE criteria. *Seizure* 2012;**21**:266–272

The Economic Impact of Medication-Resistant Epilepsy

Charles E. Begley and Shin Jeong

Introduction

The economic impact of epilepsy in the USA and other countries has been well documented in terms of direct treatment-related costs. The average annual direct cost of the disease in the USA is typically estimated by comparing the use and cost of healthcare services in large representative samples of people with an epilepsy diagnosis to similar people without epilepsy using claims or medical billing data. The latest studies, reviewed recently by Begley and Durgin [1], indicate that the average individual with epilepsy and commercial or Medicaid coverage (all ages, genders, seizure types and severity) experiences excess epilepsy-related annual costs in a range between $7659 and $11 354 in 2013 dollars. Only a few of these studies provide separate cost estimates for subpopulations among those with epilepsy, such as individuals with intractable epilepsy. This is problematic for understanding the economic impact of epilepsy because of the variability in how the disease affects people and the effectiveness of existing treatments. As noted in an Institute of Medicine report, 'Epilepsy is a spectrum of disorders – the epilepsies – with a range of severities, widely differing seizure types and causes, and varying impacts on individuals and their families' [2]. The existing studies of direct costs in the intractable population reviewed here, though limited in number and methodological rigor, suggest that they are substantially higher than in the general population, but there is no consensus on how much higher.

Only a few studies attempt to measure the economic impact of epilepsy in terms of indirect costs, i.e. lost earnings from work loss, reductions in productivity at work or at home, and premature mortality. Existing estimates indicate they exceed direct costs by a significant margin, suggesting that investing in medical care that improves the quality of life of people with epilepsy may also lead to substantial reductions in the indirect costs of the disease. In a recent systematic review of cost-of-illness studies conducted around the world, indirect costs range from 12% to 85% of total costs [3]. As with direct costs, the only studies of indirect costs in the refractory population indicate much higher figures than in the general epilepsy population and, again, the studies vary substantially in terms of the methods, data sources and components of indirect costs that were captured.

In this chapter we provide an overview of the existing literature on the direct and indirect costs of intractable epilepsy in the USA, discuss the variation in methods and estimates, and offer research questions for the future. A literature review was performed by applying pre-specified search and selection criteria to Ovid-Medline, an electronic database. The search covered publications in English for the period from 2000 to 2015 based on one or more of the following search terms: 'epilepsy', 'seizures', 'refractory/non-refractory', 'stable/non-stable', 'controllable/non-controllable' and cost-related search terms including 'cost', 'burden of illness', 'direct cost', 'indirect cost', 'economics', 'expenditures', 'healthcare cost' and 'utilization'. Among 122 studies identified in the initial screen, 21 were selected based on the potential relevance suggested by the title and abstract. Five direct-cost studies were selected for review of direct costs and two indirect cost studies based on applying the following criteria: (1) representative sample from the US population, (2) estimates of a comprehensive set of medical care costs and/or components of indirect costs for populations with intractable epilepsy, (3) acceptable design, methods, data sources and analyses for generating epilepsy-specific estimates and (4) case identification criteria and procedures consistent with recommended guidelines [4]. Our review provides separate summaries of the major characteristics and findings of the selected studies of the direct and indirect costs of intractable epilepsy.

Direct Cost

Five estimates from methodologically well-described and reasonably rigorous studies of the direct cost of

Table 4.1 Characteristics of direct-cost studies

Study	Design	Sample	Estimates
Begley et al. (2001) [5]	Epilepsy-specific direct costs using 1987–1995 billing and medical records data from two healthcare clinic systems following the bottom-up attribution approach	608 privately insured users at epilepsy clinics in Houston, Texas and Rochester, Minnesota, incident cases, all ages, seizure types, active and inactive seizures	Average annual costs in 1995 dollars for incident cases over four to six years of follow-up
Chen et al. (2013) [7]	Total and epilepsy-specific direct costs from 2004–2008 using insurance claims data and following the bottom-up attribution approach	41 640 privately insured in USA, prevalent cases, children and non-elderly adults, active, partial onset seizures, refractory and non-refractory	Average annual epilepsy-specific direct costs in 2008 dollars
Cramer et al. (2013) [8]	Total and epilepsy-specific direct costs from 2007–2009 insurance claims using the bottom-up attribution approach	10 107 privately insured adults and elderly in USA, incident and prevalent cases, active, all seizure types, controlled and uncontrolled	Annual total and epilepsy-specific direct costs in 2009 dollars
Cramer et al. (2014) [9]	Total and epilepsy-specific direct costs from 2007–2009 using insurance claims data and following the bottom-up attribution approach	2170 children under 12 with private insurance in USA, incident and prevalent cases, active, all seizure types, controlled and uncontrolled	Annual total and epilepsy-specific direct costs in 2009 dollars
Manjunath et al. (2012) [10]	Total and epilepsy-specific direct costs from 1997–2009 commercial insurance and Medicaid claims data using the comparative attribution approach	6908 Medicaid enrollees in five states and 1204 privately insured in USA, prevalent cases, adults and elderly, active, controlled and uncontrolled, all seizure types	Annual total and epilepsy-specific direct costs in 2009 dollars

intractable epilepsy in the USA have been published since 2000. The major characteristics of these studies are summarized in Table 4.1.

In 2001, Begley et al. [5] determined epilepsy-specific direct costs from onset to six years, using 1987–1995 billing and medical chart data from two healthcare systems in Minnesota and Texas. They used the bottom-up attribution approach to estimate epilepsy-specific costs, selecting only services that were epilepsy-related, as defined by ICD-9 diagnosis codes and/or medical record information [6]. To examine variation in costs by severity, patients were divided into three broad groups based on prognosis Group 1, consisting of persons with early remission, defined as cases with no additional seizures during follow-up after the first year. Group 2 were people with delayed remission (e.g. had seizures one or more years after onset but were seizure-free for at least a year at last follow-up). Group 3, intractable epilepsy, included people still having seizures in the last year of follow-up. They found substantial variation in the average annual direct cost over the follow-up period for each group. Epilepsy-related costs averaged $776 per person per year in 1995 dollars for Group 1, for Group 2, epilepsy with delayed remission, the

cost was $934 per person-year, while Group 3 costs averaged $1588, more than twice as high as Group 1 patients.

Chen et al. [7] reported the direct cost of refractory vs. non-refractory epilepsy per year from 2004 to 2008 for commercially insured individuals based on insurance claims data. They identified a refractory epilepsy case as an individual with a diagnosis of partial onset seizures and on three or more anti-seizure medications in a year. They also used the bottom-up attribution approach to estimate total direct epilepsy-specific costs at $4032 (2008 dollars) for non-refractory epilepsy vs. $10 804 for refractory epilepsy, 2.7 times higher. They determined hospital inpatient costs to be $2005 for non-refractory vs. $3887 for refractory epilepsy, outpatient costs were $2850 vs. $4432, and pharmacy costs $1443 vs. $2772. The differences were consistent across all years examined.

Cramer et al. [8] compared healthcare costs and utilization for individuals with stable vs. uncontrolled epilepsy based on 2007–2009 insurance claims data for a sample of 10 107 privately insured patients. Individuals with stable epilepsy were identified in the claims data based on having no change in their medication therapy during the study year. Individuals with uncontrolled epilepsy were identified by their need for the addition of one or more ASMs during the study year compared to the previous year. They estimated the annual direct epilepsy-specific costs using the bottom-up attribution approach at $5511 (2009 dollars) for adults with stable epilepsy and $12 399 for uncontrolled epilepsy, a 2.3-fold difference. They used the same database to estimate treatment costs for children and reported similar findings. [9]. Children with uncontrolled epilepsy had epilepsy-specific costs of $16 894 per year, while children with stable epilepsy averaged $7979, a 2.2-fold difference.

Manjunath et al. [10] estimated the direct cost of uncontrolled epilepsy using health insurance claims data from five state Medicaid programs from 1997 to 2008 and 55 private self-insured employers from 1999 to 2008. They defined uncontrolled epilepsy in the claims data as individuals with two changes in ASM therapy followed by one or more epilepsy-related ED visits or hospitalization in one year. The comparative attribution approach [1] was used to identify epilepsy-specific costs and propensity score matching was used to control for differences in population characteristics of the uncontrolled and controlled epilepsy groups. The estimated average annual epilepsy-specific cost

for Medicaid patients with controlled epilepsy was $1293 (2008 dollars), while the cost for those with uncontrolled epilepsy was $7592, almost five times higher. Privately insured patients with controlled epilepsy had epilepsy-specific cost of $903, while the cost of patients with uncontrolled epilepsy was $9590, a 10.6-fold difference. These estimates represent the difference in cost comparing the total cost of people with uncontrolled to those with controlled epilepsy, i.e. the comparative approach to calculating epilepsy-specific costs.

The cost estimates from these studies are summarized in Table 4.2, showing the reported estimates and their 2015-dollar values [11]. All indicate that service use and costs increase dramatically with more severe forms of illness, this being more marked in adults than in children. Per-person average annual epilepsy-related direct costs from these studies consistently showed that costs were higher for uncontrolled or treatment-refractory epilepsy than controlled or treatment-responsive epilepsy by a factor ranging from twice as high to 10 times higher.

Figure 4.1 compares the 2015 estimates of average annual direct cost per person with intractable epilepsy across the studies. The figure shows that the estimates range from $4909 to $18 597. The findings of the most

Table 4.2 Average annual total and epilepsy-specific direct cost per person in dollars

Study	Total cost (reported)	Adjusted (2015 US$)	Epilepsy-specific cost (reported)	Adjusted (2015 US$)
Begley et al. (2001) [5]		Commercially insured all ages		
Refractory	–	–	3157	4909
Chen et al. (2013) [7]		Commercially insured adults non-elderly		
Non-refractory	19 085	21 009	4032	4438
Refractory	33 613	37 002	10 804	11 893
Cramer et al. (2013) [8]		Commercially insured adults and elderly		
Non-refractory	13 839	15 234	5511	6066
Refractory	23 238	25 581	12 399	13 649
Cramer et al. (2014) [9]		Commercially insured children		
Non-refractory Children	18 206	20 042	7979	8783
Refractory Children	30 343	33 403	16 894	18 597
Manjunath et al. (2012) [10]		Medicaid adults		
Non-refractory	29 635	32 740	1293	1428
Refractory	38 708	42 763	7592	8387
		Commercially insured adults		
Non-refractory	9005	9948	903	997
Refractory	24 853	27 457	9590	10 594

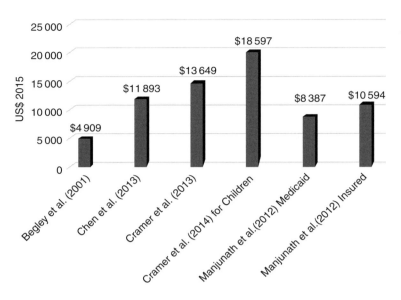

Figure 4.1 Variation in estimates of direct cost for intractable epilepsy.

Table 4.3 Indirect cost studies

Study	Method	Sample	Estimates
Manjunath et al. (2012) [10]	Total indirect costs from work loss and associated costs comprising short- and long-term disability and sick leave	183 privately insured in USA, prevalent cases, adults and elderly, active, controlled and uncontrolled all seizure types from 1997–2009 insurance claims	Indirect cost differential per year between matched sample of well-controlled vs. uncontrolled epilepsy
Begley et al. (2000) [13]	Compared the responses of the epilepsy sample on work status, annual earnings and hours if working, and hours spent in home production with similar information for general population	A survey of 1168 adult patients with active epilepsy who visited one of 18 epilepsy treatment centres in 1995 or 1996	Annual morbidity and mortality related cost for patients with active epilepsy who are in remission versus those having seizures

recent and comparable studies, basing estimates on claims data for adults and elderly, and using bottom-up ICD-9 coding for attribution, were much higher than those of Begley et al. [5] who used medical chart and billing data, and medical chart information to identify epilepsy-specific services. These studies yielded annual cost estimates ranging from $11 893 to $13 649, which exceeded the average cost in the non-refractory epilepsy population by 1.3–1.7 times.

Indirect Cost

Based on the human capital framework for estimating the costs of illness [12], indirect costs from any chronic disease are defined as lost earnings due to reduced ability to work, work loss from sickness,

reductions in productivity and premature death. The data needed to generate estimates of these costs is extensive and generally not readily available for large populations of people with epilepsy. However, some of the items can be estimated from administrative data and population surveys.

Two studies were found in the literature search that estimated the indirect costs of intractable epilepsy in the USA based on the human capital model. Table 4.3 provides a summary of the selected studies.

Manjunath et al. [10] reported indirect costs associated with work-loss from short- and long-term disability and sick leave from the employer perspective (Table 4.4). The study sample was derived from health claims of individuals with Medicaid or private insurance. Work-loss days and indirect work-loss costs

Table 4.4 Annual epilepsy-specific indirect costs for adults

Manjunath et al. (2012) [10]	Work loss (reported)	Adjusted (2015 $)	Disability Loss (reported)	Adjusted (2015 $)	Sick Leave Loss (reported)	Adjusted (2015 $)
Non-refractory	3197	3531	1055	1165	2142	2366
Refractory	7133	7879	4234	4677	2899	3202

Begley et al. (2000) [13]	Morbidity-related (reported)		Adjusted (2015 $)	Mortality-related indirect cost	Adjusted (2015 $)
Group 1	0		0	0	0
Group 2	6740		10 482	328 929	511 560
Group 3	11 031		17 196	317 877	494 878

were estimated for employees of the private insurance population, based on employer payments for sick leave due to short-term and long-term disability. Sick leave days were imputed as half-days for an out-patient visit and the number of full days of the stay for a hospitalization, and associated costs. The indirect costs due to work loss and disability was $7133 (2009 dollars) with uncontrolled epilepsy and $3197 with controlled epilepsy, a 2.2-fold difference. About 75% of the difference was due to differences in disability costs and the rest to sick leave.

In the study by Begley et al. [13], the average annual indirect cost of epilepsy for adults with intractable epilepsy was estimated in terms of morbidity- and mortality-related (Table 4.4). The morbidity-related costs were based on a survey of 1168 adult patients with active epilepsy who were patients at one of 18 epilepsy treatment centres around the country in 1995 or 1996. Estimates of indirect costs attributable to epilepsy were calculated based on comparing the responses of the epilepsy sample to the general population on work status, annual earnings, hours if working and hours spent in home production. Data from the general population was obtained from the March 1996 Current Population Survey [14] and the 1992 Panel Study of Income Dynamics [15]. Expected earnings were calculated as the probability of working and expected earnings, conditional on working. A probit regression model was used to estimate the probability of working, and a standard regression model was used to estimate expected earnings of workers. A separate home-production model was estimated that had the same independent variables plus the current unemployment rate. Estimates were made for two groups defined in the direct-cost portion of the study

described above. Group 2 people in the indirect-cost study were assumed to be patients who were seizure-free when surveyed. Group 3, intractable epilepsy, included patients who, when surveyed, were still having seizures. It was assumed that none of the patients at the treatment centres matched the profile of Group 1, consisting of persons with early remission. This subpopulation was assumed to have little or no indirect costs.

The annual morbidity-related indirect cost per adult under age 65 with intractable epilepsy (Group 3) and epilepsy with delayed remission (Group 2) was $11 031 (1995 dollars) and $6740 per person, respectively, a difference of 1.6 times. The annual mortality-related indirect cost per person for intractable epilepsy (Group 3) and epilepsy with delayed remission (Group 2) was similar, $328 929 and $317 877, respectively.

Figure 4.2 compares the 2015-dollar estimates of average annual morbidity-related indirect cost per person with intractable epilepsy across the two studies. The figure shows the estimates range from $7133 to $17 196 per case per year for adults. The study estimates are not comparable, given differences in the types of indirect costs captured and the methods and data sources used for estimation. When added to the direct cost estimates from the same studies, the indirect costs range from about 50% of total costs, just for the work-loss- and sick-leave-related items estimated by Manjunath et al. [10] to 78% of total costs when productivity reductions are considered, as reflected by Begley et al. [12]. The figure also includes the mortality-related costs associated with premature deaths, which were estimated by Begley et al. [12], but not Manjunath et al. [10].

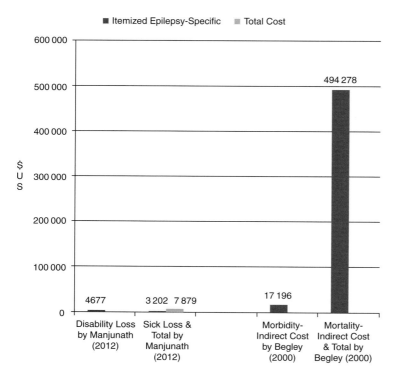

■ Itemized Epilepsy-Specific   ■ Total Cost

Figure 4.2 Variation in estimates of indirect cost for intractable epilepsy.

Conclusion and Discussion

We conducted a systematic review and comparison of published estimates of the direct and indirect costs of intractable epilepsy in the USA. Our review found only five studies with substantial variation in cost estimates, reflecting differences in methods – particularly in how costs were defined and determined – as well as in study populations and data sources. Despite the methodological differences, the direct-cost studies consistently showed that costs were higher for uncontrolled or treatment-refractory epilepsy than controlled or treatment-responsive epilepsy by a factor ranging from twice as high to 10 times higher. The most recent and comparable studies basing estimates on claims data and using ICD-9 coding for attribution yielded annual cost estimates ranging from $11 894 to $20 120 in 2015 dollars. This compares to $8412 and $9287 (2013 dollars) for the general population, reported by Begley and Durgin [1].

In our review, indirect costs ranged from 50% to 77% of total costs. This compares to a recent systematic review of 22 cost-of-illness studies conducted around the world for the general population of epilepsy indicating indirect costs ranging from 12% to 85% of the total costs [3]. The studies varied in terms of the measures of indirect costs that were captured.

The economic impact studies we reviewed contain flaws and limitations in methods, data and analysis with direct implications for understanding the burden of the disease. Flaws include, but are not limited to, different definitions used for study populations (uncontrolled vs. refractory vs. intractable epilepsy), varying inclusion of cost items, particularly regarding non-medical costs in direct-cost studies and productivity-related costs in indirect-cost studies.

More evidence is being revealed that people with severe epilepsy are also more likely to have comorbid conditions such as mental illness and injuries that significantly contribute to the cost burden [16]. The excess direct costs for people with intractable epilepsy may be underestimated when only epilepsy-specific costs are considered. Excess total costs from comparing people with epilepsy to the general population without epilepsy may be more representative of the excess costs associated with epilepsy.

Among the needs for future research identified in our review of published direct and indirect costs of intractable epilepsy is the need for understanding the cost burden of non-acute social and medical services for epilepsy populations. Such costs are frequently unidentifiable in studies based on analysis of public and private insurance claims data but may have a considerable impact on families and on society. There is a need for a current study of the indirect cost of epilepsy to update the comprehensive estimates provided by Begley et al. [12]. Better estimates of the economic impact of intractable epilepsy are needed in order to determine the potential benefits of surgery or neurosurgical interventions that may have a marked benefit to patients with refractory epilepsy, not only in terms of improving quality of life but also reducing the economic burden.

Key Points

- Variability in how the disease affects people and their responsiveness to existing treatments necessitates separate cost estimates for subpopulations of individuals with epilepsy.
- Existing studies of direct costs in the intractable epilepsy population suggest they are 30% to 70% higher than in the general epilepsy population.
- Existing studies of indirect costs in the intractable epilepsy population suggest they are 60% to 220% higher than in the general epilepsy population.

References

1. Begley CE, Durgin T. The direct cost of epilepsy in the United States: a systematic review of estimates. *Epilepsia* 2015;**56**(9):1376–1387

2. Institute of Medicine (US) Committee on the Public Health Dimensions of the Epilepsies. *Epilepsy Across the Spectrum: Promoting Health and Understanding.* Washington, DC: National Institutes of Health, 2012

3. Strzelczyk A, Reese JP, Dodel R, et al. Cost of epilepsy: a systematic review. Pharmacoeconomics 2008;**26**:463–476

4. Thurman DJ, Beghi E, Begley CE, et al. Standards for epidemiologic studies and surveillance of epilepsy. *Epilepsia* 2011;**52**(Supp 7):1–26

5. Begley CE, Lairson DR, Reynolds TF, Coan S. Early treatment cost in epilepsy and how it varies with seizure type and frequency. *Epilepsy Res* 2001;**47**:205–215

6. Frost FJ, Hurley JS, Petersen HV, et al. A comparison of two methods for estimating the health care costs of epilepsy. *Epilepsia* 2000;**41**:1020–1026

7. Chen S, Wu N, Boulanger L, Sacco P. Antiepileptic drug treatment patterns and economic burden of commercially-insured patients with refractory epilepsy with partial onset seizures in the United States. *J Med Econ* 2013;**16**:(2):240–248

8. Cramer JA, Wang ZJ, Chang E, et al. Healthcare utilization and costs in adults with stable and uncontrolled epilepsy. *Epilepsy Behav* 2013;**31**:356–362

9. Cramer JA, Wang ZJ, Chang E, et al. Healthcare utilization and costs in adults with stable and uncontrolled epilepsy. *Epilepsy Behav* 2014;**32**:135–141

10. Manjunath R, Paradis PE, Parisé H, et al. Burden of uncontrolled epilepsy in patients requiring an emergency room visit or hospitalization. *Neurology* 2012;**79**(18):1908–1916

11. United States Department of Labor, Bureau of Labor Statistics. Consumer Price Index. Available at: www.bls.gov/cpi/ (accessed March 2020)

12. Hodgson TR, Meiners MR. Cost-of-illness methodology: a guide to current practices and procedures. *Milbank Q* 1982;**60**:429–462

13. Begley CE, Famulari MF, Annegers JF, Lairson DR, Reynolds T. The cost of epilepsy in the United States: an estimate from population-based clinical and survey data. *Epilepsia* 2000;**41**:342–351

14. Hofferth S, Stafford FP, Yeung WJ, et al. *Panel Study of Income Dynamics, 1968-1992.* Ann Arbor, MI: Survey Research Center, 1995

15. US Bureau of the Census. *Current Population Survey, March 1996.* Washington, D.C.: Bureau of the Census, 1996

16. Lee WC, Arcona S, Thomas SK, et al. Effect of comorbidities on medical care use and cost among refractory patients with partial seizure disorder. *Epilepsy Behav* 2005;**7**:123–126

Social Consequences of Medication-Resistant Epilepsy

Amy Crepeau and Joseph I. Sirven

Introduction

For persons with epilepsy (PWE) who are refractory to medication, there are many health-related concerns: potential for injury, cognitive impairment, risk of sudden unexpected death in epilepsy (SUDEP). However, the social consequences of seizures that do not respond to medical therapy can have the greatest day-to-day impact.

Quality of life is a complex measure of which multiple facets are impacted by medication-resistant epilepsy. PWE are more likely to report life dissatisfaction. In a large survey of patients with and without epilepsy, PWE were more likely to be dissatisfied with their education, family life, health, social life, goal achievement and energy levels. Many factors played a role in dissatisfaction: lower incomes, lack of emotional support despite a sense of dependence on others, and increased frequency of mood disorders [1]. These findings reflect that epilepsy has a greater impact on well-being than just the discrete seizures. There are complex social consequences of epilepsy, which are magnified in those PWE who are refractory to medication.

Stigma

Stigma is defined as loss of status due to a specific characteristic, such as a chronic illness. Goffman explored the impact of stigma in epilepsy in the 1960s, describing individuals as having a sense of being 'undesirably different', and having 'an attribute that is deeply discrediting' [2]. Stigmatization may in part be due to seizures having been related to demonic or supernatural powers through ancient history and continues even today in some cultures.

Unfortunately, there is a significant lack of information, or misinformation, in the community, leading to misconceptions about epilepsy. A survey of a random sampling of adults in the United States reflected multiple negative stereotypes and beliefs about epilepsy. There was high prevalence of beliefs that PWE were not as intelligent as those without, and that they should not marry or have children. Many survey participants also endorsed the belief that PWE are not likely to be successful and should not work 40 hours per week [3]. Misconceptions such as these can result in enacted stigma. Enacted stigma relates to the real prejudices that people with epilepsy face in the community. Among patients with refractory epilepsy, nearly 90% reported experiencing stigma due to their epilepsy. The experiences of discrimination were particularly likely to occur in public administration institutions and education, and to be experienced by younger patients. Those patients with greater intellectual impairment were also more likely to experience discrimination [4]. There are also very real limitations to PWE: exclusion from military services, and often, police or fire forces. Driving limitations, for both personal and commercial licenses, result in greater limitations. Although these restrictions are in place for the safety of the individual and the community, they can result in enacted stigma.

Stigma may also be internal, that which is felt by the individual, or external, other people's perceptions of epilepsy and limitations that go along with it. Internal, or felt, stigma reflects the discrimination a person perceives due to epilepsy. Individuals with lower socioeconomic status and more severe depressive symptoms are more likely to experience felt stigma [5]. The challenge of stigma is magnified in patients with uncontrolled epilepsy, as these patients are more likely to feel stigmatized and to have a greater frequency of depressive symptoms [6].

Impact on Childbearing

The diagnosis of epilepsy impacts on the perception of PWE being able to parent successfully. A study of pregnant women with epilepsy in India demonstrated poorer coping skills relying on religion/faith more than problem-solving strategies compared to women with migraine. Less frequent seizures, better education and remission sustained for at least six months were associated with improved functional status [7].

Employment

Employment for PWE refractory to medical therapy can be a significant issue. In estimates of the economic impact that epilepsy has on society, employment-related costs account for 85% of the total $10.8 billion per year [8]. PWE are less likely to be employed [9] and have lower household incomes compared to the general population [10]. In particular, refractory epilepsy is related to lower rates of employment and reduced income [11,12].

PWE also deal with discrimination at work and may have more difficulty being hired. A survey of young adults in a work training program in Ireland revealed that 50% felt as though they were actively discriminated against when seeking employment [13]. Whether this represents enacted or felt stigma, these feelings can impact the job search and maintaining employment.

PWE should have protection in the United States, as epilepsy is covered under the Americans with Disabilities Act (ADA). The ADA states that an individual cannot be discriminated against if 'reasonable accommodations' can be made to allow the individual to remain in a specific position. There are limitations, however. The ADA does not apply to employers with fewer than 15 employees and 'reasonable accommodations' remains open to interpretation. The United States Equal Employment Opportunity Commission (EEOC) has created guidelines for individuals with epilepsy and specific activities covered under the ADA, which are detailed in Table 5.1.

Driving

For many adults in communities that expect individuals to drive their personal automobile, the ability to drive represents autonomy, and the loss of that privilege has a significant impact on day-to-day living. In surveys assessing quality of life in PWE, driving ranks as a top factor [14]. In the United States, driving laws are determined by each state and are dependent upon medication compliance and seizure control. These laws are created to protect the individual with epilepsy, and society at large. The American Academy of Neurology, the American Epilepsy Society and the Epilepsy Foundation of America collectively issued

Table 5.1 Americans with Disabilities Act Amendments Act of 2008: Life activities that must be impaired by seizures to be considered for disability

- Walking
- Seeing
- Speaking
- Breathing
- Thinking
- Performing manual tasks
- Concentrating
- Learning
- Social interactions
- Reproduction
- Sleeping

recommendations regarding driving restrictions in 1994. These included a seizure-free period of three months, and allowances for purely nocturnal seizures or an established pattern of a prolonged and consistent aura [15].

It is difficult to determine the accident rate in PWE, since most studies rely on self-reporting and likely underestimate the risk. It is estimated that PWE account for 0.02–0.04% of accidents [16,17]. Features that are likely protective against accidents are epilepsy surgery, longer periods of seizure freedom, more frequent medication changes and few non-seizure-related crashes [18]. Despite earlier recommendations, reliable auras do not seem to have a protective effect against accidents [19]. Despite restrictions, many PWE, even with uncontrolled epilepsy, continue to drive. Factors that are associated with continued driving despite restrictions include male gender, focal seizures without loss of awareness, onset of epilepsy after age 18, ASM monotherapy and employment [20,21].

Financial Impact

Refractory epilepsy has significant direct and indirect cost on individuals, with the financial burden contributing to their struggles and potentially limiting access to healthcare. Direct costs to PWE can be difficult to estimate. In the United States, the Affordable Health Care Act enacted in 2010 requires that insurance companies cover individuals with pre-existing conditions, such as epilepsy. In practice, however, these plans may be expensive and have variable contracts with comprehensive epilepsy centres where these patients are best served. Without good health-care coverage, many medications, and certainly pre-surgical evaluations, devices and epilepsy surgery are out of reach for the vast majority of patients.

A systematic review used pooled data to estimate the cost of epilepsy to individuals in the United States. A wide range of direct healthcare cost was found, ranging from $10 192 to $47 862 per patient. Though results varied amongst different studies, there was consistently an increased cost in association with medication-resistant epilepsy [22]. These findings have been corroborated in additional studies, with a clear association found between seizure frequency and increased medical costs [23]. Costs are high in countries with nationalized healthcare. A prospective study of PWE refractory to medical therapy in Italy found the average per person cost to be €4677. However, the average does not reflect the wide range per centre and per individual (€109–100 436) found in the survey [24].

The increased cost associated with medication-resistant epilepsy may also be associated with the greater incidence of status epilepticus in this population. Penberthy et al. estimated the hospital reimbursement of an episode of status epilepticus to be $8417, though this figure does not directly reflect the cost to the patient [25]. The inpatient costs of status epilepticus are higher than inpatient costs associated with newly diagnosed or established epilepsy [26].

Quality of Life After Epilepsy Surgery

The primary goal of surgery for medication-resistant epilepsy is seizure freedom. When this goal is achieved, or there is a significant improvement in seizure frequency or severity, PWE typically will have improvements in quality of life as well, and in general, quality of life after surgery correlates with seizure freedom. In addition to the factors discussed above that impact quality of life, driving and employment have potential to improve after surgery as well.

In long-term follow-up after epilepsy surgery, it was found that PWE had improved health-related quality of life (HRQOL) compared to matched patients who had not undergone surgery. The specific dimensions which demonstrated a significant improvement included health perceptions, physical limitations, pain, energy/fatigue, emotional well-being and social isolation [27]. Among PWE undergoing anterior temporal lobe resection for mesial temporal sclerosis, overall quality of life significantly

correlated with post-operative seizure freedom at greater than two years follow-up [28].

In surveys of PWE with a mean follow-up of 10.3 years after epilepsy surgery, the most frequent advantage of surgery cited was seizure freedom, followed by psychosocial advantages. The 50% of patients that reported such advantages included increased independence and confidence, ability to work and drive, and being able to live a 'normal life' contributing to the overall psychosocial advantages. The quality of life gains were significantly greater in those PWE who were seizure-free [29].

PWE can make gains in regard to employment following epilepsy surgery. Among 86 patients who underwent temporal lobe epilepsy surgery, Sperling et al. found an increase in employment and decrease in underemployment [30]. In concordance with other data, improvement followed seizure outcome. Those patients rendered seizure-free were most likely to improve their employment status. However, those patients with more variable outcomes still demonstrated improvement. Employment was not always immediate, and in some patients, took two years after surgery [30].

Improvements in quality of life are sustained in older individuals undergoing epilepsy surgery after age 50. In a comparison of older and younger patients after surgery, Sirven et al. found that older individuals had similar seizure-freedom rates, neuropsychological outcomes and return to driving [31].

Improved quality of life is a long-term goal with continued gains for years after surgery. Markand compared health-related quality of life in PWE undergoing anterior temporal lobe resection, compared to a control group [32]. There was an overall improvement in HRQOL at one and two years after surgery, with gains in each follow-up. Five scales showed greater improvement at two years than at one year: overall QOL, emotional well-being, attention/concentration, language and social isolation. Five additional scales also showed significant improvement independent of the time frame: health perceptions, limitations (physical, work/drive/social), health discouragement and seizure worry. Again, PWE who achieved seizure freedom were most likely to have improvement in QOL, but this study illustrates that improvements continue for years after surgery [32].

Summary

Medication-resistant epilepsy has wide-ranging implications beyond breakthrough seizures. The social implications have tremendous impact on quality of life, through social stigma, employment and driving restrictions, and financial considerations. These considerations need to be a part of the overall care of PWE and to assist in ultimately guiding treatment.

Key Points

- The social consequences of medication-resistant epilepsy are due to the direct effect of the seizures as well as the diagnosis of epilepsy.
- Persons with epilepsy struggle with both internal, that which they perceive, and external, that which they experience, stigma.
- PWE face greater struggles in obtaining and maintaining employment and need to be aware of their rights under the Americans with Disability Act.
- Driving limitations are present to protect the individual with epilepsy and the general populations.
- Many of the social factors can improve after successful epilepsy surgery, with subsequent gains in overall quality of life.

References

1. Kobau R, Luncheon C, Zack MM, Shegog R, Price PH. Satisfaction with life domains in people with epilepsy. *Epilepsy Behav* 2012;**25**:546–551

2. Goffman E. *Stigma: Notes on the Management of Spoiled Identity*. Englewood Cliffs, NJ: Prentice-Hall, 1963.

3. Diiorio CA, Kobau R, Holden EW, et al. Developing a measure to assess attitudes toward epilepsy in the US population. *Epilepsy Behav* 2004;**5**:965–975

4. Viteva E, Semerdjieva M. Enacted stigma among patients with epilepsy and intellectual impairment. *Epilepsy Behav* 2015;**42**:66–70

5. Leaffer EB, Hesdorffer DC, Begley C. Psychosocial and sociodemographic associates of felt stigma in epilepsy. *Epilepsy Behav* 2014;**37**:104–109

6. Ridsdale L, Robins D, Fitzgerald A, Jeffery S, McGee L. Epilepsy in general practice: patients' psychological symptoms and their perception of stigma. *Br J Gen Pract* 1996;**46**:365–366

7. Sachin S, Padma MV, Bhatia R, et al. Psychosocial impact of epilepsy in women of childbearing age in India. *Epileptic Disord* 2008;**10**:282–289

8. Begley CE, Annegers JF, Lairson DR, Reynolds TF. Estimating the cost of epilepsy. *Epilepsia* 1999;**40** Suppl 8:8–13

9. Korchounov A, Tabatadze T, Spivak D, Rossy W. Epilepsy-related employment prevalence and retirement incidence in the German working population: 1994–2009. *Epilepsy Behav* 2012;**23**:162–167

10. Fisher RS, Vickrey BG, Gibson P, et al. The impact of epilepsy from the patient's perspective II: views about therapy and health care. *Epilepsy Res* 2000;**41**:53–61

11. Salgado PC, Souza EA. [Impact of epilepsy at work: evaluation of quality of life]. *Arq Neuropsiquiatr* 2002;**60**:442–445

12. Lindsten H, Stenlund H, Edlund C, Forsgren L. Socioeconomic prognosis after a newly diagnosed unprovoked epileptic seizure in adults: a population-based case-control study. *Epilepsia* 2002;**43**:1239–1250

13. Carroll D. Employment among young people with epilepsy. *Seizure* 1992;**1**:127–131

14. Gilliam F, Kuzniecky R, Faught E, et al. Patient-validated content of epilepsy-specific quality-of-life measurement. *Epilepsia* 1997;**38**:233–236

15. Consensus conference on driver licensing and epilepsy: American Academy of Neurology, American Epilepsy Society, and Epilepsy Foundation of America. Washington, D.C., May 31–June 2, 1991. Proceedings. *Epilepsia* 1994;**35**:662–705

16. Millingen KS. Epilepsy and driving. *Proc Aust Assoc Neurol* 1976;**13**:67–72

17. Drazkowski JF, Fisher RS, Sirven JI, et al. Seizure-related motor vehicle crashes in Arizona before and after reducing the driving restriction from 12 to 3 months. *Mayo Clin Proc* 2003;**78**:819–825

18. Classen S, Crizzle AM, Winter SM, Silver W, Eisenschenk S. Evidence-based review on epilepsy and driving. *Epilepsy Behav* 2012;**23**:103–112

19. Punia V, Farooque P, Chen W, et al. Epileptic auras and their role in driving safety in people with epilepsy. *Epilepsia* 2015;**56**:e182–185

20. Bicalho MA, Sukys-Claudino L, Guarnieri R, Lin K, Walz R. Socio-demographic and clinical characteristics of Brazilian patients with epilepsy who drive and their association with traffic accidents. *Epilepsy Behav* 2012;**24**:216–220

21. No YJ, Lee SJ, Park HK, Lee SA. Factors contributing to driving by people with uncontrolled seizures. *Seizure* 2011;**20**:491–493

22. Begley CE, Durgin TL. The direct cost of epilepsy in the United States: a systematic review of estimates. *Epilepsia* 2015;**56**:1376–1387

23. van Hout B, Gagnon D, Souetre E, et al. Relationship between seizure frequency and costs and quality of life of outpatients with partial epilepsy in France,

Germany, and the United Kingdom. *Epilepsia* 1997;**38**:1221–1226

24. Luoni C, Canevini MP, Capovilla G, et al. A prospective study of direct medical costs in a large cohort of consecutively enrolled patients with refractory epilepsy in Italy. *Epilepsia* 2015;**56**:1162–1173

25. Penberthy LT, Towne A, Garnett LK, Perlin JB, DeLorenzo RJ. Estimating the economic burden of status epilepticus to the health care system. *Seizure* 2005;**14**:46–51

26. Strzelczyk A, Knake S, Oertel WH, Rosenow F, Hamer HM. Inpatient treatment costs of status epilepticus in adults in Germany. *Seizure* 2013;**22**:882–885

27. Stavem K, Bjornaes H, Langmoen IA. Long-term seizures and quality of life after epilepsy surgery compared with matched controls. *Neurosurgery* 2008;**62**:326–334; discussion 334–325

28. Lowe AJ, David E, Kilpatrick CJ, et al. Epilepsy surgery for pathologically proven hippocampal sclerosis provides long-term seizure control and improved quality of life. *Epilepsia* 2004;**45**:237–242

29. Reid K, Herbert A, Baker GA. Epilepsy surgery: patient-perceived long-term costs and benefits. *Epilepsy Behav* 2004;**5**:81–87

30. Sperling MR, Saykin AJ, Roberts FD, French JA, O'Connor MJ. Occupational outcome after temporal lobectomy for refractory epilepsy. *Neurology* 1995;**45**:970–977

31. Sirven JI, Malamut BL, O'Connor MJ, Sperling MR. Temporal lobectomy outcome in older versus younger adults. *Neurology* 2000;**54**:2166–2170

32. Markand ON, Salanova V, Whelihan E, Emsley CL. Health-related quality of life outcome in medically refractory epilepsy treated with anterior temporal lobectomy. *Epilepsia* 2000;**41**:749–759

Chapter

6

Mortality and Morbidity of Medication-Resistant Epilepsy

Nuria Lacuey and Samden D. Lhatoo

Introduction

There is significant mortality and morbidity associated with medication-resistant epilepsy, with attendant major impact on physical, psychological, emotional, socioeconomic and other aspects of the lives of persons with epilepsy and their families. Emphasis on these issues is an imperative that is often underappreciated or overlooked, with subsequent far-reaching consequences that may be avoidable. Young adults with active epilepsy from low socioeconomic groups are more likely to die prematurely, and important contributors to mortality include comorbid disorders, such as cardiovascular diseases, cancer and unintentional injuries [1]. Notably, deaths from direct epilepsy-related causes occur in about 10% of cases, but are likely to be underestimated [2]. In this chapter, we examine the risks, types, impact and governing factors of mortality and morbidity in the population of persons with intractable epilepsy. We also discuss the commonest

category of death in the intractable population – sudden unexpected death in epilepsy (SUDEP).

Mortality: the Scale of the Problem

The preferred metric in mortality studies in epilepsy is the standardized mortality ratio (SMR), which is the ratio of the number of observed deaths in a study population to the number of expected deaths in the age- and sex-matched general population in the same time period. In the epilepsy population overall, SMRs are two to three times that of the general population [3]. In the more selected cohorts, where intractability is more likely, SMRs range from 1.9 [4] to 15.9 [5]. It is important to note however, that lower figures approaching general epilepsy population SMRs are likely to be the result of compensating biases rather than true similarity, whereas those at the high end of the range are likely to represent intractable epilepsy cohorts (Table 6.1). The highest mortality, with an almost 16-fold elevation, has been reported in the

Table 6.1 Mortality in selected epilepsy cohorts

Author	Country	Population studied	SMR (95% CI)
Alstrom 1950 [6]	Sweden	Hospital-based	2.4 (2.0–2.8)
Henriksen 1970 [7]	Denmark	Hospital-based	2.7 (2.3–3.2)
White 1979 [8]	UK	Residential care	3.0 (2.8–3.3)
Klenerman 1993 [4]	UK	Residential care	1.9 (1.6–2.3)
Nashef 1995 [9]	UK	Hospital-based	5.1 (3.3–7.6)
Nashef 1995 [5]	UK	Learning disabled	15.9 (10.6–23)
Forsgren 1996 [10]	Sweden	Learning disabled	5.0 (3.3–7.5)
Nilsson 1997 [11]	Sweden	Hospital-based	3.6 (3.5–3.7)
Shackleton 1999 [12]	Netherlands	Hospital-based	3.2 (2.9–3.5)
Sperling 1999 [13]	USA	Epilepsy surgery	4.69 (2.33–7.87)
Callenbach 2001 [14]	Netherlands	Hospital-based	7 (2.4–11.5)
Sperling 2005 [15]	USA	Epilepsy surgery	3.56 (2.21–5.67)
Granbichler 2015 [16]	Austria	Hospital-based	1.7 (1.6–1.9)
Sperling 2016 [17]	USA	Epilepsy surgery	1.82 (1.38–2.34)

young, learning disabled population, where over a 23-year observation period, 71% of deaths were epilepsy related and more than half of all deaths were due to SUDEP [5].

Causes of Mortality

Causes (Table 6.2) and frequency of mortality vary according to the populations studied and case ascertainment techniques. Reliance on death certificates and population-based studies may underestimate direct epilepsy-related deaths. For example, SUDEP deaths account for between 0.1–30% of proportional mortality, depending on the study. SUDEP is considered to be the commonest direct epilepsy-related cause of mortality and is discussed below. Drowning on the other hand, can represent up to 14% of epilepsy-related mortality in some cohorts [18]. One study derived data from 51 cohorts of people with epilepsy in whom the number of deaths by drowning and the number of person-years at risk could be estimated; 88 drowning deaths were observed as compared to the 4.70 expected deaths (SMR 18.7 [95% CI 15.0 to 23.1]). As opposed to community-based incident studies (SMR 5.4), SMRs were significantly raised in prevalent epilepsy (SMR 18.0), in people with epilepsy and learning disability (SMR 25.7), in institutionalized patients (SMR 96.9) and in those who had undergone temporal lobe epilepsy surgery (SMR 41.1).

Accidents due to seizures are responsible for 2.68 deaths per 100 000 person-years [19], and SMRs for accidental deaths in epilepsy range from 2.4–10.4 [12,20]. Suicide risk is increased ninefold in epilepsy patients and may be more likely to occur in those with higher seizure frequency [21].

Status epilepticus is a significant cause of mortality in intractable epilepsy. Death due to status epilepticus is a relatively uncommon event in the general epilepsy population, but, overall, 20% of patients who develop this condition die. When acute causes of status epilepticus are excluded and mortality in the chronic epilepsy population is studied, mortality is comparatively lower. Mortality from status epilepticus due to low anti-seizure medication concentrations, for example, is 4%. Remote symptomatic status epilepticus is associated with higher mortality of approximately 14% [22].

Table 6.2 Causes of mortality in intractable epilepsy

Epilepsy-related deaths	
Directly related	SUDEP
	Status epilepticus
Indirectly related	Drowning
	Traumatic accidents due to seizures
	Burns
	Aspiration due to seizures
	Drug toxicity
	Idiosyncratic drug reactions
	Suicides
Underlying disease-related deaths	
	Primary brain tumours
	Metastatic brain tumours
	Cerebrovascular disease
	Central nervous system infection/inflammation
	Inherited neurodegenerative diseases
	Inherited metabolic diseases
Unrelated deaths	
	Other (non-brain) neoplasia
	Ischaemic heart disease
	Pneumonia
	Homicide
	Accidents unrelated to seizures

Mortality Risk

Intractability appears to confer significant risk of mortality, and patients who are seizure-free after epilepsy surgery, for example, have significantly less risk of mortality than those who continue to have seizures [17] (Figure 6.1). In one important study of mortality in 1110 patients with intractable epilepsy (1006 surgically and 104 non-surgically treated) followed for 8126.62 person-years, 89 deaths were observed [17]. Non-surgically treated patients had a threefold higher mortality rate compared to those surgically treated. Seizure-free patients had a mortality rate (5.2 per 1000 person-years [95% CI 2.67–9.02]) that was half that of non-seizure-free patients (10.4 per 1000 person-years [95% CI 7.67–13.89] p = 0.03). More frequent post-operative tonic–clonic seizures (more than two per year) were associated with increased mortality (p = 0.006) whereas complex partial seizure frequency was not related to death rate. Mortality was similar in temporal and extra-temporal epilepsy patients (p = 0.7).

Results

Seizure type may play an important role in mortality overall. The same study examined mortality risk in

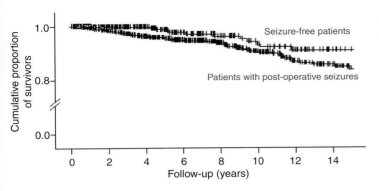

Figure 6.1 Comparison of mortality in seizure-free and non-seizure-free patients treated with focal resection or transection. From [17].

relation to generalized tonic–clonic seizures (GTCS). Out of 300 patients with post-operative GTCS, 179 (59.7%) patients had <1 post-operative GTCS after surgery per year (death rate = 3.8 per 1000 person-years [95% CI 1.4–8.3}), 39 patients had 1–2 GTCS seizures per year (death rate = 3.3 per 1000 person-years [95% CI 0.1–19.2]) and 82 patients had >2 GTCS per year (death rate = 15.3 per 1000 person-years [95% CI 6.9–28.9]). Post-operative GTCS frequency was increased in direct proportion to mortality (p = 0.006).

Sudden Unexpected Death in Epilepsy

Definition

SUDEP is defined as a sudden, unexpected, witnessed or unwitnessed, non-traumatic and non-drowning death, in an individual with epilepsy, with or without evidence of a seizure having occurred and excluding documented status epilepticus, in which post-mortem examination does not reveal an anatomical, toxicological or other cause of death [23]. Deaths are classified into definite, probable and possible categories, depending on the meeting of the definition (definite), absence of post-mortem (probable) and both absence of post-mortem as well as insufficient clinical evidence, where SUDEP cannot be ruled out (possible) [24]. Since the original definitions, a number of additional categories have been proposed to incorporate caveats that are routinely encountered in practice as well as in the research setting (Table 6.3) [25]. A pragmatic, biologically intuitive example includes the presence of long QT (LQT) genes in a patient with SUDEP, where tachyarrhythmic death (sudden cardiac death) may have occurred, regardless of epilepsy, and therefore representing a group distinct from those without LQT. The proposal to include patients who survive a near-SUDEP incident for more than an hour, but later succumb to severe hypoxic ischaemic brain injury as a direct result, as near-SUDEP rather than SUDEP, may be artificial.

A number of grey areas exist, including a potential overlap between sudden unexplained death in childhood (SUDC) and SUDEP, since more than half of SUDC cases may have hippocampal malformations or febrile seizures. The current definition of SUDEP excludes patients with febrile seizures; patients with provoked seizures and single unprovoked seizures are also excluded, and in unwitnessed cases where large time lags exist between death and discovery, status epilepticus cannot be completely excluded.

Incidence

SUDEP risk is highest in epilepsy surgery cohorts, approaching 6.3/1000 cases per year in epilepsy surgery candidates, and 9.3/1000 cases per year in surgical failures [26] (Figure 6.2). Data pooled from level 2 studies (studies with relatively good sensitivity of case ascertainment, reasonably high positive predictive value and relatively low risk of bias) suggest an overall crude rate of 0.81/100 000 population and, assuming an overall epilepsy prevalence of 7.1/100 000 population, a crude annual SUDEP incidence of 1.16/1000 persons with epilepsy [27]. Epilepsy cohorts with mainly intractable epilepsy have higher incidences of 1.1–5.9/1000 persons per year [28].

SUDEP incidence appears to vary with age (Figure 6.3). Age-adjusted annual SUDEP incidence suggests that deaths are commonest in those between 21 and 50

Table 6.3 Proposed unified SUDEP definition and classification

1. Definite SUDEP[a]	Sudden, unexpected, witnessed or unwitnessed. non-traumatic and non-drowning death, occurring in benign circumstances, in an individual with or without evidence of a seizure and excluding documented status epilepticus (seizure duration ≥30 min or seizures without recovery in between), in which post-mortem examination does not reveal a cause of death
1a. Definite SUDEP Plus[a]	Satisfying the definition of definite SUDEP, if a concomitant condition other than epilepsy is identified before or after death, if the death may have been due to the combined effect of both conditions and if autopsy or direct observations/recordings of the terminal event did not prove the concomitant condititon to be the cause of death
2. Probable SUDEP/ Probable SUDEP Plus[a]	Same as definite SUDEP but without autopsy. The victim should have died unexpectedly while in a reasonable state of health, during normal activities and in benign circumstances, without a known structural cause of death
3. Possible SUDEP[a]	A competing cause of death is present
4. Near-SUDEP/ Near-SUDEP Plus	A patient with epilepsy survives resuscitation for more than 1 h after a cardiorespiratory arrest that has no structural cause identified after investigation
5. Not SUDEP	A clear cause of death is known
6. Unclassified	Incomplete information available; not possible to classify

[a] If a death is witnessed, an arbitrary cutoff of death within 1 h from acute collapse is suggested.

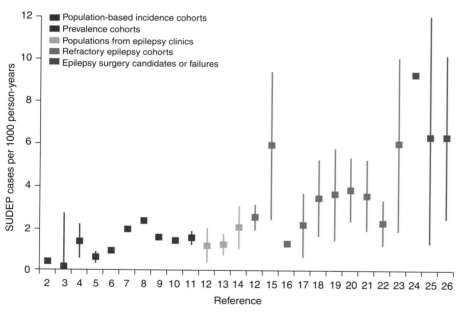

Figure 6.2 Incidence rates of SUDEP in 26 studies in different epilepsy populations. 95% CIs are shown where data were available. Reproduced from [28].

years of age. Depending on the age of onset of epilepsy, cumulative risk of SUDEP can be substantial. Assuming age of onset of subsequently intractable epilepsy at 1, 15 and 30 years, the cumulative ('lifetime') risk of SUDEP is 8.0%, 7.2% and 4.6% by age 70 [27] (Figure 6.4).

Risk Factors

The consistently strongest SUDEP risk factor across a majority of studies is frequent generalized tonic–clonic seizures (GTCS) in persons with long-standing, intractable epilepsy. Case-control studies are relatively few, and interpretation of results is constrained

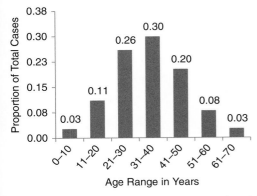

Figure 6.3 Age distribution of SUDEP cases: combined data from four population-based studies.

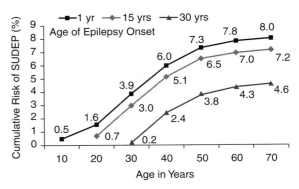

Figure 6.4 Estimated cumulative risk of death from SUDEP among people with epilepsy by age, assuming age of onset at 1, 15, and 30 years. Proportions are shown as percentages.

by the small number of deaths in each. Pooled data from case-control studies suggest that male gender, epilepsy onset before age 16 years and epilepsy duration greater than 15 years are all significantly associated with SUDEP [29]. However, odds ratios for these risk factors (1.42 to 1.95) are considerably lower than those for GTCS (15.46 for three or more GTCS/year). No anti-seizure medication has proved to be significantly associated with SUDEP and polytherapy, when controlled for GTCS, is also not significantly associated [30]. Children with intellectual disability, structural brain lesions or abnormal neurological examinations may have higher SUDEP incidence (73/100 000 person-years) than patients without such abnormalities (9/100 000) [31]. Learning difficulties, mental illness and alcohol abuse, have not consistently emerged as risk factors [29,32–37]. Some epilepsy syndromes may predispose to death; SUDEP risk in Dravet syndrome can be as high as 10.8%[38]. Dup15q patients may also have increased risk [39].

SUDEP occurs during sleep hours in 58% of deaths [40]. Such patients had a greater than threefold likelihood of having a history of nocturnal seizures than those with non-sleep-related SUDEP. SUDEP cases were also four times more likely to have a history of nocturnal seizures than controls. After correction for established SUDEP risk factors, the presence of nocturnal seizures was still significant (OR 2.6, 95% CI 1.3–5.0). Sleeping in the prone position has been reported as a risk factor although the prone finding in many SUDEP cases is more likely consequence than risk factor [41].

Genetic Factors

Few large-scale SUDEP genetic studies exist [42,43]. Exome sequencing suggested an excess of mutations in cardiac channel genes in one [42] and a higher overall burden of pathogenic variants in another [43]. Any reported mutations have not been consistent across cases, although a number of candidate 'SUDEP' genes have been reported (Table 6.4). Whether and what genetic influences directly impact ictal and post-ictal cardio-respiratory and brain homeostasis, or simply enhance intractability and epilepsy severity is unknown.

SUDEP Mechanisms

SUDEP is likely to be a heterogeneous phenomenon, usually occurring in the critically obtunded post-ictal state, but also as an ictal or inter-ictal phenomenon. Heart rate and breathing abnormalities are common after both GTCS and partial seizures, although death is rare after seizures. The final common pathway of death mandates cardiac and/or respiratory failure, although upstream mechanisms that lead to this agonal state are poorly understood.

SUDEP usually occurs in the critically obtunded post-ictal phase of a GTCS but may occur after complex partial seizures and sometimes in the absence of seizures. It is characterized by a combination of disordered respiration, arousal failure and non-tachyarrhythmic cardiac dysfunction, along with profound post-ictal generalized EEG suppression (PGES). The Mortality in Epilepsy Monitoring Unit Study (MORTEMUS) is perhaps the most important source of information on SUDEP pathomechanisms. It recorded 11 SUDEPs during EMU admissions, all

Table 6.4 Potential genetic markers of SUDEP

Gene	Clinical disorder or disease	Potential SUDEP mechanisms
SCN1A	Dravet, epileptic encephalopathy, GEFS+	Post-ictal parasympathetic hyperactivity; epilepsy severity?
SCN2A	Epileptic encephalopathy	Increased epilepsy severity?
SCN5A	Long QT syndrome	Combined epilepsy and arrhythmia?
SCN8A	Epileptic encephalopathy	Increased epilepsy severity
PRRT2	Benign familial infantile seizures	Uncertain
DEPDC5	Focal epilepsy (multiple types)	Increased epilepsy severity?
CSTB	Unverricht–Lundborg disease	Increased epilepsy severity?
TSC1/2	Tuberous sclerosis complex	Increased epilepsy severity?
HCN2	Generalized epilepsy	Uncertain
KCNQ1	Long QT syndrome	Combined epilepsy and arrhythmia?
KCNH2	Long QT syndrome	Combined epilepsy and arrhythmia?
NOS1AP	Long QT syndrome	Combined epilepsy and arrhythmia?
RYR2	Sudden cardiac death	Combined epilepsy and arrhythmia?
HCN4	Bradycardia; sick sinus syndrome	Combined epilepsy and arrhythmia?
Dup15q11	Epilepsy encephalopathy	Increased epilepsy severity?
5q14.3	Epilepsy and learning difficulties	Increased epilepsy severity?

Modified from [2].

occurring after terminal GTCS [44]. Patients had EEG and ECG recorded, whilst breathing information was derived from video evidence and breathing artifact in EEG channels. A consistent pattern of immediate post-ictal tachypnoea (>18 breaths/min) and non-tachyarrhythmic (bradycardia/bigeminy, irregular) cardiac dysfunction was observed. This was followed (within 3 minutes) by transient/terminal apnoea and bradycardia, and then asystole. When apnoea/bradycardia were transient, subsequent terminal dysfunction occurred within 11 minutes of seizure end (Figure 6.5). This study provides strong evidence that deaths are not primary cardiac events, that breathing dysfunction is not peripheral and that a combination of cardiac and respiratory dysfunction is necessary to produce death. All patients had profound PGES immediately after seizure cessation, and continued until death, suggesting severe obtundation from 'electrocerebral shutdown' and arousal failure. Vagal hypertonia (bradycardia/asystole) [45,46] and central hypoventilation may be responsible, as seen in Scn1a animal models. Severe hypotension is logical in this scenario and has been reported [47] to contribute to PGES although larger-scale studies are currently lacking.

Prolonged PGES, as observed in MORTEMUS, is considered a potential SUDEP biomarker [48]. SUDEP is produced by the one seizure that is fatally different from all others that precede it; PGES is seen in only some GTCS [49], varying even in the same patient [50], and durations can vary widely [28]. It is most likely to be produced by GTCS that have symmetrical, 'decerebrate' type posturing during the tonic phase of the GTCS, thereby indicating pontomedullary involvement during this seizure phase. PGES is associated with greater autonomic dysregulation [51,52], greater respiratory distress [53–55] and greater arousal impairment [56,57]. The association between PGES and peri-ictal autonomic dysregulation has varied, however [58], and reports of non-significant association between PGES and SUDEP [49] or even a protective association [59] emphasize the need for a large-scale prospective study [60]. Prolonged PGES is uncommon in children [61,62], a low-risk SUDEP group, but occurs in direct proportion to the duration of the tonic phase of the GTCS [61,63], another uncommon childhood seizure feature [61,64].

Several types of seizure-related arrhythmias can be seen, including asystole, bradycardia, AV nodal block

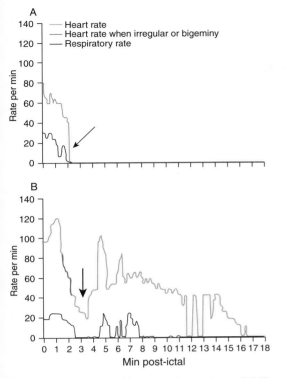

Figure 6.5 Breathing and heart rate changes in two SUDEP patients showing characteristic progression to terminal apnoea and asystole after seizure end. Patient A has rapid breathing followed by progressive breathing failure and bradycardia/asystole resulting in early death. Patient B has a similar initial pattern which is transient, and onset of terminal breathing and cardiac failure appears later.

and atrial or ventricular tachyarrhythmias [65]. However, peri-ictal primary cardiac tachyarrhythmias rarely cause near-SUDEP or SUDEP. The presence of LQT genetic mutations in some SUDEP cases is therefore not completely explained, and the fact that LQT genes are expressed in brain tissue may or may not be of relevance.

Evidence from monitored SUDEP cases suggest that a seizure may not always precede SUDEP [66], but that critical cardio-respiratory dysfunction may be similar to that observed in seizure-related SUDEP. Post-ictal brainstem dysfunction in the form of brainstem spreading depolarization, with or without preceding seizures, is postulated as a mechanism in animal SUDEP, namely mice with mutations in either Kcna1 or Scn1a [67]. This is a plausible scenario in humans, causing fatal malfunction of pontomedullary breathing and cardiac control structures, although there is no evidence to prove this hypothesis yet. At a molecular level, abnormalities in serotonergic and purinergic mechanisms have also been postulated, supported by some animal models of SUDEP although, again, human evidence is lacking.

Neuropathology

Other than possible epilepsy aetiologies, gross pathological abnormalities to which death is attributable are absent in SUDEP cases and no pathognomonic lesion has been described. However, mild cerebral oedema may be observed in a minority of cases [68]. Acute hypoxic neuronal changes, particularly in the hippocampus can be seen in approximately half of all cases, more often when a seizure occurred within the 24 hours preceding death. This is consistent with the detection of HSP-70-positive hippocampal neurons in SUDEP, suggesting seizure-induced neuronal injury prior to death [69]. Whether hypoxic ischaemic changes in the brainstem induced by seizures exist, as has been described in sudden infant death syndrome, is unknown, although imaging studies have pointed to structural changes in the dorsal mesencephalon in some SUDEP cases [70].

Prevention

At the current time, there is little by way of evidence as far as SUDEP prevention is concerned. It can be indirectly surmised that seizure freedom through medication changes, epilepsy surgery or similar interventions provides the best reduction of SUDEP risk. This may be particularly true of generalized tonic–clonic seizures. SUDEP information and education is therefore an important aspect of care in medication-resistant epilepsy, since medication compliance, avoidance of excessive alcohol, sleep hygiene and the pursuit of seizure freedom have to be emphasized to patients and carers. Additionally, there is a medico-legal imperative, and bereaved relatives have consistently voiced their view that SUDEP information at the outset is highly desirable. The role of devices is currently mostly limited to seizure detection devices, seizure alerts and smother-proof pillows. The evidence base for their efficacy in SUDEP prevention is sparse. In large part, the expense and scale of SUDEP intervention studies is due to the relative rarity of the phenomenon, and the lack of concrete biomarkers upon which to base intervention, suggest that such studies may be some way away in the future.

The Morbidity of Epilepsy

It is generally believed that persons with epilepsy carry a higher risk of morbidity as compared to those without a seizure disorder. Morbidity (distinct from comorbidity, where illness coexists with epilepsy) causes vary from cognitive dysfunction to accident-related injuries (Table 6.5).

Some aspects of epilepsy morbidity were addressed in part by a large collaborative European study that prospectively followed 951 patients and 909 controls [71]. At entry, 468 illnesses were recorded in 282 cases and 189 in 159 controls, as opposed to 2491 illnesses in 644 patients with epilepsy, compared to 1665 illnesses in 508 controls during the study period. Inevitably, neurologic disorders were commonest; ENT, cardiovascular, respiratory disorders, gastrointestinal and eye problems were all seen in epilepsy and control patients. Seizure frequency was less than one per month in the majority, although 83% had suffered seizures within the two years prior to enrollment. Differences between cases and controls were greatest in nervous system and ENT problems, which predominated in epilepsy patients. Cumulative time-dependent chances of illness in patients were 49% and 86% by 12 months and 24 months, respectively (Figure 6.6) as opposed to 39% and 75% in controls (p <0.0001). Even after excluding seizure-related events, chances of illness in epilepsy patients were significantly higher; the hazard ratio for illness in epilepsy patients after adjusting for age, sex, disability and country was 1.3 [95% CI 1.2–1.4].

A distinct correlation between seizure frequency and chance of illness, as well as the number of illnesses was noted. Hazard ratios in comparison to patients with no seizures were 1.3 (95% CI, 0.9–1.8) in those with rare seizures (less than one seizure/six months), 1.6 (95% CI, 1.1–2.0) in those with less than one seizure/month, and 1.7 (95% CI, 1.2–2.1) in those with more than one seizure/month.

Two hundred and seventy accidents were reported by 199 patients, compared to 149 accidents in 124 controls. Both of the two accidental deaths during the study period occurred in epilepsy patients (electrocution and accidental poisoning). Wounds, concussions and abrasions were significantly more incident in epilepsy patients. Apart from brain concussion, no disease characteristics were significantly associated with accident risk. Cumulative probabilities of accidents in cases were 17% and 27% by 12 and 24 months, respectively, compared to 12% and 17% in controls (p < 0.0001). The hazard ratio for accidents in epilepsy patients after adjusting for age, sex, disability and country was 1.6 (95% CI, 1.3–2.1), remaining significant even when seizure-related accidents were excluded. Disease characteristics had no effect on cumulative risk of accidents.

Cognitive Morbidity in Epilepsy

Patients with epilepsy can suffer a variety of cognitive difficulties, including memory, concentration, language and other intellectual issues. These may be influenced by epilepsy genotype, and phenotypic features including certain aetiology, seizure frequency, age of onset, duration and laterality of epilepsy, EEG epileptiform discharge frequency and duration, medication effects and loss of cognitive ability from eloquent cortex resection. The role of EEG discharges in cognitive impairment is interesting, and their adverse impact has been demonstrated in generalized spike wave discharge disorders, as well as with focal discharges such as with benign focal epilepsy of childhood. These have been postulated to be due to epileptic activity interfering with normal physiological function of neuronal circuitry involved in cognition, or perhaps prolonged neuronal hyperpolarization subsequent to epileptiform activity. Seizures themselves are obviously disruptive

Table 6.5 Morbidity caused by intractable epilepsy

Neurological	Cognitive/memory impairment
	Learning difficulties
	Traumatic brain injury and consequences
	Brain atrophy e.g. cerebellar
Psychiatric	Depression
	Psychosis
	Anxiety
Social and Economic	Stigmatization
	Poverty
	Unemployment
	Homelessness
Other Systemic	Poor bone health (osteoporosis, osteomalacia)
	Consequences of traumatic bone and joint injury
	Consequences of burns
	Aspiration pneumonia
	Poor dental health
	Organ damage due to seizure medication

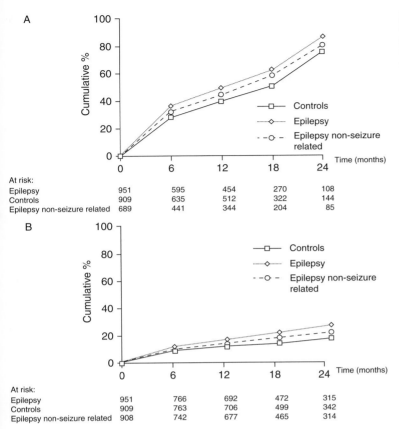

Figure 6.6 (A) Cumulative probability of having an illness in 951 patients with epilepsy and 909 controls. **(B)** Cumulative probability of having an accident in 951 patients with epilepsy and 909 controls.

At risk:

Epilepsy	951	595	454	270	108
Controls	909	635	512	322	144
Epilepsy non-seizure related	689	441	344	204	85

At risk:

Epilepsy	951	766	692	472	315
Controls	909	763	706	499	342
Epilepsy non-seizure related	908	742	677	465	314

to cognitive processes and a generalized tonic–clonic seizure can affect attention and concentration for days to weeks afterwards. Anti-seizure medications, by virtue of their neuronal effects, often adversely impact cognition, perhaps more so with older or conventional medications compared to newer anti-seizure medications. Memory difficulties are often prevalent in temporal lobe epilepsy, where the functional deficit zone encompasses mesial temporal lobe structures critical to memory function. Laterality of temporal lobe epilepsy may have an important influence, whereby patients with non-dominant temporal lobe epilepsy have greater likelihood of visual memory issues, for example. However, patients with generalized epilepsies may be as likely to complain of memory problems as patients with focal epilepsy. It has also been suggested that patients with secondarily generalized tonic–clonic seizures have more difficulty with concentration and mental flexibility compared to patients with complex partial seizures.

Whether such cognitive morbidity in epilepsy is progressive is controversial. Some studies have reported progressive volume loss in brain structures.

In one prospective study of 179 patients with epilepsy, MRI scans carried out 3.5 years later showed significant atrophy of hippocampus, neocortex or cerebellum in 17% of patients compared with 6.7% of control subjects. There were no identifiable risk factors for the development of atrophy, and patients with and without significant volume reduction were comparable in terms of seizure frequency, anti-seizure medication use and epilepsy duration [72].

References

1. Kaiboriboon K, Schiltz NK, Bakaki PM, et al. Premature mortality in poor health and low income adults with epilepsy. *Epilepsia* 2014;**55**:1781–1788

2. Devinsky O, Spruill T, Thurman D, et al. Recognizing and preventing epilepsy-related mortality: a call for action. *Neurology* 2016;**86**:779–786

3. Lhatoo SD, Johnson AL, Goodridge DM, et al. Mortality in epilepsy in the first 11 to 14 years after diagnosis: multivariate analysis of a long-term, prospective, population-based cohort. *Ann Neurol* 2001;**49**:336–344

4. Klenerman P, Sander JW, Shorvon SD. Mortality in patients with epilepsy: a study of patients in long term residential care. *J Neurol Neurosurg Psychiatry* 1993;**56**:149–152

5. Nashef L, Fish DR, Garner S, et al. Sudden death in epilepsy: a study of incidence in a young cohort with epilepsy and learning difficulty. *Epilepsia* 1995;**36**:1187–1194

6. Alstrom CH. A study of epilepsy in its clinical, social and genetic aspects. *Acta Psychiatr Neurol Suppl* 1950;**63**:1–284

7. Henriksen B, Juul-Jensen P, Lund M. The mortality of epilepsy. In: RDC Brackenridge (ed), *Proceedings of the 10th International Conference on Life Insurance Medicine*, London:Pitman, 1970:139–148.

8. White SJ, McLean AE, Howland C. Anticonvulsant drugs and cancer: a cohort study in patients with severe epilepsy. *Lancet* 1979;**2**:458–461

9. Nashef L, Fish DR, Sander JW, et al. Incidence of sudden unexpected death in an adult outpatient cohort with epilepsy at a tertiary referral centre. *J Neurol Neurosurg Psychiatry* 1995;**58**:462–464

10. Forsgren L, Edvinsson SO, Nystrom L, et al. Influence of epilepsy on mortality in mental retardation: an epidemiologic study. *Epilepsia* 1996;**37**:956–963

11. Nilsson L, Tomson T, Farahmand BY, et al. Cause-specific mortality in epilepsy: a cohort study of more than 9,000 patients once hospitalized for epilepsy. *Epilepsia* 1997;**38**:1062–1068

12. Shackleton DP, Westendorp RG, Trenite DG, Vandenbroucke JP. Mortality in patients with epilepsy: 40 years of follow up in a Dutch cohort study. *J Neurol Neurosurg Psychiatry* 1999;**66**:636–640

13. Sperling MR, Feldman H, Kinman J, Liporace JD, O'Connor MJ. Seizure control and mortality in epilepsy. *Ann Neurol* 1999;**46**:45–50

14. Callenbach PM, Westendorp RG, Geerts AT, et al. Mortality risk in children with epilepsy: the Dutch study of epilepsy in childhood. *Pediatrics* 2001;**107**:1259–1263

15. Sperling MR, Harris A, Nei M, et al. Mortality after epilepsy surgery. *Epilepsia* 2005;**46** Suppl 11:49–53

16. Granbichler CA, Oberaigner W, Kuchukhidze G, et al. Cause-specific mortality in adult epilepsy patients from Tyrol, Austria: hospital-based study. *J Neurol* 2015;**262**:126–133

17. Sperling MR, Barshow S, Nei M, et al. A reappraisal of mortality after epilepsy surgery. *Neurology* 2016;**86**:1938–1944

18. Ding D, Wang W, Wu J, et al. Premature mortality risk in people with convulsive epilepsy: long follow-up of a cohort in rural China. *Epilepsia* 2013;**54**:512–517

19. Kirby S, Sadler RM. Injury and death as a result of seizures. *Epilepsia* 1995;**36**:25–28

20. Hauser WA, Annegers JF, Elveback LR. Mortality in patients with epilepsy. *Epilepsia* 1980;**21**:399–412

21. Nilsson L, Ahlbom A, Farahmand BY, et al. Risk factors for suicide in epilepsy: a case control study. *Epilepsia* 2002;**43**:644–651

22. DeLorenzo RJ, Kirmani B, Deshpande LS, et al. Comparisons of the mortality and clinical presentations of status epilepticus in private practice community and university hospital settings in Richmond, Virginia. *Seizure* 2009;**18**:405–411

23. Nashef L. Sudden unexpected death in epilepsy: terminology and definitions. *Epilepsia* 1997;**38**:S6–S8

24. Annegers JF, Coan SP. SUDEP: overview of definitions and review of incidence data. *Seizure* 1999;**8**:347–352

25. Nashef L, So EL, Ryvlin P, et al. Unifying the definitions of sudden unexpected death in epilepsy. *Epilepsia* 2012;**53**:227–233

26. Dasheiff RM. Sudden unexpected death in epilepsy: a series from an epilepsy surgery program and speculation on the relationship to sudden cardiac death. *J Clin Neurophysiol* 1991;**8**:216–222

27. Thurman DJ, Hesdorffer DC, French JA. Sudden unexpected death in epilepsy: assessing the public health burden. *Epilepsia* 2014;**55**:1479–1485

28. Shorvon S, Tomson T. Sudden unexpected death in epilepsy. *Lancet* 2011;**378**:2028–2038

29. Hesdorffer DC, Tomson T, Benn E, et al. Combined analysis of risk factors for SUDEP. *Epilepsia* 2011;**52**:1150–1159

30. Hesdorffer DC, Tomson T, Benn E, et al. Do antiepileptic drugs or generalized tonic–clonic seizure frequency increase SUDEP risk?: a combined analysis. *Epilepsia* 2012;**53**:249–252

31. Berg AT, Nickels K, Wirrell EC, et al. Mortality risks in new-onset childhood epilepsy. *Pediatrics* 2013;**132**:124–131

32. Walczak TS, Leppik IE, D'Amelio M, et al. Incidence and risk factors in sudden unexpected death in epilepsy: a prospective cohort study. *Neurology* 2001;**56**:519–525

33. Jick SS, Cole TB, Mesher RA, et al. Sudden unexplained death in young persons with primary epilepsy. *Pharmacoepidemiol Drug Saf* 1992;**1**:59–64

34. Young C, Shankar R, Palmer J, et al. Does intellectual disability increase sudden unexpected death in epilepsy (SUDEP) risk? *Seizure* 2015;**25**:112–116

35. Langan Y, Nashef L, Sander JW. Case-control study of SUDEP. *Neurology* 2005;**64**:1131–1133

36. McKee JR, Bodfish JW. Sudden unexpected death in epilepsy in adults with mental retardation. *Am J Ment Retard* 2000;**105**:229–235

37. Nilsson L, Farahmand BY, Persson PG, et al. Risk factors for sudden unexpected death in epilepsy: a case-control study. *Lancet* 1999;**353**:888–893

38. Akiyama M, Kobayashi K, Yoshinaga H, et al. A long-term follow-up study of Dravet syndrome up to adulthood. *Epilepsia* 2010;**51**:1043–1052

39. Wegiel J, Schanen NC, Cook EH, et al. Differences between the pattern of developmental abnormalities in autism associated with duplications 15q11.2-q13 and idiopathic autism. *J Neuropathol Exp Neurol* 2012;**71**:382–397

40. Lamberts RJ, Thijs RD, Laffan A, et al. Sudden unexpected death in epilepsy: people with nocturnal seizures may be at highest risk. *Epilepsia* 2012;**53**:253–257

41. Liebenthal JA, Wu S, Rose S, et al. Association of prone position with sudden unexpected death in epilepsy. *Neurology* 2015;**84**:703–709

42. Bagnall RD, Crompton DE, Petrovski S, et al. Exome-based analysis of cardiac arrhythmia, respiratory control and epilepsy genes in sudden unexpected death in epilepsy. *Ann Neurol* 2015;**79**(4):522–534

43. Leu C, Balestrini S, Maher B, et al. Genome-wide polygenic burden of rare deleterious variants in sudden unexpected death in epilepsy. *EBioMedicine* 2015;**2**(9):1063–1070

44. Ryvlin P, Nashef L, Lhatoo SD, et al. Incidence and mechanisms of cardiorespiratory arrests in epilepsy monitoring units (MORTEMUS): a retrospective study. *Lancet Neurol* 2013;**12**:966–977

45. Lacuey N, Zonjy B, Theerannaew W, et al. Left insular damage, cardiac instability, and sudden unexpected death in epilepsy. *Epilepsy Behav* 2016;**55**:170–173

46. Jeppesen J, Fuglsang-Frederiksen A, Brugada R, et al. Heart rate variability analysis indicates preictal parasympathetic overdrive preceding seizure-induced cardiac dysrhythmias leading to sudden unexpected death in a patient with epilepsy. *Epilepsia* 2014;**55**:e67–e71

47. Bozorgi A, Chung S, Kaffashi F, et al. Significant post-ictal hypotension: expanding the spectrum of seizure induced autonomic dysregulation. *Epilepsia* 2013;**54**(9):e127–e130

48. Lhatoo SD, Faulkner HJ, Dembny K, et al. An electroclinical case-control study of sudden unexpected death in epilepsy. *Ann Neurol* 2010;**68**:787–796

49. Surges R, Strzelczyk A, Scott CA, et al. Postictal generalized electroencephalographic suppression is associated with generalized seizures. *Epilepsy & behavior* 2011;**21**:271–274

50. Lamberts RJ, Gaitatzis A, Sander JW, et al. Postictal generalized EEG suppression: an inconsistent finding in people with multiple seizures. *Neurology* 2013;**81**:1252–1256

51. Sarkis RA, Thome-Souza S, Poh MZ, et al. Autonomic changes following generalized tonic clonic seizures: an analysis of adult and pediatric patients with epilepsy. *Epilepsy Res* 2015;**115**:113–118

52. Poh MZ, Loddenkemper T, Reinsberger C, et al. Autonomic changes with seizures correlate with postictal EEG suppression. *Neurology* 2012;**78**:1868–1876

53. Seyal M, Hardin KA, Bateman LM. Postictal generalized EEG suppression is linked to seizure-associated respiratory dysfunction but not postictal apnea. *Epilepsia* 2012;**53**:825–831

54. Alexandre V, Mercedes B, Valton L, et al. Risk factors of postictal generalized EEG suppression in generalized convulsive seizures. *Neurology* 2015;**85**:1598–1603

55. Moseley BD, So E, Wirrell EC, et al. Characteristics of postictal generalized EEG suppression in children. *Epilepsy Res* 2013;**106**:123–127

56. Seyal M, Bateman LM, Li CS. Impact of periictal interventions on respiratory dysfunction, postictal EEG suppression, and postictal immobility. *Epilepsia* 2013;**54**:377–382

57. Semmelroch M, Elwes RD, Lozsadi DA, et al. Retrospective audit of postictal generalized EEG suppression in telemetry. *Epilepsia* 2012;**53**:e21–e24

58. Lamberts RJ, Laranjo S, Kalitzin SN, et al. Postictal generalized EEG suppression is not associated with periictal cardiac autonomic instability in people with convulsive seizures. *Epilepsia* 2013;**54**:523–529

59. Rabiei A, Kang J, Nei M. *Is There an EEG Marker of Increased SUDEP risk?* Philadelphia, PA: American Epilepsy Society, 2015

60. Lhatoo S, Noebels J, Whittemore V. Sudden unexpected death in epilepsy: identifying risk and preventing mortality. *Epilepsia* 2015;**56**:1700–1706

61. Freitas J, Kaur G, Fernandez GB, et al. Age-specific periictal electroclinical features of generalized tonic–clonic seizures and potential risk of sudden unexpected death in epilepsy (SUDEP). *Epilepsy Behav* 2013;**29**(2):289–294

62. Pavlova M, Singh K, Abdennadher M, et al. Comparison of cardiorespiratory and EEG abnormalities with seizures in adults and children. *Epilepsy Behav* 2013;**29**:537–541

63. Tao JX, Yung I, Lee A, et al. Tonic phase of a generalized convulsive seizure is an independent predictor of postictal generalized EEG suppression. *Epilepsia* 2013;**54**:858–865

64. Korff C, Nordli DR, Jr. Do generalized tonic–clonic seizures in infancy exist? *Neurology* 2005;**65**:1750–1753

65. van der Lende M, Surges R, Sander JW, et al. Cardiac arrhythmias during or after epileptic seizures. *J Neurol Neurosurg Psychiatry* 2016;**87**:69–74

66. Lhatoo SD, Nei M, Raghavan M, et al. Nonseizure SUDEP: sudden unexpected death in epilepsy without preceding epileptic seizures. *Epilepsia* 2016;**57**:1161–1168

67. Aiba I, Noebels JL. Spreading depolarization in the brainstem mediates sudden cardiorespiratory arrest in mouse SUDEP models. *Sci Transl Med* 2015;**7** (282):282ra46

68. Thom M, Michalak Z, Wright G, et al. Audit of practice in sudden unexpected death in epilepsy (SUDEP) post mortems and neuropathological findings. *Neuropath Appl Neurobiol* 2016;**42** (5):463–476

69. Thom M, Seetah S, Sisodiya S, et al. Sudden and unexpected death in epilepsy (SUDEP): evidence of acute neuronal injury using HSP-70 and c-Jun immunohistochemistry. *Neuropath Appl Neurobiol* 2003;**29**:132–143

70. Mueller SG, Bateman LM, Laxer KD. Evidence for brainstem network disruption in temporal lobe epilepsy and sudden unexplained death in epilepsy. *Neuroimage Clin* 2014;**5**:208–216

71. Beghi E, Cornaggia C. Morbidity and accidents in patients with epilepsy: results of a European cohort study. *Epilepsia* 2002;**43**:1076–1083

72. Liu RS, Lemieux L, Bell GS, et al. Cerebral damage in epilepsy: a population-based longitudinal quantitative MRI study. *Epilepsia* 2005;**46**:1482–1494

Models for Medication-Resistant Epilepsy

Raman Sankar

Introduction and Historic Perspectives

The earliest effective therapies for the treatment of epilepsy emerged in the nineteenth and early twentieth centuries without the use of any model systems. As documented engrossingly by Professor Martin Brodie [1], the description of the utility of bromides in the treatment of 'hysterical' epilepsy in young women by Sir Charles Locock in 1857, and the serendipitous discovery of the anti-convulsant properties of phenobarbital by Alfred Hauptman in 1912 [2] stemmed directly from human observations. It was Tracy Putnam who first set up a laboratory with electroencephalographic (EEG) equipment and studied the ability of compounds to protect cats from electroconvulsive seizures. The compounds were related to phenobarbital, and represented a portfolio of molecules developed by Parke, Davis & Company to create nonsedative anti-seizure drugs. Using the feline electroshock model (maximal electroshock seizures, MES), Putnam identified phenytoin (PHT) as a suitable candidate for clinical evaluation. Houston Merritt, his assistant, successfully used it to treat seizures in patients who were refractory to available treatments at that time [3].

Everett and Richards reported in 1944 [4] that seizures induced by subcutaneous pentylenetetrazol (PTZ) were, in fact, exacerbated by phenytoin and related drugs, but were ameliorated by trimethadione. It was William Lennox who first demonstrated that the findings of Everett and Richards were predictive of the efficacy of trimethadione in petit mal epilepsies, in which phenytoin had proved to be ineffective [5]. Parke, Davis & Company continued to develop other congeners of barbiturates and discovered that a large number of succinimide derivatives were also effective against seizures induced by subcutaneous PTZ in rats [6]. Goldensohn and colleagues published the successful use of ethosuximide in patients who suffered from petit mal (now called absence) seizures [7].

Indeed, the value of ethosuximide in the treatment of childhood absence epilepsy (CAE) has been validated in a robust randomized controlled trial in modern times [8]. This trial demonstrated the superiority of ethosuximide over valproic acid and lamotrigine for CAE, validating Goldensohn's observations nearly half a century earlier, and serves as a testament to the utility of the classic PTZ model in rodents in affording a simple and inexpensive means to screen compounds against generalized spike-wave epilepsy.

In a review of the pharmacological basis of anti-seizure medication action nearly two decades ago, we pointed out the correspondence among drug effects against animal models of seizures, human epilepsy/seizure types and what had later emerged to be mechanisms of action of effective drugs at the membrane receptor–ion channel level [9]. Knowledge at that time suggested that compounds active against MES were typically use-dependent voltage-gated sodium channel blockers, while those that were especially against scPTZ seizures were antagonists of low-threshold calcium channels (T-calcium channel). While the MES and the scPTZ seizures in rodents have been widely used as pharmacologic screens in the development of anti-seizure medications, and have resulted in the successful development of numerous ASMs, many limitations have become obvious. First, these models represent acute and induced seizures rather than epilepsy, a chronic disorder of abnormal neuronal excitability and synchronization that results in spontaneous and unprovoked seizures. Second, the faithfulness in correspondence between acute animal models and human epilepsies, as we had pointed out previously [9], is imperfect. Thus, while gabapentin is effective against PTZ-induced seizures in rodents, it is not useful in the treatment of generalized spike-waves in either rodents or human CAE [10]. It should also be noted that the successful development of levetiracetam against both focal and generalized epilepsies despite its lack of efficacy against both MES and PTZ seizures in rodents [11] provides a strong warning about the limitations of these easy-to-execute and cost-effective screening tests [10]; the same finding also raises the concern that many useful molecules for the treatment of epilepsy may have been discarded during screening on the basis of failure in the MES and PTZ tests.

The Problem of Medication-Resistant Epilepsy and its Biology

Scope of the Clinical Problem

A large body of literature exists on the prevalence of medication-resistant epilepsy, which is estimated to be in the range of 20–30%. This topic is covered extensively in several chapters of this book and this section will limit itself to the consideration of approaches to modeling categories of medication-resistant epilepsy. In approaching this topic, the following considerations should be recognized. The existence of recurrent and unprovoked seizures characterizes a number of disorders, some attributed to genetics, others representing the development of a network featuring abnormal excitability as a result of aberrant plasticity in response to various types of injuries, such as status epilepticus (SE), traumatic brain injury, strokes, etc. What complicates this dichotomous view of genetics vs. acquired aetiologies is that genetics likely contributes to why some people develop epilepsy after an injury while others seem to be protected after a similar injury. Likewise, prolonged seizures from a genetic disorder may produce secondary injury in vulnerable structures such as the hippocampus after several bouts of prolonged seizures or SE.

It is also recognized that many patients show good response to medications initially, but develop resistance over time; institution of therapy with a new medication provides a 'honeymoon' period of response, only to fade over time. Such phenomena, in the short term, can be theoretically attributed to changes in the subject's ability to metabolize and eliminate the drug. One could also hypothesize the induction over time of transport mechanisms that exclude the drug from the brain. The other reason responses to medications may change over time is the possibility that the chronic epileptic state is accompanied by changes in subunit composition of ion channels and neurotransmitter receptors, as well as altered networks. Some proposed models for refractory epilepsy that are reviewed below demonstrate alterations in targets such as sodium channels, gamma-aminobutyric acid (GABA) receptors due to subunit changes, etc.; many models of temporal lobe epilepsy (TLE) show sprouting of mossy fibre axons of dentate granule cells, which provide recurrent excitation as well as synchronization of the dentate gyrus granule cells. This phenomenon has been observed in resected human hippocampi, as well as in the hippocampi from a number of animal models of TLE.

The foregoing can thus be broadly grouped into categorical hypotheses to explain the development of medication resistance. Remy and Beck grouped them as the transporter hypothesis and the target hypothesis [12]. The former focuses on the impairment of access of the medication to the target of action in the brain, while the latter focuses on the epilepsy-associated modifications of the drug targets themselves that compromise the sensitivity to drugs.

The other type of situation is represented by those medication-resistant epilepsies that show refractoriness to pharmacotherapy right at the outset, reflecting unique genetically determined problems that are not directly attributable to defective neurotransmitter pathways, receptors, ion channels or distinctly abnormal circuits.

Findings in Humans

Transport Problems

The ABCB1 gene codes for the P-glycoprotein (multiple drug resistance protein 1, Pgp, MDR1) that transports many drugs out of the brain. An association between the ABCB1 genotype (C3435T polymorphism) and drug-resistant epilepsy, proposed based on studies of polymorphisms in the ABCB1 gene [13,14], has not been confirmed in multiple populations [15–17]. Further, a number of ASMs such as lacosamide [18], as well as rufinamide, pregabalin and zonisamide [19] are not significant substrates for the Pgp. Clearly, these ASMs have not resolved the problem of medication-resistant epilepsy. An in vitro study of slices obtained from resected cortical or hippocampal tissue from patients who underwent epilepsy surgery for treatment-resistant epilepsy did not confirm a role for Pgp in their medical refractoriness. In a slice preparation there is no blood–brain barrier (BBB). Moreover, recordings of seizure-like events that were resistant to carbamazepine or valproate remained resistant even when competitive inhibitors to Pgp such as verapamil or probenecid were added to the preparation [20]. The weight of evidence seems to suggest that pursuing transport problems to help us model treatment-resistant epilepsy may not be very fruitful.

Cellular and/or Synaptic Plasticity

A consistent finding in resected hippocampi from patients with medication-resistant TLE with hippocampal sclerosis is the abnormal sprouting of dentate granule cell axons, the mossy fibres, back to the hilus and the dentate granule cells [21,22]. Interestingly, enhanced mossy fibre input to the granule cells may result in excessive zinc release by these axon terminals. Zinc released in this manner has been shown to interfere with the GABA-mediated chloride currents, contributing to yet another mechanism of failure of inhibition in chronic epilepsy [23]. Changes in dynorphin immunoreactivity suggestive of mossy fibre reorganization have also been observed in human hippocampi from patients who had undergone surgery [24]. Studies of resected tissue from epileptic patients who had Ammon's horn sclerosis and mossy fibre sprouting exhibited compromises in dynorphin-mediated inhibition of voltage-dependent calcium channels [25], suggesting that mossy fibre reorganization may contribute to compromises in GABAergic inhibition due to enhanced zinc release, while also resulting in diminished inhibition of voltage-dependent calcium channels by downregulation of the κ-opiate receptors to dynorphin on the granule cells.

Dentate gyrus granule cell neurons isolated from resected human epileptic hippocampi demonstrated large sodium current densities and slow recovery from inactivation [26]. Large, persistent sodium currents produce paroxysmal depolarization shifts (PDS) and give rise to abnormal bursting of action potentials. An interesting study compared sodium channel function in resected hippocampal tissue from patients who became seizure-free to that from therapy-resistant patients [27]. The ability of carbamazepine to produce a use-dependent block of voltage-dependent sodium channels was completely lost in hippocampal slices from treatment-resistant patients, while it was preserved in the slices obtained from patients responsive to treatment.

Inherited Genetic Defects and Medication-Resistant Epilepsy

We alluded earlier to epilepsies that are medication-resistant right at the onset. This phenomenon exists in a number of inherited disorders, including, but not limited to channelopathies. A particularly interesting situation is exemplified by patients who carry a mutation in the SLC2A1 gene that codes for the GLUT1 glucose transporter [28]. In this condition, there is a shortage of substrate for energy metabolism in the brain, resulting in epilepsy. The seizures are refractory to medications, but the seizures in these patients respond to the provision of an alternate energy substrate that overcomes the limitations of transport of glucose across the BBB. The use of the ketogenic diet is the therapy of choice for this syndrome [29]. The metabolism of fats yields the ketone bodies β-hydroxybutyrate and acetoacetate which can be transported across the BBB by the monocarboxylate transporter MCT1 and become a source for acetate moieties to enter the Krebs cycle. Thus, even though GLUT1-deficient mice are available, they have not been used for screening ASMs; rather, treatment of the brain energy substrate deficiency turns out to be the most practical way to address medication-resistant epilepsy in this case. Other such examples include exclusion of phenylalanine in patients with phenylketonuria.

Findings in Animal Models

Transport Problems

Increased expression of Pgp was demonstrated in the brain of rats subjected to two different models (lithium–pilocarpine, electrical stimulation) of SE after 48 hours [30]. Thus, Pgp expression could not explain the acute refractoriness self-sustaining SE. The same group had shown earlier that the increase in Pgp expression after convulsive SE produced by kainic acid was transient [31]. Another laboratory demonstrated improved reduction in seizures by phenytoin when it was combined with the Pgp inhibitor tariquidar following electrically induced SE [32]; however, this effect was quite transient. Given the discrepant human data from studies on the role of ABCB1 gene polymorphisms in medication-resistant epilepsy, and the in vitro studies described earlier on cells obtained from resected human tissue, there is diminished enthusiasm to pursue this phenomenon as a significant explanation for medically refractory epilepsy, and in generating models for screening ASM candidates for the treatment of refractory epilepsy.

Modified Targets of Anti-Convulsant Action

A number of changes in ion-channels that mediate excitation or inhibition have been identified in chronic, drug-resistant epilepsy in rodents. Both dental granule cells and CA1 pyramidal neurons isolated from epileptic rats exhibited significantly reduced chloride conductance response to GABA at all doses tested [33]. A subsequent study from that laboratory demonstrated several changes in the expression of GABA receptor subunits [34]; further, the granule cells also showed enhanced sensitivity to block of chloride conductance by zinc [34], which is especially significant since in the epileptic brain significant zinc release occurs at the neosynapses formed by the sprouted mossy fibres. In a murine model of TLE produced by pilocarpine-induced SE, gradual loss of δ-subunit labeling was observed, seen in the dentate gyrus [35]. The δ-subunit is associated with extrasynaptic GABA receptors that mediate tonic inhibition and are activated by neurosteroids. In the hippocampal slices obtained from these mice, tetrahydrodeoxycorticosterone (THDOC), was less effective in reducing excitability in stimulus-response experiments [35]. Numerous changes in a number of GABA receptor subunits, including an upregulation of $\alpha 4$ subunits in the CA1 was documented by Bethmann et al. [36] in epileptic rats that were non-responders to phenobarbital compared to responders or control rats.

In addition to changes in inhibitory neurotransmission, alterations in ion channels relevant to mediating excitation have also been found in animal models of TLE. In the rat pilocarpine model, there was an increased expression of low-threshold (T-type) calcium channels in the apical dendrites, and they seemed to contribute to burst firing of CA1 pyramidal neurons [37]. Subsequent studies revealed that there were also intrinsic changes in the sodium channels per se, such that even when low-threshold bursting mediated by T-Ca^{2+} channels was blocked by Ni^{2+}, the cells were capable of high-threshold bursting driven by persistent sodium currents (I_{NaP}) at or near the soma [38]. Studies of kindling epileptogenesis also showed an increase in Nav1.6 expression in the CA3 pyramidal neurons, giving rise to augmented I_{NaP}, while heterozygous loss of the gene for that channel interfered with kindling development [39]; such a model gives rise to speculations about whether selective blockers of Nav1.6 channels may offer possibilities for the treatment of a subset of medication-resistant epilepsy.

Empiric Animal Models of Medication-Resistant Epilepsy

In creating animal models for developing drugs that may benefit patients with medication-resistant epilepsy, one must recognize that many of the changes described above in resected human tissue and mirrored in animal models occur in a parallel manner and may all contribute to diminishing response to medications over time. In this regard, creating, for example, chronic TLE in rodents would seem a fruitful approach to identify drugs, regardless of the candidate drug's performance in the MES and PTZ drug screens. At the same time, the kindling models, as well as the post-SE epilepsy models cannot serve as primary screens since they involve considerable labour and time to produce the animals, and hence cost. The 6 Hz psychomotor seizure model, on the other hand, is executed as readily as the MES and PTZ models, and correctly identified levetiracetam as an entity worth pursuing [40]. Varying the stimulus current intensity in this method was useful in identifying ASMs with a different activity profile from phenytoin. The NINDS supported Anticonvulsant Screening Project at the University of Utah adopted the 6 Hz model as a secondary screen for evaluating compounds that may be inactive in the MES and PTZ models. An overview of the available models summarized in Figure 7.1 is taken from Professor Löscher's review on this topic [41].

In the early nineties, Professor Löscher's group identified that subsets of kindled rats were phenytoin-resistant, and proposed those as offering a model to study the mechanisms of drug resistance in epilepsy [42]. It was also discovered that low level exposure of rats to lamotrigine during amygdala kindling gave rise to epileptic rats with diminished responsiveness to lamotrigine [43], providing another animal model for drug-resistant epilepsy. Brandt and Löscher found that one-third of the rats that developed spontaneous recurrent seizures after SE induced by sustained electrical stimulation of the basolateral amygdala were not sensitive to phenobarbital [44]. In these rats, lamotrigine was more effective in suppressing seizures than phenytoin. Many characteristics of these specific ASM-resistant rats have been summarized by Löscher in his review. Despite the identification of such models, which seem helpful in identifying ASMs with a somewhat different pharmacological profile, such as levetiracetam or lamotrigine,

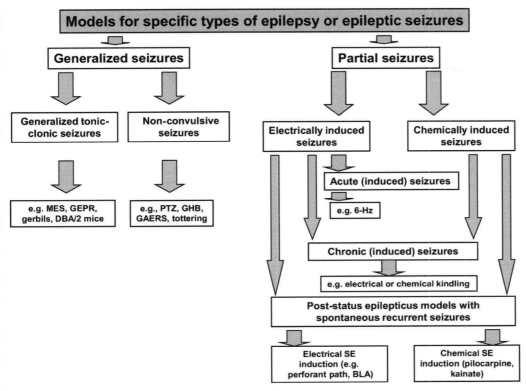

Figure 7.1 Overview of models for major categories of epilepsy emphasizing early screens for compounds. Specific aetiologies such as traumatic brain injury or stroke are not addressed [40].

medication-resistant epilepsy remains a significant problem, and its prevalence has not diminished discernibly.

Patients with focal cortical dysplasia represent a significant proportion of medically refractory epilepsy that undergo surgical treatment. Cortical dysplasia can be induced by exposure to methylazoxymethanol acetate (MAM) or ionizing radiation during the time of neuroblast division and migration, or freeze lesions created on the cortex of newborn rats. These models have been extensively studied in terms of aberrant neurotransmitter balances and connectivity [45], but have seen limited application for ASM development. Smyth and colleagues [46] studied hippocampal slices from rats exposed to MAM in utero and found that the bursting produced by the potassium channel blocker 4-aminopyridine (4-AP) were insensitive to several ASMs (phenobarbital, carbamazepine, valproic acid, ethosuximide and lamotrigine) at concentrations highly effective in slices from control rats. These models have not been exploited further in the development of novel ASMs.

In the past decade, zebrafish-based models have been advanced as efficient paradigms for both early stage screening of compounds [47] and specific seizure types. It is possible to induce seizure-type behaviour in zebrafish with conventional convulsants such as PTZ or kainic acid. Despite their significant genetic differences from the human compared to rodents, they represent a system more amenable to high-speed screening. A hyperthermia-induced seizure model in zebrafish has been described [48]. It is also possible to produce specific genetic models of medication-resistant epilepsy in this model, and a zebrafish model for Dravet syndrome has been described [49]. In the next section, which describes mechanism-based models, we shall briefly describe the promising results of a recent study for the sodium channel mutation associated with Dravet syndrome.

Inbred rat species that are subsets of Wistar rats, such as the Genetic Absence Epilepsy Rat from Strasbourg (GAERS) and the Wistar Albino Glaxo rat developed at Radbound University, Nijmegen, Netherlands (WAG/Rij) exhibit spontaneous staring spells and generalized spike-waves that have been useful in the development of anti-absence medications. No viable model for drug-resistant CAE has been described.

Medication-Resistant Epilepsy with Known Mechanisms

The burgeoning era of genomics and stem-cell technologies offer both opportunities and challenges. It is feasible to knock in mutations in mice and it is also feasible to produce induced pluripotent stem cells. While cells with mutations knocked in are readily studied by patch clamp techniques for currents and pharmacology, such a screening system lacks the complex circuitry underlying the epilepsy. Studying brain slices from mutant mice permits inclusion of some levels of circuitry, but cannot bring into focus the diversity of genetic backgrounds in patients that confound genotype–phenotype correlations, as well as predictability of response to drug treatment.

Griffin and colleagues utilized zebrafish with a mutation in SCN1A homologue and undertook phenotypic screening of drug libraries to identify clemizole and other drugs interacting with the serotonergic system as potentially useful therapeutic agents [50]. Encouraged by the findings they treated a few patients with Dravet syndrome with some available serotonergic drugs, found promising results and reported this approach as a rapid pathway to targeted drug discovery.

The importance of the network context is illustrated nicely in Figure 7.2. Several mutations have been associated with a common and phenotypically highly variable epilepsy syndrome of genetic epilepsy with febrile seizures plus (GEFS+). Interestingly, GEFS+ patients with SCN1A loss-of-function mutations do not respond favourably to classic Na^+ channel blockers, and indeed experience exacerbation of their condition. This makes sense, since the channels coded by SCN1A are associated with GABAergic interneurons, and blocking the channel in these cells adversely affects the release of GABA at synapses with principal neurons. However, patients who present phenotypically with GEFS+ but carry a mutation in SCN2A respond quite differently, and benefit from Na^+ channel blocking drugs! It turns out the gain-of-function mutations in SCN2A are expressed in the axon initial segment (AIS, Figure 7.2) of principal neurons. This is an especially simple illustration to highlight the impact of the context of the mutation in a network.

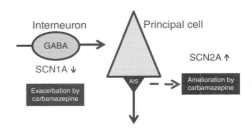

Figure 7.2 Genetic heterogeneity complicates our understanding of drug response. The syndrome of GEFS+ can be caused by a number of different genes. Patients with SCN1A mutations (typically loss of function) do not respond well to voltage-dependent sodium channel blocking drugs, because they already have an impairment of GABA release, since the mutation is expressed in interneurons. SCN2A is mainly expressed in the axon initial segment of the principal cells and the mutations typically represent a gain of function. In such cases a voltage-dependent channel blocker like carbamazepine can be quite useful.

Mutations in KCNT1 can present with a number of phenotypes, and one that has received considerable attention of late is the very difficult to treat syndrome of malignant migrating partial seizures of infancy (MMPSI). The KCNT1 mutations are associated with significant gain of function in the 'slack' potassium channels. Steven Petrou's laboratory reported that those currents could be moderated by application of quinidine in patch clamp experiments [51]. This finding created considerable excitement about the possibility of repurposing known drugs. However, experience has shown that results in patients are quite variable [52]. Especially striking is the fact that two children with the identical mutation in the KCNT1 gene (p.Arg428Gln, R428Q) discovered by whole-exome scanning responded quite differently to quinidine therapy. This example highlights the impact of genetic background in modifying response.

As specific molecular targets and signaling cascades aberrant in some highly refractory types of epilepsy are being unraveled, we are able to forego traditional screening models, and consider a shorter pathway to drug development. Table 7.1 shows some examples. We have already alluded to the success of the ketogenic diet, as well as the challenges about targeting KCNT1 channels.

A well-recognized type of highly treatment-resistant epilepsy is commonly encounterd in patients with tuberous sclerosis, a disease attributed to mutations in TSC1 or TSC2. The proteins coded by these genes comprise the mammalian target of rapamycin (mTOR). This pathway was initially selected for the treatment of subependymal giant-cell astrocytomas

Table 7.1 Knowledge of specific targets or molecular cascades has shortened the path to drug discovery in specific instances [53]

Target	ASM
NKCC1	Bumetanide
ICE/Caspase-1	VX-765
KCNT1 (SLACK)	Quinidine
mtor	Everolimus
Glycolysis	2-DG
PCDH19	Ganaxolone
Refractory SE	Allopregnanolone

(SEGAs) in patients with tuberous sclerosis. The role played by this signaling pathway (which also involves PTEN, DEPDC5 and a host of other players) is not only in growth and proliferation, but also in neural plasticity involving regulation of ion channel expression, neurotransmitter receptor expression, neurite outgrowth and overall synaptic plasticity. These considerations led investigators to examine its role in epileptogenesis. It appeared likely that pharmacologic modulation of this pathway could influence epileptogenesis as well as treat seizures. Investigations in the laboratory of Michael Wong demonstrated that early treatment with rapamycin prevented the development of epilepsy and premature death observed in a mouse model of TSC generated by a conditional knock-out of the TSC1 gene in glial fibrillary acidic protein (GFAP)-expressing cells [54]. When rapamycin treatment was applied to mice that had already developed epilepsy, the treatment still suppressed seizures and prolonged survival of those mice. The same laboratory showed that rapamycin treatment also interfered with the development of limbic epilepsy after kainic acid-induced status epilepticus in Sprague Dawley rats [55]. However, in the pilocarpine-induced status epilepicus model of temporal lobe epilepsy (TLE), treatment with high-dose rapamycin abolished mossy fibre sprouting (a feature seen in both human and rodent models of TLE), but did not protect the animals from developing recurrent spontaneous seizures [56]. Nevertheless, when the rapamycin analogue, everolimus, was used to treat SEGAs in children, the results showed that many children enjoyed a reduction in seizure frequency in addition to a reduction in the volume of tumours [57]. These results encouraged Krueger and colleagues to undertake a prospective trial of everolimus specifically for

the evaluation of seizure reduction [58]. They enrolled 20 patients who were treated with everolimus; 12 of 20 subjects attained a reduction in seizure frequency by ≥50%. Overall, seizures were reduced in 17 of the 20 by a median reduction of 73% (p <0.001) and families reported an improvement in behaviour and quality of life [58]. Similar encouraging results have been reported by Cardamone et al., based on treatment with either rapamycin (sirolimus) or everolimus [59]. Much remains to be explored to see if such treatment can be applied safely to very young infants diagnosed with TSC, even before they develop infantile spasms, or begin to exhibit traits of autism. So far, the emerging applications of mTOR inhibitors appear to represent a translational success story. The business risk of investments in everolimus for epilepsy-related disorders is mitigated by the promise for that drug in a very wide range of tumours.

An example of a translational approach that began at first with findings in patients, but culminated in the initiation of trials after the untying of a perplexing genetic knot involves the story of the discovery of the role of neurosteroids in Protocadherin 19 female limited epilepsy (PCDH19-FE) [60]. This is an unusual X-linked disorder, with clinical expression seen only in females, while male carriers are typically asymptomatic. Tan et al. undertook a study of genes with gender-biased expression in a population of patients with this disorder, female controls, as well as male carriers and male controls [61]. They narrowed their findings to the aldo-keto reductase gene AKR1C3 involved in steroid metabolism. They identified reduced mRNA and protein levels of AKR1C3 and coincident reductions in the blood levels of allopregnanolone [61]. Allopregnanolone can enhance GABA-mediated Cl^- currents at γ-subunit containing synaptic GABA receptors that mediate phasic inhibition as well as δ-subunit containing extrasynaptic GABA receptors that mediate tonic inhibition [62,63]. Based on those findings and the extensive studies summarized by Reddy [64], Tan et al. [61] proposed a possible therapeutic role for neurosteroids in PCDH19-FE. Ganaxolone (3α-hydroxy-3β-methyl-5α-pregnan-20-one), which results from the addition of a 3β-methyl group to allopregnanolone has undergone many trials over the years, with varying success [65], but has now been selected for a targeted trial in patients with PCDH19-FE.

Another interesting facet to the neurosteroids story is the emergence of allopregnanolone itself being studied for super refractory SE [66]. It has been suggested that the progressive internalization of synaptic GABA receptors is a mechanism underlying the medication resistance in SE [67,68]. Since neuroactive steroids are potent positive allosteric modulators at the α6 and δ-subunit containing extrasynaptic GABA receptors that mediate tonic inhibition, and because these receptors have not been observed to undergo internalization with ongoing seizure activity, treating refractory SE with this class of compound would seem a very logical choice. Based on that concept, and a few encouraging clinical reports of success in terminating SE after failure of numerous available medications [69,70], a clinical trial of allopregnanolone for refractory SE is under way.

If trials like this prove to be successful, such achievements will reinforce the notion that the much touted ideas about the refractoriness of epilepsy in up to one-third of all patients is, at least in part, an artifact of the entry criteria used in most studies. Most clinical trial designs for regulatory approval are based only on seizure types and seizure counts, the underlying molecular pathologies are seldom used as considerations. This is a less acknowledged problem, while the limitations of existing animal models are frequently blamed for the lack of truly new solutions for patients with refractory epilepsy. Such a selection of trial subjects serves commercial interests by offering a broad population in which a new drug might prove efficacious, tantalizing the developer with a large market. However, ignoring a more refined selection process based on aetiology has condemned us to develop ASMs that will be predictably unhelpful to a sizeable population of patients with chronic and refractory epilepsy. The above examples suggest that we are beginning to enter patients in clinical trials based on aetiologic understanding without going through traditional screens, where feasible. Much progress remains to be made in this regard.

Key Points

- Models for medication-resistant epilepsy evolved from classic models of acute seizures, and selected resistant strains of animals without exploration of mechanisms of resistance.
- Increasing understanding of the neurobiology of epilepsies focused attention on the pharmacokinetic and pharmacodynamic aspects

(ranging from changes in clearance due to enzyme induction, MDR proteins to receptor plasticity) of the development of drug resistance.

- The most recent approaches are targeting specific mechanisms underlying the epilepsies – general mechanisms such as glucose transporter defect to specific channelopathies, pathways such as the mTOR signaling pathway. This paradigm may not be applicable to all situations at this time, while it can form a basis for the introduction of 'precision medicine in epilepsy'.

References

1. Brodie MJ. Antiepileptic drug therapy the story so far. *Seizure* 2010;**19**:650–655

2. Hauptmann A. Luminal bei epilepsie. *Munch Med Wochenshr* 1912;**59**:1907–1909

3. Merritt HH, Putnam TJ. Sodium diphenylhydantonate in the treatment of convulsive disorders. *J Am Med Assoc* 1938;**111**:1068–1075

4. Everett GM, Richards RK. Comparative anticonvulsive action of 3,5,5-trimethyloxazolidine-2,4-dione (Tridione), Dilantin, and phenobarbital. *J Pharmacol Exp Ther* 1944;**81**:402–407

5. Lennox WG. The petit mal epilepsies: their treatment with Tridione. *J Am Med Assoc* 1945;**129**:1069–1074

6. Chen G, Portman R, Ensor CR, Bratton AC, Jr. The anticonvulsant activity of a-phenyl succinimides. *J Pharmacol Exp Ther* 1951;**103**:54–61

7. Goldensohn ES, Hardie J, Borea ED. Ethosuximide in the treatment of epilepsy. *J Am Med Assoc* 1962;**180**:840–842

8. Childhood Absence Epilepsy Study Group, Glauser TA, Cnaan A, Shinnar S, et al. Ethosuximide, valproic acid, and lamotrigine in childhood absence epilepsy. *N Engl J Med* 2010;**362**:790–799

9. Rho JM, Sankar R. The pharmacologic basis of antiepileptic drug action. *Epilepsia* 1999;**40**:1471–1483

10. White HS. Clinical significance of animal seizure models and mechanism of action studies of potential antiepileptic drugs. *Epilepsia* 1997;**38** Suppl 1:S9–S17

11. Klitgaard H, Matagne A, Gobert J, Wülfert E. Evidence for a unique profile of levetiracetam in rodent models of seizures and epilepsy. *Eur J Pharmacol* 1998;**353**:191–206

12. Remy S, Beck H. Molecular and cellular mechanisms of pharmacoresistance in epilepsy. *Brain* 2006;**129**(Pt 1):18–35

13. Sisodiya SM, Lin WG, Harding BN, Squier MV, Thom M. Drug resistance in epilepsy: expression of

drug resistance proteins in common causes of refractory epilepsy. *Brain* 2002;**125**:22–31

14. Siddiqui A, Kerb R, Weale ME, et al. Association of multidrug resistance in epilepsy with a polymorphism in the drug-transporter gene ABCB1. *N Engl J Med* 2003;**348**:1442–1448

15. Tan NC, Heron SE, Scheffer IE, et al. Failure to confirm association of a polymorphism in ABCB1 with multidrug-resistant epilepsy. *Neurology* 2004;**63**:1090–1092

16. Sills GJ, Mohanraj R, Butler E, et al. Lack of association between the C3435T polymorphism in the human multidrug resistance (MDR1) gene and response to antiepileptic drug treatment. *Epilepsia* 2005;**46**:643–647

17. Manna I, Gambardella A, Labate A, et al. Polymorphism of the multidrug resistance 1 gene MDR1/ABCB1 C3435T and response to antiepileptic drug treatment in temporal lobe epilepsy. *Seizure* 2015;**24**:124–126

18. Zhang C, Chanteux H, Zuo Z, Kwan P, Baum L. Potential role for human P-glycoprotein in the transport of lacosamide. *Epilepsia* 2013;**54**:1154–1160

19. Chan PS, Zhang C, Zuo Z, Kwan P, Baum L. In vitro transport assays of rufinamide, pregabalin, and zonisamide by human P-glycoprotein. *Epilepsy Res* 2014;**108**:359–366

20. Sandow N, Kim S, Raue C, et al. Drug resistance in cortical and hippocampal slices from resected tissue of epilepsy patients: no significant impact of p-glycoprotein and multidrug resistance-associated proteins. *Front Neurol* 2015;**6**:30

21. Sutula T, Cascino G, Cavazos J, Parada I, Ramirez L. Mossy fiber synaptic reorganization in the epileptic human temporal lobe. *Ann Neurol* 1989;**26**:321–330

22. Babb TL, Kupfer WR, Pretorius JK, Crandall PH, Levesque MF. Synaptic reorganization by mossy fibers in human epileptic fascia dentata. *Neuroscience* 1991;**42**:351–363

23. Buhl EH, Otis TS, Mody I. Zinc-induced collapse of augmented inhibition by GABA in a temporal lobe epilepsy model. *Science* 1996;**271**(5247):369–373

24. Houser CR, Miyashiro JE, Swartz BE, et al. Altered patterns of dynorphin immunoreactivity suggest mossy fiber reorganization in human hippocampal epilepsy. *J Neurosci* 1990;**10**:267–282

25. Jeub M, Lie A, Blümcke I, Elger CE, Beck H. Loss of dynorphin-mediated inhibition of voltage-dependent Ca2+ currents in hippocampal granule cells isolated from epilepsy patients is associated with mossy fiber sprouting. *Neuroscience* 1999;**94**:465–471

26. Reckziegel G, Beck H, Schramm J, Elger CE, Urban BW. Electrophysiological characterization of

Na+ currents in acutely isolated human hippocampal dentate granule cells. *J Physiol* 1998;**509**(Pt 1):139–150

27. Remy S, Gabriel S, Urban BW, et al. A novel mechanism underlying drug resistance in chronic epilepsy. *Ann Neurol* 2003;**53**:469–479

28. De Vivo DC, Trifiletti RR, Jacobson RI, et al. Defective glucose transport across the blood-brain barrier as a cause of persistent hypoglycorrhachia, seizures, and developmental delay. *N Engl J Med* 1991;**325**:703–709

29. Klepper J. Glucose transporter deficiency syndrome (GLUT1DS) and the ketogenic diet. *Epilepsia* 2008;**49** (Suppl 8):46–49

30. Bankstahl JP, Löscher W. Resistance to antiepileptic drugs and expression of P-glycoprotein in two rat models of status epilepticus. *Epilepsy Res* 2008;**82**:70–85

31. Seegers U, Potschka H, Löscher W. Transient increase of P-glycoprotein expression in endothelium and parenchyma of limbic brain regions in the kainate model of temporal lobe epilepsy. *Epilepsy Res* 2002;**51**:257–268

32. van Vliet EA, van Schaik R, Edelbroek PM, et al. Inhibition of the multidrug transporter P-glycoprotein improves seizure control in phenytoin-treated chronic epileptic rats. *Epilepsia* 2006;**47**:672–680

33. Gibbs JW 3rd, Shumate MD, Coulter DA. Differential epilepsy-associated alterations in postsynaptic GABA(A) receptor function in dentate granule and CA1 neurons. *J Neurophysiol* 1997;**77**:1924–1938

34. Brooks-Kayal AR, Shumate MD, Jin H, Rikhter TY, Coulter DA. Selective changes in single cell GABA(A) receptor subunit expression and function in temporal lobe epilepsy. *Nat Med* 1998;**4**:1166–1172

35. Peng Z, Huang CS, Stell BM, Mody I, Houser CR. Altered expression of the delta subunit of the GABA$_A$ receptor in a mouse model of temporal lobe epilepsy. *J Neurosci* 2004;**24**:8629–8639

36. Bethmann K, Fritschy JM, Brandt C, Löscher W. Antiepileptic drug resistant rats differ from drug responsive rats in GABA A receptor subunit expression in a model of temporal lobe epilepsy. *Neurobiol Dis* 2008;**31**:169–187

37. Su H, Sochivko D, Becker A, et al. Upregulation of a T-type Ca2+ channel causes a long-lasting modification of neuronal firing mode after status epilepticus. *J Neurosci* 2002;**22**:3645–3655

38. Chen S, Su H, Yue C, et al. An increase in persistent sodium current contributes to intrinsic neuronal bursting after status epilepticus. *J Neurophysiol* 2011;**105**:117–129

39. Blumenfeld H, Lampert A, Klein JP, et al. Role of hippocampal sodium channel Nav1.6 in kindling epileptogenesis. *Epilepsia* 2009;**50**:44–55

40. Barton ME, Klein BD, Wolf HH, White HS. Pharmacological characterization of the 6 Hz psychomotor seizure model of partial epilepsy. *Epilepsy Res* 2001;**47**:217–227

41. Löscher W. Critical review of current animal models of seizures and epilepsy used in the discovery and development of new antiepileptic drugs. *Seizure* 2011;**20**:359–368

42. Löscher W, Rundfeldt C. Kindling as a model of drug-resistant partial epilepsy: selection of phenytoin-resistant and nonresistant rats. *J Pharmacol Exp Ther* 1991;**258**:483–489

43. Postma T, Krupp E, Li XL, Post RM, Weiss SR. Lamotrigine treatment during amygdala-kindled seizure development fails to inhibit seizures and diminishes subsequent anticonvulsant efficacy. *Epilepsia* 2000;**41**:1514–1521

44. Brandt C, Löscher W. Antiepileptic efficacy of lamotrigine in phenobarbital-resistant and -responsive epileptic rats: a pilot study. *Epilepsy Res* 2014;**108**:1145–1157

45. Jacobs KM, Kharazia VN, Prince DA. Mechanisms underlying epileptogenesis in cortical malformations. *Epilepsy Res* 1999;**36**:165–188

46. Smyth MD, Barbaro NM, Baraban SC. Effects of antiepileptic drugs on induced epileptiform activity in a rat model of dysplasia. *Epilepsy Res* 2002;**50**:251–264

47. Berghmans S, Hunt J, Roach A, Goldsmith P. Zebrafish offer the potential for a primary screen to identify a wide variety of potential anticonvulsants. *Epilepsy Res* 2007;**75**:18–28

48. Hunt RF, Hortopan GA, Gillespie A, Baraban SC. A novel zebrafish model of hyperthermia-induced seizures reveals a role for TRPV4 channels and NMDA-type glutamate receptors. *Exp Neurol* 2012;**237**:199–206

49. Hortopan GA, Dinday MT, Baraban SC. Zebrafish as a model for studying genetic aspects of epilepsy. *Dis Model Mech* 2010;**3**:144–148

50. Griffin A, Hamling KR, Knupp K, et al. Clemizole and modulators of serotonin signalling suppress seizures in Dravet syndrome. *Brain* 2017;**140**(3):669–683

51. Milligan CJ, Li M, Gazina EV, et al. KCNT1 gain of function in 2 epilepsy phenotypes is reversed by quinidine. *Ann Neurol* 2014;**75**:581–590

52. Bearden D, DiGiovine M, Dlugos D, Goldberg E. (Reply to: Chong PF, Nakamura R, Saitsu H, Matsumoto N, Kira R. Ineffective quinidine therapy in early onset epileptic encephalopathy with KCNT1 mutation. Ann Neurol 2016;79:502–503). *Ann Neurol* 2016;**79**:503–504

53. Chang E, Sankar R. Drug development for epilepsy: past, present and future. In: JM Pellock, DB Nordli, R Sankar, J Wheless (eds.) *Pellock's Pediatric Epilepsy: Diagnosis and Therapy, 4th edn.* New York: Demos Publishing, 2017.

54. Zeng LH, Xu L, Gutmann DH, Wong M. Rapamycin prevents epilepsy in a mouse model of tuberous sclerosis complex. *Ann Neurol* 2008;**63**:444–453

55. Zeng LH, Rensing NR, Wong M. The mammalian target of rapamycin signaling pathway mediates epileptogenesis in a model of temporal lobe epilepsy. *J Neurosci* 2009;**29**:6964–6972

56. Heng K, Haney MM, Buckmaster PS. High-dose rapamycin blocks mossy fiber sprouting but not seizures in a mouse model of temporal lobe epilepsy. *Epilepsia* 2013;**54**:1535–1541

57. Krueger DA, Care MM, Holland K, Agricola K, Tudor C, et al. Everolimus for subependymal giant-cell astrocytomas in tuberous sclerosis. *N Engl J Med* 2010;**363**:1801–11

58. Krueger DA, Wilfong AA, Holland-Bouley K, Anderson AE, Agricola K, et al. Everolimus treatment of refractory epilepsy in tuberous sclerosis complex. *Ann Neurol* 2013;**74**:679–687

59. Cardamone M, Flanagan D, Mowat D, et al. Mammalian target of rapamycin inhibitors for intractable epilepsy and subependymal giant cell astrocytomas in tuberous sclerosis complex. *J Pediatr* 2014;**164**:1195–1200

60. Dibbens LM, Tarpey PS, Hynes K, et al. X-linked protocadherin 19 mutations cause female-limited epilepsy and cognitive impairment. *Nat Genet* 2008;**40**:776–781

61. Tan C, Shard C, Ranieri E, Hynes K, Pham DH, et al. Mutations of protocadherin 19 in female epilepsy (PCDH19-FE) lead to allopregnanolone deficiency. *Hum Mol Genet* 2015;**24**:5250–5259

62. Belelli D, Bolger MB, Gee KW. Anticonvulsant profile of the progesterone metabolite 5a-pregnan-3a-ol-20-one. *Eur J Pharmacol* 1989;**166**:325–329

63. Stell BM, Brickley SG, Tang CY, Farrant M, Mody I. Neuroactive steroids reduce neuronal excitability by selectively enhancing tonic inhibition mediated by d subunit-containing GABAA receptors. *Proc Natl Acad Sci USA* 2003;**100**:14439–14444

64. Reddy DS. Neurosteroids: endogenous role in the human brain and therapeutic potentials. *Prog Brain Res* 2010;**186**:113–137

65. Bialer M, Johannessen SI, Levy RH, et al. Progress report on new antiepileptic drugs: a summary of the Twelfth Eilat Conference (EILAT XII). *Epilepsy Res* 2015;**111**:85–141

66. Rogawski MA, Loya CM, Reddy K, Zolkowska D, Lossin C. Neuroactive steroids for the treatment of status epilepticus. *Epilepsia* 2013;**54**(Suppl 6):93–98

67. Naylor DE, Liu H, Wasterlain CG. Trafficking of GABA(A) receptors, loss of inhibition, and a mechanism for pharmacoresistance in status epilepticus. *J Neurosci* 2005;**25**: 7724–7733

68. Goodkin HP, Joshi S, Mtchedlishvili Z, Brar J, Kapur J. Subunit-specific trafficking of GABA(A) receptors during status epilepticus. *J Neurosci* 2008;**28**:2527–2538

69. Vaitkevicius H, Ng M, Moura L, Rosenthal E, Westove MB, et al. Successful allopregnanolone treatment of new onset refractory status epilepticus (NORSE) syndrome: first in man experience. *Epilepsia* 2013;**54**(Suppl 6):106–124

70. Broomall E, Natale JE, Grimason M, Goldstein J, Smith CM, et al. Pediatric super-refractory status epilepticus treated with allopregnanolone. *Ann Neurol* 2014;**76**:911–915

Neurobiology of Medication-Resistant Epilepsy

Jerome Engel Jr

The commonly stated figure throughout this volume that 30–40% of people with epilepsy have medication-resistant epilepsy (MRE) deserves qualification. Because patients who are seizure-free on anti-seizure medication over a given interval may not remain seizure-free indefinitely, we really do not know the percentage who are truly seizure-free. On the other hand, the term MRE generally is taken to mean that seizures persist despite anti-seizure treatment, although often seizure frequency or severity is improved by medication. Medication resistance, therefore, is a relative, rather than an absolute concept. Furthermore, it is important to note that the essential conceptual definition of MRE, which implies that available anti-seizure medications are incapable of controlling epileptic seizures in a given patient, is not the same as the practical diagnosis based on the observation that two or more anti-seizure medications have not worked. There are several reasons why patients may be diagnosed with MRE when their seizures are not, in fact, medication resistant. Pseudo-MRE results when patients do not take their drugs, were prescribed the wrong drugs, took the wrong dose, or had lifestyle choices promoting seizure occurrence. A common cause of pseudo-MRE, constituting approximately one-third of admissions for video-EEG monitoring at most epilepsy centers, is non-epileptic events that have been misdiagnosed as epileptic seizures. There are many systemic, neurologic, and psychiatric conditions associated with recurrent transient phenomena that can be mistaken for epileptic seizures. Discussion of these causes of apparent MRE is beyond the scope of this chapter, which is specifically concerned with the neurobiology of epileptic seizures that are not completely controlled by anti-seizure medications.

Types of Medication-Resistant Epilepsy

There are undoubtedly multiple reasons for MRE. The fact that some epilepsy syndromes, for instance

childhood absence epilepsy, are easily treated with anti-seizure medication, while others, such as West syndrome, are not, is largely attributable to the manner in which the pharmaceutical industry validates potential anti-seizure compounds. In order to screen tens of thousands of compounds with potential anti-seizure properties, it is necessary to have cost-effective, rapid-throughput, approaches. For many years, these involved two mouse models, maximal electro-shock (MES), which is a model for generalized tonic–clonic seizures, and subcutaneous pentylenetetrazol (PTZ), which causes events that model typical absence seizures [1]. As a result, all new anti-seizure medications were highly effective against either generalized tonic–clonic seizures or absences, seizure types for which adequate medications already existed, and were not as effective against many other seizure types, such as limbic seizures, focal neocortical seizures, infantile spasms and drop attacks. Although several excellent animal models of limbic seizures, such as amygdala kindling and post-status epilepticus epilepsy, have been developed in rodents, these are labour-intensive and not cost-effective for screening potential anti-seizure compounds [1]. Eventually, however, one compound that failed MES and PTZ screening was found to be effective against amygdala kindling, and levetiracetam became commercially available [2]. There is a great need for cost-effective rapid-throughput models that would allow potential anti-seizure compounds to be screened for effectiveness against focal neocortical and limbic seizures, and there are, as yet, no reliable screening models for other highly medication-resistant seizure types, such as infantile spasms and drop attacks [3].

The best predictor of medication resistance is failure of the first anti-seizure medication to control the ictal events. According to one classic paper, when the first anti-seizure medication failed due to inefficacy, not intolerance, only 11% of patients responded to a second, and only 3% to a third [4]. This is evidence that many patients with MRE have this condition at outset. On the other hand, however, there is considerable evidence that some patients are initially medication-responsive and develop MRE over time. For instance, a retrospective study of a large population of patients who underwent surgical treatment for medication-resistant focal seizures indicated that it took an average of nine years before patients met criteria for MRE [5].

MRE at Outset

Many different epilepsy syndromes have been well documented, and these represent a variety of different fundamental neuronal mechanisms of epileptogenesis (the development of epilepsy) and ictogenesis (the generation of spontaneous seizures). Some of these mechanisms have been well described and others have not. Most epilepsy syndromes that are medication-resistant from onset begin in infancy and early childhood, and are often associated with diffuse severe structural or metabolic abnormalities. Although the so-called genetic epilepsies were historically considered easy to treat, there are exceptions, the most notable being Dravet syndrome, now known to most often result from a mutation of the sodium channel gene *SCN1A* [6]. The historic impression of the medication responsiveness of genetic epilepsies is based overwhelmingly on familial 'idiopathic' epilepsies, while the use of widespread gene panel testing has revealed several more channel mutations, many that are de novo and not Mendelian, that result in MRE [7].

Genetics contributes to the development of epilepsy, and its medication responsiveness, in three different ways. In addition to epilepsy genes, which are responsible for specific epilepsy syndromes, there are genetic diseases, such as tuberous sclerosis, in which mutations in the *TSC1* and *TSC2* genes result in hyperactivation of the mTOR pathway and the abnormal growth of tubers in the brain [8]. In this situation, the seizures are caused by the tubers, as well as other effects of aberrant neural plasticity [9]. Finally, an individual's propensity to develop epilepsy, given a potential epileptogenic insult, the threshold, is also genetically determined. Identification of susceptibility genes for the acquired epilepsies would greatly help to understand the fundamental neuronal mechanisms of medication resistance in patients who are have medication resistance at the outset. Not only could this result in the development of novel treatments for medication-resistant epilepsy, but it would enable the development of more accurate experimental animal models, because the introduction of an epileptogenic insult into a normal rodent brain may not result in the same phenotype as the introduction of the same insult into the brain of a rodent with the susceptibility gene profile of patients who manifest the epilepsy syndrome in question.

Epileptic seizures due to specific causes that are unresponsive to anti-seizure medications may be responsive to other medical treatments. Two examples of this are focal seizures due to non-ketogenic hyperglycaemia, which are treated with insulin, and focal seizures due to autoantibodies to NMDA, GABA and AMPA receptors, as well as the voltage-gated potassium channel complex, which are treated with anti-inflammatory therapies such as steroids, IVIg, plasmapheresis, and rituximab. These conditions would be considered MRE according to the ILAE definition; however, they are not medically refractory in the sense that these other medical treatments are effective.

Progressive Development of MRE

The most common, and most medically refractory, epilepsy syndrome, at least in adults, is mesial temporal lobe epilepsy (MTLE) with hippocampal sclerosis (HS) [10]. Many of these patients have a history of a prolonged febrile seizure, or another brain insult, within the first five years of life, and a family history of epilepsy, suggesting a genetic predisposition to develop epilepsy following a specific epileptogenic injury during a critical phase of development. Seizures can begin at any age, but most commonly begin in late childhood, before puberty. At this stage, anti-seizure treatment is usually successful and patients may remain seizure-free on, or even off, medication for several years. The medically refractory form of this syndrome begins later in life when seizures recur, and all attempts at further medical control fail, suggesting a progressive condition [11]. Although progression has been best documented for patients with MTLE with HS [12], similar scenarios can be seen with focal neocortical seizures caused by a variety of lesions, suggesting that other forms of acquired epilepsy, with focal seizures, are progressive as well [5]. In addition to progressive changes that lead to medication resistance, it is important to note that there is also considerable evidence supporting the notion that epileptic seizures can contribute to developmental delay in infants and small children, and cognitive disturbances later in life, as in the so-called epileptic encephalopathies, which can be prevented or reversed if seizures are controlled [13].

Two theories are being pursued to determine why seizures in some patients are initially pharmacoresponsive but over time become medication-resistant [14]. One theory is that the target epileptogenic mechanism gradually becomes refractory to the effects of the anti-seizure drug. How this might happen is unknown, and presumably there could be multiple mechanisms of progressive insensitivity that vary from one seizure type to another. The second theory concerns increased expression of a multi-drug resistance (MDR) gene responsible for transporters such as P-glycoprotein (PGP) that move molecules across the blood–brain barrier and expel toxins from the brain [15]. It has been suggested that this process is progressively increased in some patients in the epileptogenic region, selectively reducing access of anti-seizure drugs to the target.

Treatment of MRE

It is likely that many more potential mechanisms will be identified to explain why some patients have MRE at outset, and why others slowly develop MRE over time. It is anticipated that research in this area will eventually result in pharmacological interventions that selectively prevent or reverse different types of MRE. Just as approaches to anti-seizure drug discovery and validation with animal models is problematic and partially explains the prevalence of MRE, current approaches to clinical trials are inadequate to reveal effective treatments for many patients with MRE. Most clinical trials are conducted on populations of patients with 'complex partial seizures, with or without secondarily generalized seizures'. This is a highly non-specific designation, undoubtedly including patients with many different types of epilepsy. The persistent difficulty in creating a pathophysiologically based classification of epileptic seizures, particularly focal seizures [16–18], has made it impossible to carry out clinical trials on populations of patients whose seizures represent the same, or similar, fundamental neuronal ictogenic mechanisms. As a result, during any given clinical trial, if there is a subset of patients with MRE who would respond to a specific potential anti-seizure compound under investigation, and their numbers are relatively small compared to the total population, this selective success would likely go undetected. Clearly, more basic research is necessary to create a pathophysiologic classification of epilepsy, before more rational clinical trials of potential anti-seizure compounds can be carried out.

Biomarkers

Biomarkers are defined as dynamic biological changes that indicate the presence of an epileptogenic process with a sufficiently high degree of reliability to warrant intervention. Biomarkers of epileptogenesis would not only indicate the presence of processes that lead to the development of epilepsy, but also processes that cause the progression of epilepsy after it has developed. Biomarkers of epileptogenicity, or ictogenicity, that identify the propensity to generate spontaneous seizures, would be useful to diagnose epilepsy or, conversely, to document prevention or cure, either after an effective anti-epileptogenic intervention or spontaneously. Biomarkers of ictogenicity could also be used to tailor individual pharmacotherapy, and to diagnose medication resistance by rapidly assessing large numbers of anti-seizure medications, rather than assuming that trials of two drugs are sufficient to indicate MRE in every patient. Biomarkers of epileptogenesis that identify progression and biomarkers of ictogenicity that identify medication resistance could be used to determine which patients with MRE deserve aggressive treatment, such as surgery, sooner rather than later. Biomarkers of ictogenicity that identify brain tissue capable of generating spontaneous seizures could be used to identify the epileptogenic region and facilitate evaluation prior to resective surgical therapy. Finally, biomarkers of epileptogenesis and ictogenicity might be used to develop cost-effective rapid-throughput screening models for validating novel potentially anti-epileptogenic and anti-seizure compounds.

Figure 8.1 illustrates three important components of the multi-factorial basis of epilepsy: threshold, specific epileptogenic abnormality and precipitating factors [19]. Anti-seizure drugs act to elevate threshold, identification of the epileptogenic abnormality can lead to specific targeted treatments, such as surgical removal, and identification of precipitating factors can suggest avoidance strategies. MRE could result from a chronically low threshold and/or a particularly virulent epileptogenic substrate, and/or frequent unavoidable precipitating factors. Figures 8.2 and 8.3 demonstrate how biomarkers that could identify changes in threshold, as well as the underlying epileptogenic and ictogenic abnormalities, could be used to identify patients at risk for developing epilepsy, diagnose progressive disorders, distinguish remission from cure, and document the effectiveness of preventive interventions.

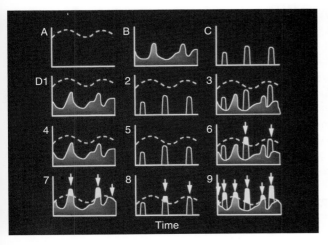

Figure 8.1 Multi-factorial basis of epilepsy. (A) The dashed line indicates seizure threshold; it is wavy to acknowledge that seizure threshold is not static. Seizure threshold or probability is defined as the propensity or likelihood for a seizure to occur; it also represents *epileptogenicity*, but what might more accurately be called *ictogenicity*. (B) This represents a specific epileptogenic abnormality that could be structural metabolic or genetic. Specific epileptogenic abnormalities are also not necessarily static, and the degree of epileptogenicity can change from one time to another. (C) This illustrates precipitating factors, which can be external, for instance for reflex seizures, or internal and usually not detectable. Precipitating factors determine when seizures occur. The subsequent panels (D1–9) illustrate how these three factors interact. Someone with a high threshold may have epileptogenic abnormalities and precipitating factors and never have seizures, whereas someone with a low threshold could have seizures due to epileptogenic abnormalities without precipitating factors, seizures due to precipitating factors without an epileptogenic abnormality (provoked seizures), or both. From [19], with permission.

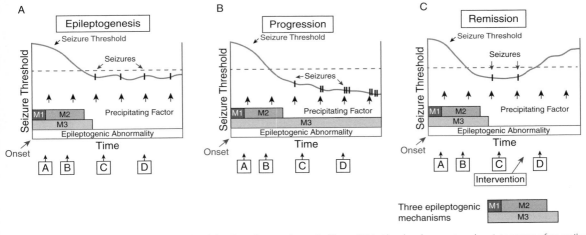

Figure 8.2 (A) This figure illustrates the role of the three factors shown in Figure 8.1 in the development and maintenance of an epilepsy condition. At the bottom there is a cascade of mechanisms that begin, continue, and maintain the epileptogenic process. These last for varying periods of time. Some may invariably lead to epilepsy and others not. The top line illustrates changes in threshold. A lower threshold indicates an increased propensity for seizure generation related to the epileptogenic process illustrated on the bottom line. Once the threshold goes below a certain level (dashed line), seizures occur, in response to precipitating factors illustrated in the middle. The threshold level could be considered ictogenicity and the bottom boxes could represent epileptogenesis. Measures taken at point A might reveal biomarkers of epileptogenic processes with a predictive value for development of epilepsy, whereas biomarkers of ictogenicity would have no predictive value. Measures taken at point B might reveal biomarkers of different epileptogenic mechanisms that have a different predictive value than those at A, and could permit staging of the epileptogenic process, whereas measures of ictogenicity could reveal a change suggestive of a developing epileptogenic process. Measures taken at point C could reveal biomarkers of epileptogenic processes that document that an epilepsy condition exists, and perhaps determine whether it was stable or progressive. Biomarkers of ictogenicity at this point might also reveal that an epilepsy condition exists, but would provide no information regarding potential progression. Measures that are taken at point D could also yield biomarkers indicating whether epileptogenesis is persistent or progressive, whereas changes in biomarkers of ictogenicity from point C to point D could indicate progression or improvement, but not determine whether this reflects changes in epileptogenic processes. Repeated measures could document reduction in epileptogenic processes as a result of antiepileptogenic interventions, and fluctuations in ictogenicity due to anti-seizure drugs, or circumstances such as illness or stress that might increase the propensity for seizures to occur. Measures taken at any point in time after the development of epilepsy might reveal biomarkers of the onset of a precipitating factor, which could be used for seizure prediction. Such biomarkers would be necessary for the development of interventions that abort seizures. (B) This figure illustrates progression. In this case, more of the epileptogenic processes continue after seizures begin and the threshold continues to be reduced, resulting in more frequent or more severe seizures with precipitating factors. Measures at D could indicate biomarkers of epileptogenic processes that document progression as well as a further lowering of the threshold or increased ictogenicity. (C) This figure illustrates remission where an intervention results in an increase in threshold and freedom from seizures, but the underlying epileptogenic abnormality persists. Measures taken at D in this situation could reveal biomarkers indicating that the epileptogenic process persists, although the threshold is elevated so that ictogenicity is decreased, perhaps even to a 'normal' level. From [26], with permission.

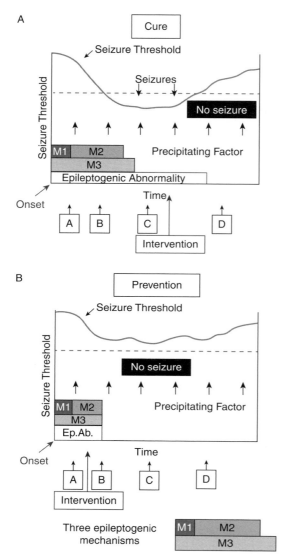

Figure 8.3 (A) This figure illustrates cure. In this instance, the intervention after epilepsy is established eliminates the underlying epileptogenic abnormality so that a measure taken at C would be the same as in Figure 8.2B, but a measure taken at D would show that biomarkers for the underlying epileptogenic abnormality are now resolved, thereby confirming cure. (B) This figure illustrates prevention. In this case, an intervention shortly after the epileptogenic process begins results in the elimination of the underlying epileptogenic abnormality before seizures occur, and the threshold returns to baseline. Measures at B would indicate loss of some biomarkers of the epileptogenic abnormality, whereas measures at C and D would indicate absence of biomarkers for the epileptogenic abnormality and a return of threshold, or ictogenicity, to baseline levels, thereby confirming prevention. From [26], with permission.

A variety of mechanisms of epileptogenesis and ictogenicity have been identified that could serve as targets for the development of biomarkers, including cell loss (e.g. hippocampal atrophy), axonal sprouting, synaptic reorganization, altered neuronal function (e.g. gene expression profiles and protein products), neurogenesis, altered glial function and gliosis, inflammatory changes, angiogenesis, alterations in the blood–brain barrier, and altered excitability and synchrony [20]. Potential biomarkers currently under investigation include hippocampal changes on MRI [21], interictal spike features, including changes during fMRI [22], pathological high-frequency oscillations (pHFOs) [23,24], excitability determined by transcranial magnetic stimulation [25], alpha-methyl-tryptophan positron emission tomography (AMT-PET) imaging [27] and blood–brain barrier integrity [28]. It would be ideal to identify alterations in gene expression profiles associated with epileptogenesis and ictogenesis, and specifically with MRE. If such profiles were present in white blood cells, a simple finger stick would suffice to definitively diagnose MRE, avoid the cost and risk of additional drug trials, and permit rapid institution of more effective alternative treatments such as surgery.

The search for biomarkers of epileptogenesis, epileptogenicity and MRE, using translational reiterative parallel human and animal research paradigms, should also lead to elucidation of fundamental mechanisms, which in turn would inform more rational novel treatments.

Summary

Medication-resistant epilepsy (MRE) is operationally defined as epilepsy in which seizures have not been controlled by trials of two appropriate anti-seizure medications. This does not necessarily mean, however, that seizures are medication-resistant. There are many types of pseudo-MRE, ranging from failure to take medication properly for various reasons, to paroxysmal events that mimic epileptic seizures but are not. Furthermore, some patients who fail two appropriate medications will ultimately respond to the third or fourth. MRE, as clinically defined, therefore, does not indicate absolute medication resistance.

Approximately 40% of patients with epilepsy have seizures that do not respond to anti-seizure medications, and the exact percentage of these who are truly medication-resistant has not been determined. Of these, however, there are undoubtedly multiple types of MRE. Some seizures are medication-resistant from the start, and most of these reflect the fact that approaches to anti-seizure drug discovery and validation do not use screening models of most medication-resistant seizure types. Other types of epilepsy, particularly those with acquired focal seizures, develop medication resistance over time, either because the target epileptogenic mechanism eventually becomes refractory to anti-seizure drugs, or because MDR genes are overexpressed, resulting in increased removal of drug from the epileptogenic region. Failure to develop a pathophysiologic classification of seizure types and epilepsy syndromes contributes to the inability of clinical trials to identify medications that may be effective in a small percentage of patients who are non-specifically categorized as having 'complex partial seizures with or without secondarily generalized seizures'.

Fortunately, there are alternative non-pharmacological treatments that can be effective for MRE, including surgical therapy, neuromodulation, the ketogenic diet and a variety of complementary and alternative therapies. Biomarkers that can be used to assess the effectiveness of treatment and definitively diagnose MRE early would greatly facilitate rapid identification of the best drug for individual patients, and a timely referral for non-pharmacological treatment.

Key Points

- Many patients who appear to have MRE, after further diagnosis at an epilepsy centre, are found to have pseudo-MRE for a variety of reasons, including non-epileptic seizures, non-adherence and lifestyle issues.
- The development of new, targeted anti-seizure medications has not altered the percentage of patients with MRE, indicating unrecognized underlying mechanisms of epilepsy.
- There must be a variety of different causes of MRE, some exist at onset and others develop over time.
- More information is needed to define the various neurobiological causes of MRE, and to identify biomarkers that could inform treatment or prevention

Acknowledgments

Original research reported by the author was supported in part by Grants NS-02808, NS-15654, NS-33310, NS-80181 and NS-100064.

References

1. Löscher W, Schmidt D. Modern antiepileptic drug development has failed to deliver ways out of the current dilemma. *Epilepsia* 2011;**52**:657–678
2. Klitgaard H, Matagne A, Gobert J, et al. Evidence for a unique profile of levetiracetam in rodent models of seizures and epilepsy. *Eur J Pharmacol* 1998;**353**:191–206
3. Galanopoulou, AS, Buckmaster, PS, Staley, KJ, et al. Identification of new epilepsy treatments: issues in preclinical methodology. *Epilepsia* 2012;**53**:571–582
4. Kwan P, Brodie MJ. Early identification of refractory epilepsy. *New Engl J Med* 2000;**342**:314–319
5. Berg AT, Langfitt J, Shinnar S, et al. How long does it take for partial epilepsy to become intractable? *Neurology* 2003;**60**:186–190
6. Brunklaus A, Zuberi SM. Dravet syndrome–from epileptic encephalopathy to channelopathy. *Epilepsia* 2014;**55**:979–984
7. Helbig I, Heinzen EL, Mefford HC; ILAE Genetics Commission. Primer Part 1-The building blocks of epilepsy genetics. *Epilepsia* 2016;**57**:861–868
8. DiMario FJ, Jr, Sahin M, Ebrahimi-Fakhari D. Tuberous sclerosis complex. *Pediatr Clin North Am* 2015;**62**:633–648
9. Wong M. mTOR as a potential treatment target for epilepsy. *Future Neurol* 2012;7:537–545
10. Semah F, Picot MC, Adam C, et al. Is the underlying cause of epilepsy a major prognostic factor for recurrence? *Neurology* 1998;**51**:1256–1262
11. Engel J Jr, Williamson PD, Wieser HG. Mesial temporal lobe epilepsy with hippocampal sclerosis. In: J Engel Jr, TA Pedley (eds.), *Epilepsy: A Comprehensive Textbook, 2nd edn.* Philadelphia, PA: Lippincott-Raven, 2008:2479–2486
12. Cendes F. Progressive hippocampal and extrahippocampal atrophy in drug resistant epilepsy. *Curr Opin Neurol* 2005;**18**:173–177
13. Shields WD, Shewmon DA, Chugani HT, Peacock WJ. The role of surgery in the treatment of infantile spasms. *J Epilepsy* 1990;(Suppl 3):321–324
14. Löscher W, Schmidt D. Mechanisms of tolerance and drug resistance. In S Shorvon, E Perucca, J Engel Jr (eds.), *The Treatment of Epilepsy, 3rd edn.* Oxford: Wiley-Blackwell, 2009:109–118
15. Sisodiya SM, Beck H, Löscher W, Vezzani A. Mechanisms of drug resistance. In: J Engel Jr, TA Pedley (eds.), *Epilepsy: A Comprehensive Textbook, 2nd edn.* Philadelphia, PA: Lippincott-Raven, 2008:1279–1289

16. Engel J, Jr. A proposed diagnostic scheme for people with epileptic seizures and with epilepsy: report of the ILAE Task Force on Classification and Terminology. *Epilepsia* 2001;**42**:796–803

17. Engel J, Jr. Report of the ILAE Classification Core Group. *Epilepsia* 2006;**47**:1558–1568

18. Berg AT, Berkovic SF, Brodie MJ, et al. Revised terminology and concepts for organization of seizures and epilepsies: report of the ILAE Commission on Classification and Terminology, 2005–2009. *Epilepsia* 2010;**51**:676–685

19. Engel J, Jr. *Seizures and Epilepsy, 2nd edn.* Oxford: Oxford University Press, 2013:706

20. Engel J, Jr. Progress in epilepsy: reducing the treatment gap and the promise of biomarkers. *Curr Opin Neurol* 2008;**21**:150–154

21. Lewis DV, Shinnar S, Hesdorffer DC, et al. Hippocampal sclerosis after febrile status epilepticus: the FEBSTAT study. *Ann Neurol* 2014;**75**:178–185

22. Coan AC, Chaudhary UJ, Grouiller F, et al. EEG-fMRI in the presurgical evaluation of temporal lobe epilepsy. *J Neurol Neurosurg Psychiatry* 2015;**87**(6):642–649

23. Worrell G, Gotman J. High-frequency oscillations and other electrophysiological biomarkers of epilepsy: clinical studies. *Biomark Med* 2011;**5** (5):557–566

24. Engel J Jr, Bragin A, Staba R, Mody I. High-frequency oscillations: what is normal and what is not? *Epilepsia* 2009;**50**:598–604

25. Valentin A, Arunachalam R, Mesquita-Rodrigues A, et al. Late EEG responses triggered by transcranial magnetic stimulation (TMS) in the evaluation of focal epilepsy. *Epilepsia* 2008;**49**:470–480

26. Engel J, Jr, Pitkänen A, Loeb JA, et al. Epilepsy biomarkers. *Epilepsia* 2013;**54**(Suppl 4):61–69

27. Kumar A, Asano E, Chugani HT. α-[^{11}C]-methyl-L-tryptophan PET for tracer localization of epileptogenic brain regions: clinical studies. *Biomark Med* 2011;**5**:577–584

28. Weissberg I, Wood L, Kamintsky L, et al. Albumin induces excitatory synaptogenesis through astrocytic TGF-β/ALK5 signaling in a model of acquired epilepsy following blood–brain barrier dysfunction. *Neurobiol Dis* 2015;**78**:115–125

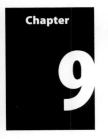

Genetic Causes of Medication-Resistant Epilepsy

Thomas N. Ferraro, Bradford D. Fischer and Russell J. Buono

Introduction: Genetics and Medication Resistant Epilepsy

The pharmacotherapy of epilepsy is a complex process guided by evidence-based research and clinical experience. Some patients achieve seizure freedom upon treatment with the first anti-seizure medication (ASM) prescribed, whereas others may be treated with two or three medications before one (or a combination) is found that reduces seizure frequency and/or severity with minimal side effects. Many patients demonstrate a partial response to treatment, leading to reduced seizure frequency and/or severity, but do not become completely seizure-free. It is often stated that ~30% of epilepsy patients have seizures that cannot be controlled pharmacologically, and these patients are defined as having medication-resistant epilepsy (MRE). The International League Against Epilepsy (ILAE) published the following definition of MRE: 'drug resistant epilepsy may be defined as failure of adequate trials of two tolerated and appropriately chosen and used ASM schedules (whether as monotherapies or in combination) to achieve sustained seizure freedom'[1]. Treatment success or sustained seizure freedom is defined as one year without seizures or three times the inter-seizure interval (whichever is longer). The ILAE definition provides a useful standard from which to work, and MRE can be clinically identified in patients that fail to achieve seizure freedom after multiple ASM trials. However, the ILAE definition of successful treatment does not account for partial response to pharmacotherapy. Indeed, many partial responders have improved quality of life, even if they are not seizure-free for one year or more.

There is currently no laboratory test to predict MRE. Thus, over the past two decades, a substantial research effort has been expended on elucidating the pharmacogenetics of ASMs in an attempt to better understand the nature of the phenomenon, as well as to advance the concept of personalized medicine with

regard to the treatment of epilepsy. Most studies focused on identifying genetic variation associated with ASM pharmacokinetics (PK) or pharmacodynamics (PD) [2]. Based on data from this approach, we hypothesize that MRE is caused by variations or mutations in genes that encode proteins critical for final common pathways of neural system activity and/or variations in genes that act as epileptogenesis susceptibility factors. We further hypothesize that ASM partial response (or response to one ASM but not another) is related to genomic variation regulating PK and/or PD mechanisms of action of specific ASMs (Figure 9.1). Some success has been achieved in discovering genetic variants associated with ASM

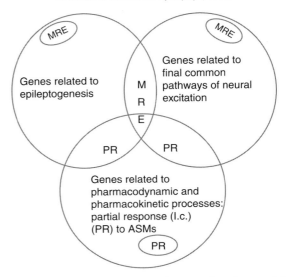

Gene variations Interact Increasing Susceptibility to Medication-Resistant Epilepsy (MRE)

Figure 9.1 Venn diagram depicts the interaction of gene variation likely to cause MRE. We hypothesize that variation in genes that cause epilepsy or variation in genes related to final common pathways of neural excitability can be sufficient by themselves to cause MRE. Some overlap of these variations is also suspected to contribute to MRE. Variation in PK/PD genes is hypothesized to play a larger role in partial response to ASMs, but can also contribute to MRE.

metabolism rates and adverse effects; however, the field has struggled to identify genetic or other biomarkers that can predict MRE in patients with epilepsy.

In this chapter, we discuss research findings supporting the concept that genetic variation causes altered function of proteins regulating neural system activity and ASM PK/PD leading to MRE or partial ASM response. We suggest that epilepsy susceptibility alleles aggregate in specific patients, causing increased levels of genetic burden that contribute to MRE. Finally, we describe potential new methods for biomarker discovery of molecular patterns that may predict MRE.

Epilepsy

Epilepsy is an umbrella term for a disease that includes many types of human seizure disorders. Rare familial forms caused by single gene mutations and inherited in Mendelian fashion are thought of as 'simple traits'. These rare monogenic epilepsies yielded early results as classic linkage analysis allowed for mapping and identification of several 'epilepsy genes'. Mutations in ion channel genes were first to be discovered, and two decades ago epilepsy was considered to be primarily an 'ion channelopathy' [3]. However, subsequent work documented that mutations in non-ion channel genes were also linked to monogenic human epilepsies [4]. Genes discovered as causes of rare forms of epilepsy provide insight into the potential causes of common forms, and establish a rationale for development of new treatment strategies.

In contrast to monogenic familial forms of epilepsy, most patients have polygenic forms caused by multiple gene variations interacting with environmental factors and defining these forms as complex traits [5]. Identifying complex trait epilepsy genes is a major challenge for researchers, in part because very large numbers of patients must be studied in order to attain the statistical power required to document *bona fide* allelic effects. Recent genome-wide association studies (GWAS) and current large-scale genomic sequencing projects are being used to identify complex trait genes. Over time, these techniques may identify genetic variants that will be useful biomarkers of MRE. Adding to the complexity is the effect of the environment on the epigenome with respect to methylation and other modification of DNA or histone proteins. Gene expression may be affected by mechanisms that include both inherited static DNA

structure and epigenetic modifications. The epigenetics of ASM response are not well studied, but may represent an important source of individual variation and potential biomarkers for MRE [6].

Genetic Influences on ASM Pharmacokinetics

Pharmocokinetics (PK) refers to the molecular mechanisms regulating drug absorption, distribution, metabolism and excretion (ADME). Each of these processes is complex, potentially involving dozens of proteins to accomplish any given function. Many PK proteins undergo post-translational modification, such as phosphorylation or glycosylation to become fully functional, and non-PK proteins regulate these modifications. Thus, it is possible that variation or mutation in literally hundreds of genes could cause dysfunction in ASM ADME processes and contribute to or cause partial ASM response or even MRE. Given the fundamental role of kinetic processes in determining the therapeutic effects of drugs, MRE may hypothetically be related to variants that decrease or prevent ASM absorption, prevent ASM entry into the brain or accelerate ASM metabolism or excretion. However, there are no examples of monogenic forms of MRE, suggesting MRE is a complex trait.

PK parameters are typically defined through serum or plasma measurements in healthy human volunteers during phase I clinical trials. These studies document PK differences between healthy individuals and support the notion that genetic variation accounts for some of these differences. Gender, age, body weight, diet, smoking history and other data should be taken into account for PK analysis, as a combination of environmental signals and genetic background ultimately determines ASM PK. Phase II clinical studies include patients with different levels of disease severity, presumably from different levels of genetic susceptibility. Ideally, patients in a phase II study would be naïve to ASMs, be placed on ASM monotherapy and have no other drug use. PK parameters measured in these patients could be associated with response rate, and genetic variation with predictive value could be identified. However, this ideal situation is difficult to achieve in practice. Inclusion criteria are often relaxed to increase patient participation and statistical power to detect endpoint measures. In studies of ASMs, many patients are taking more than one drug for epilepsy and/or are taking other drugs for comorbid disease. Lack of control of individual patient differences in environmental exposures, gender, age, percentage body fat and other factors have led to limited success in identifying genetic variants with predictive value with regards to MRE.

Cytochrome P450 Enzymes

Cytochrome P450 (CYP) enzymes comprise a large, highly polymorphic family of which a subset of members is critically involved in the metabolism of the majority of standard ASMs [7]. CYP enzymes participate predominantly in phase I of drug metabolism, and genetic variations that lead to enzymes with impaired activity are often associated with relatively higher plasma drug levels. In a number of studies, this has been linked to increased drug toxicity and a requirement for dosage reduction. It is not uncommon for toxicity to be the major cause of treatment failure for some drugs in some patients. Studies of the influence of genetic variation in ASM-metabolizing enzymes on therapeutic responses to ASMs are less frequent and the results less clear with regard to clinical relevance.

Drug metabolism varies between individuals, and genetic variation in specific CYP genes has been identified that can predict these metabolic rates for certain drugs. Potentially, this information could be useful in determination of initial starting doses of first-generation ASMs in specific populations [8]. Indeed, the Clinical Pharmacogenetics Implementation Consortium (CPIC) periodically publishes guidelines to support use of genotyping specific allelic variants before initiating therapy. CPIC issued recommendations for genotyping CYP2C9 prior to using phenytoin or carbamazepine in patients with newly diagnosed epilepsy (see Box 9.1).

The CYP2C family is the most extensively studied enzyme system in relation to ASMs. CYP2C family genes are highly expressed in liver and various isoforms exhibit polymorphisms, including some that are clinically relevant to drug biotransformation. Seminal research showed that the ratio of the plasma concentration of the active metabolite of clobazam, N-desmethylclobazam, to the administered dose of clobazam (the so-called CD ratio) was significantly greater in patients harboring CYP2C19 variants [9]. In a related study, the concomitant use of phenytoin and carbamazepine, both hepatic enzyme inducers, reduced the CD ratio of clobazam independent of CYP2C19 genotype; however, ratios for N-desmethylclobazam were only elevated in patients harbouring variant alleles [10]. This latter study showed that when the cut-off

---

Box 9.1 Online Pharmacogenetics Resources

A number of online resources exist to enhance appreciation of the clinical relevance of pharmacogenomics and to promote its application. The US Food and Drug Administration curates one such resource: www.fda.gov/Drugs/ScienceResearch/ResearchAreas/Pharmacogenetics/ucm083378.htm. This site provides a list of drugs for which there are biomarkers that help to guide physicians with regard to medication selection and dosage. Drugs may be sorted alphabetically or by therapeutic area. Additional information is provided on each drug with regards to the patient genotypes that are relevant to the given pharmacogenomic effect and the FDA labeling category.

Another major resource for accessing pharmacogenetic information on drugs is the PharmGKB website (www.pharmgkb.org/). This site may be used to gain an appreciation of the complexity of the issue and as a first stop for reviewing the current literature on pharmacogenomics. The site includes a database that can be queried by drug or phenotype and that leads to detailed information on PK and PD parameters, as well as pharmacogenetic influences, known drug–drug interactions, pathway diagrams, references and more. The database is also searchable by gene name and it links back to literature regarding the pharmacological relevance of the protein product. In addition, the Clinical Pharmocogenetic Implementation Consortium (CPIC) guidelines on genotype–phenotype correlations for drugs with known pharmacogenomic data are also housed on this site. CPIC is dedicated to getting more clinicians to order genotype information where well-documented pharmacogenomics research data can inform the process of choosing the right drug and the right dose for initial and maintenance pharmacotherapy.

---

value of the CD ratio for N-desmethylclobazam was set as 10.0 (μg/mL)/(mg/kg) for predicting the CYP2C19 variant status, the sensitivity and specificity were 94.4% and 95.7%, respectively [10]. Screening tests such as this that allow better management of ASM polypharmacy have high potential clinical utility.

CYP2C9 is involved in metabolism of phenytoin and carbamazepine and other drugs used to treat epilepsy, including several benzodiazepines [11,12]. The gene has over 50 alleles in humans; however, three of the most common alleles can distinguish between rapid, intermediate and poor metabolizers of phenytoin. Analysis of CYP2C9 genotypes could lead to initial starting does that are 25–50% lower for intermediate and poor metabolizers, respectively, compared to rapid metabolizers [13, 42]. Such refinements reduce the likelihood of adverse drug side effects and help facilitate patient compliance. Despite the body of evidence documenting the effect of CYP2C9 and CYP2C19 polymorphisms on the metabolism of several standard ASMs, and the related impact on dosing, both starting and maintenance, genotyping the CYP2C9 is not frequently performed. For first generation ASMs, it is more common for physicians to start patients on a low dose and escalate it slowly using therapeutic drug monitoring and/or clinical efficacy to determine maintenance dosing schemes. Thus, even when reliable biomarkers are available, integration into clinical practice is not always certain.

P-Glycoprotein

Early work on the development of drugs to treat cancer revealed that some cancer cells were resistant to multiple agents. The search for a 'multi-drug resistance' (MDR) factor led to the discovery of a family of ATP-dependent proteins which act as drug efflux transporters. These proteins are able to move exogenous molecules out of cells and into the extracellular space for ultimate metabolism and/or excretion. The genes encoding this class of transport proteins belong to the ATP-binding cassette (ABC) gene family and likely evolved to protect cells from xenobiotic agents. One gene in particular, ABCB1, encodes the MDR1 protein or the P-glycoprotein-1 and has been studied extensively with respect to ASM distribution in the brain. ABC genes belong to a larger gene family of solute transport carrier (SLC) genes and other members of this family have also been investigated based on the hypothesis that altered SLC function reduces ASM access to the brain.

A major point of contention with regards to the potential role for MDR1 in the treatment of epilepsy is related to the specific ASMs that are substrates for it [14]. Analysis of prior work suggests that of currently available ASMs, phenytoin, phenobarbital, oxcarbazepine and lamotrigine are highly likely to serve as substrates for ABC transport proteins [15,16]. There is also evidence that levetiracetam, carbamazepine, felbamate, topiramate, valproate and gabapentin interact with ABC transporters, although there are

conflicting data on these agents [15,16]. The potential importance of a role for the MDR1 protein in refractory epilepsy was highlighted by studies that found it to be upregulated in the brain of epilepsy patients and in experimental models of epilepsy. However, it was later discovered that MDR1 upregulation in animal models is short lived and returns to baseline levels after a few weeks of chronic seizure activity. In humans, it is unclear if the relatively high levels of MDR1 found in resected brain tissue from temporal lobe epilepsy patients are transient or constant. Recent work using an ABCB1 knockout mouse documents no difference between knockout and wild-type controls with regard to the effectiveness of ASMs against chemically induced seizures [17]; however, in a separate study brain levels of certain ASMs are higher in knockout compared to wild-type mice [18]. Thus, the putative role of the ABCB1 gene product in ASM efflux or its effects is not fully elucidated and its clinical relevance is still unknown.

Finally, there are a large number of studies that examined a possible genetic association between ABCB1 variants and response to ASMs in epilepsy patients. Not surprisingly, both positive and negative reports have been published. In general, the limitations of this work reflect problems inherent in most candidate gene association studies. Specifically, they are hampered by heterogeneous patient profiles and treatment paradigms, as well as by the relatively small numbers of patients and controls included. Thus, replication of ABCB1 genetic association studies has been problematic and studies from across the world show conflicting results. Similarly, several large meta-analyses of ABCB1 variation in association with ASM response have also led to conflicting results, but the most recent work continues to suggest that variants in this gene may ultimately be developed into a biomarker for ASM resistance in epilepsy [19].

Genetic Influences on ASM Pharmacodynamics

Pharmacodynamics (PD) refers to the mechanism of action of a drug and to those molecules that are its targets in the body. ASMs interact with a wide variety of brain molecules, but their ability to directly modulate sodium or calcium channels, facilitate the function of GABA receptors or block the metabolism of GABA are believed to be of prime importance with regard to their usefulness in treating epilepsy. A key concept with regard to the mechanism of ASMs is that most drugs have multiple actions and it is generally not clear which action or subset of actions is relevant to their ability to inhibit seizure activity. For example, valproate is a common ASM used to treat generalized epilepsy and is a first-line, first-generation drug. PD targets of valproate lead to actions that include: inhibition of sodium and calcium channels, inhibition of GABA degradation, and both inhibition and induction of histone deacetylase [20]. All of these mechanisms could potentially contribute to the therapeutic efficacy of valproate in treating epilepsy patients, and genetic variation in any or all the molecules that mediate these mechanisms may contribute to individual differences in response. Detailed discussion of the mechanism of action for all ASMs is beyond the scope of this chapter. We refer the reader to the PharmGBK website as an initial starting point for investigating any specific ASM and its PK/PD characteristics (see Box 9.1).

With regard to MRE, the role of genetic influences on the PD targets of ASMs, although highly plausible and extensively studied, is not well established. Theoretically, genetic variation in an ASM target could alter interaction between the drug and the target such that there is no resulting pharmacologic action or therapeutic effect. However, this would not explain resistance to multiple ASMs, assuming drugs with different mechanisms of action are tried. Alternatively, the existence of a final common pathway of seizure abrogation impacted by all ASMs may, if altered appropriately, hinder ASM efficacy in a much more general way.

SCN1A

Of all drugs that are approved to treat epilepsy, the most common mechanism of action among them involves inhibition of voltage-dependent sodium channels [20]. SCN1A is the gene that encodes the major subunit of the primary neuronal voltage-dependent sodium channel, NaV1.1, and this has spurred extensive investigation into the possibility that genetic variation in SCN1A may affect the action and efficacy of ASMs as a general class. An intronic single nucleotide polymorphism (SNP), denoted as rs3812718, disrupts the consensus sequence of the 5′ donor splice site of the highly-conserved 5 N alternative exon, thereby altering the ratio between the 5 N (fetal) isoform and the 5 A (adult) isoform [21]. Initial genetic association analyses using this SNP revealed that it was associated with maximum doses of carbamazepine and phenytoin [21]; however, despite some positive follow-up studies, most attempts at replication have failed to confirm the association of this variant with response to ASMs [22, 23].

Whereas statistical genetic studies on the SCN1A splicing SNP have been equivocal, functional studies have been more consistently positive. For example, sodium channels containing an expressed 5 N (fetal) exon exhibited enhanced tonic block and enhanced use-dependent block by both phenytoin and lamotrigine compared to channels expressing the adult exon [24]. Phenytoin and lamotrigine also both induced shifts in steady-state inactivation and recovery from fast inactivation for both splice isoforms [24]. Functional evidence for an effect of the splicing SNP on carbamazepine comes from a recent in vivo study in humans in which the SCN1A splicing SNP genotype was associated with the level of carbamazepine-induced increase in the duration of the 'cortical silent period', as measured by transcranial magnetic stimulation, reflecting a genetic influence on GABAergic inhibition by cortical interneurons [25]. Thus, whereas results of genetic association studies have led to significant conflicts in the literature with regard to the influence of the SCN1A splicing polymorphism on ASM response in epilepsy patients, provocative functional findings provide an impetus to further examine the potential impact of the SCN1A splicing polymorphism on ASM action and therapeutic effects.

In addition to the SCN1A intronic splicing SNP, several other SCN1A variants have been studied in relation to ASMs, including the A3184G SNP which predicts an A1056T amino acid substitution. In an initial investigation, this SNP was shown to be without effect on a multi-drug resistance phenotype [26]; however, a follow-up revealed that the proportion of AA genotype carriers exhibiting seizure freedom was significantly higher than that of AG plus GG genotype carriers [23]. An SNP in SCN1B has also been studied in regard to multi-drug resistance and was reported to have an effect in a gene-by-gene interaction model involving variants in SCN2A [27].

SCN2A and SCN3A

Other sodium channel subunit genes whose variation has been investigated in relation to ASMs include SCN2A and SCN3A. One potentially relevant variant in SCN2A is rs17183814, a non-synonymous SNP,

G61478A, that predicts an R19K amino acid substitution. In one study, it was reported that the A allele was associated with lack of therapeutic response to carbamazepine, phenytoin and valproic acid [28]. However, an independent study was unable to confirm this result [29]. Another SCN2A variant that has been studied in relation to ASMs is the intronic SNP rs2304016 that has been reported to be associated with lack of therapeutic response to carbamazepine, lamotrigine, oxcarbazepine, phenytoin and topiramate [30, 43]. The SNP is located within the putative splicing branch site for splicing exons 7 and 9; thus, PCR of reverse-transcribed RNA from blood or brain of patients with different IVS7-32A>G genotypes was performed using primers in exons 7 and 9, but results showed no skipping of exon 8, and real-time PCR showed no difference in SCN2A mRNA levels among genotypes, leaving the significance of this SCN2A variant in question [30].

Epilepsy Susceptibility Genes and MRE

Common forms of human epilepsy are complex traits involving polygenic inheritance. The exact genes and the types of variations in them that account for an increased genetic burden driving epileptogenesis are largely unknown. Current theories suggest that rare and common variants across the genome act in combination to modify the clinical phenotype in each individual. It is reasonable to hypothesize that individuals with greater numbers of more deleterious variations have an increased genetic burden, leading to increased severity of disease and an increased chance of being medication resistant.

In support of this notion, examples of epilepsy genes can be cited that are also targets of ASMs. The best studied of these is the SCN1A gene, which was discussed above. The SCN1A sodium channel subunit is a PD target for phenytoin, carbamazepine and valproate [31]. Mutations in the SCN1A gene have been linked to Dravet syndrome, a rare and disabling epilepsy that presents in infancy, as well as more common epilepsy syndromes, including generalized epilepsy with febrile seizures plus (GEFS+) [32]. In addition, a large meta-analysis of genome-wide association data that included 15 512 patients with common forms of epilepsy and 29 677 controls identified variation in the SCN1A channel as being associated with generalized epilepsy [33]. Thus, the SCN1A gene is both an epilepsy susceptibility gene and a PD target of ASMs. Another example is the alpha-1 subunit of the GABA-A receptor, a gene that harbors mutations

that can cause epilepsy [34]. Given that the multimeric GABA-A receptor is a target for ASMs in the benzodiazepine and barbiturate classes [20], it is possible that specific variants in GABA-A receptor subunit genes, either the same or different from those that cause epilepsy per se, can influence response to ASMs and contribute to MRE.

Taken together, these data suggest that MRE may be caused by genetic variation in epilepsy susceptibility genes. These genes impact ASM efficacy because they are ASM PD targets as well as susceptibility genes encoding proteins that are involved in driving common final pathways of neuronal system activity. Clinically, it appears that seizure frequency and severity are prognostic indicators for ASM resistance. Those patients with frequent and severe seizure episodes are often the same patients who are most resistant to medication [31]. Thus, it is reasonable to suggest that continued research to identify alleles that either cause or predispose individuals to epilepsy will be important for both understanding the process of epileptogenesis and elucidating mechanisms of MRE.

Biomarkers

Several areas of focus have emerged as being potentially important with regard to the development of biomarkers that can predict epilepsy and MRE. A biomarker would ideally be collected from a patient in a minimally invasive way from blood, saliva or urine, and analyzed biochemically. In addition, imaging techniques, transcranial magnetic stimulation profiles and expanded power EEG recordings have all been explored as biomarkers for predicting epilepsy and MRE. Potential biochemical markers include growth factors, vitamins and molecules that reflect cellular metabolism and redox state. There is also evidence that molecules reflecting function of the blood–brain barrier and molecules that reflect signaling pathways involved in inflammatory processes may be useful biomarkers in epilepsy as well [35]. The presence of autoantibodies in sera from epilepsy patients also provides compelling evidence for immune-system-mediated inflammatory processes, and biomarkers that predict MRE may include inflammatory proteins, circulating antibodies and/or variation in the genetic sequences encoding them [36].

Genetic Biomarkers

In addition to next-generation sequencing data, there are other nucleic acid markers that hold promise for

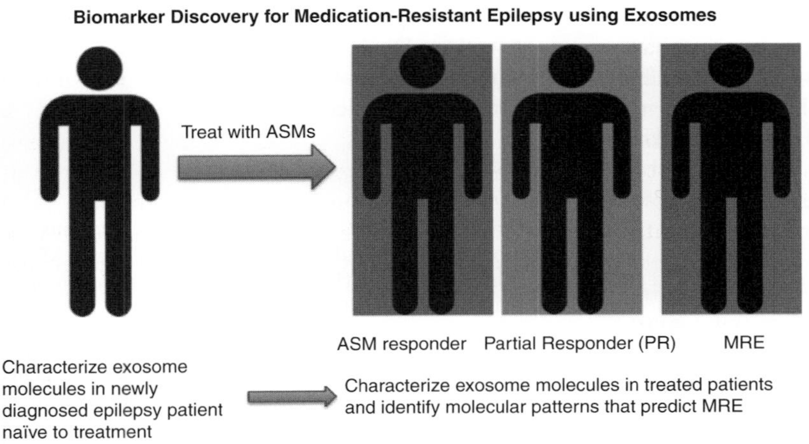

Biomarker Discovery for Medication-Resistant Epilepsy using Exosomes

Treat with ASMs

ASM responder   Partial Responder (PR)   MRE

Characterize exosome molecules in newly diagnosed epilepsy patient naïve to treatment

Characterize exosome molecules in treated patients and identify molecular patterns that predict MRE

Figure 9.2 Exosomes are small (20–150 nm) micro-vessicles secreted by most all cells and are used for autocrine, paracrine and endocrine cell-to-cell communication. They can be isolated from saliva, blood and/or urine and have been found to contain proteins, mRNA, miRNA, DNA and lipids. MRE biomarker discovery could be accomplished by collecting exosome-encapsulated molecules before ASM treatment and at intervals post-treatment. The goal would be to identify specific molecular patterns within exosomes that predict MRE (i.e. RNA/DNA sequences or differential methylation of DNA). Additional data from genome sequencing, genome-wide association studies and RNA expression profiles would be utilized to identify convergence of gene variations related to MRE.

biomarker development. Using resected brain tissue, it has been recently documented that MRE in temporal lobe epilepsy may be characterized by unique signatures of gene expression in dysfunctional neurons, suggesting that genes identified in this manner may represent biomarkers of ASM response [37]. The expression of such genes may be monitored via sequence or methylation patterns in freely circulating DNA and/or in nucleic acids encapsulated in exosomes that can be isolated from blood, urine and saliva. Recent work has also shown differences between microRNA molecules isolated from exosomes of refractory temporal lobe epilepsy patients compared to healthy controls [38]. Thus, it is reasonable to suggest that mRNA expression profiles or methylated DNA fragments may be different in the exosomes of MRE patients compared to those patients that respond to ASMs (Figure 9.2).

Development of New ASMs

One obvious approach to MRE is to develop new ASMs that have different mechanisms of action compared to the drugs currently used. Although the FDA-approved ASMs differ to some extent with regard to PK and PD properties, many of them were discovered using the same experimental models. Paradigms for testing potential ASMs have not changed appreciably for decades and typically use chemically or electrically induced seizures in otherwise normal rodents. Potential ASMs are screened by their ability to increase threshold levels of stimuli that induce acute seizures. Critics argue that drugs identified in this way do not treat the cause of epilepsy or affect the epileptogenic process; rather they only reduce the major

symptom of seizures. Further, they argue that since these same models continue to be used to search for new ASMs, no new mechanisms of action will be discovered as compounds identified will continue to target known molecules such as ion channels or proteins related to GABA neurotransmission. One approved ASM, levetiracetam, was not discovered using traditional models, but rather with a kindling model that is not standard in ASM development. The major PD target for this ASM appears to be a synaptic vesicle protein (SV2A) involved in synaptic vesicle transport and membrane fusion [39]. Thus, alternate models have the potential to discover new mechanisms of ASM function. However, the kindling model is time-consuming and not fully amenable to high-throughput screening. In addition, it still relies on seizure threshold induced by exogenous delivery of electricity to the brain of a normal animal. Thus, the field continues to search for new models to screen potential ASMs. The main problem is that, because markers of epileptogenesis have not been identified, seizures continue to be the endpoint measure used for drug development. As long as model systems use this paradigm for discovery, it is unlikely that molecules with novel mechanisms of action and improved treatment efficacy will be identified.

Anecdotal evidence that human epilepsy can be effectively treated with cannabis and its phytocannabinoid extracts has led to recent research that supports this hypothesis, including the identification of cannabidiol's efficacy for Dravet syndrome and Lennox–Gastaut syndrome. As such, modulation of the endogenous cannabinoid system with one or more phytocannabinoids appears to be an effective treatment for epilepsy, thereby identifying new mechanisms of action for seizure reduction and a possible alternative treatment strategy for those who do not respond to currently available ASMs [40]. It is likely that, as with all ASMs, some epilepsy patients will be resistant to phytocannabinoids, but it is unknown whether phytocannabinoid treatment will reduce the prevalence of MRE.

Non-Pharmacological Treatments and Genetics

When ASMs fail to control seizures, other options are often explored. Some individuals are surgical candidates, but the vast majority of refractory patients are not. Vagus nerve, trigeminal nerve and deep brain stimulation, ketogenic diet, synchronotron X-rays and other non-pharmacological methods have been used as treatment options for MRE patients [41]. As expected, none of these options is successful in all patients and trials invariably reveal patients that respond to the treatment, partially or entirely, and those that do not. Again, it is reasonable to suggest that these differences are caused by variation in the genome and epigenome, which, when elucidated, will lead to significant improvements in the treatment of epilepsy.

Summary

We hypothesize that MRE is related to variation in genes encoding proteins that regulate final common pathways of neural system activity. We suggest that partial response to ASMs, or response to one ASM but not another, is related to genetic variation at the level of specific ASM PK and PD. We further suggest that biomarker development using next-generation DNA sequencing and exosome-encapsulated or free circulating molecules will lead to identification of specific patterns that can predict MRE in new and existing patients.

Key Points

- MRE is caused in part by genetic variation.
- Gene variation in ASM PK and PD targets is suspected to cause partial response or response to specific ASMs.
- Gene variations that affect proteins important for final common pathways of neural activity are suspected to cause MRE.

- Biomarkers of MRE could be identified by next-generation DNA sequencing and/or characterization of free circulating or exosome-encapsulated molecules.

References

1. Kwan P, Arzimanoglou A, Berg AT, et al. Definition of drug resistant epilepsy: consensus proposal by the ad hoc Task Force of the ILAE Commission on Therapeutic Strategies. *Epilepsia* 2010;**51**:1069–1077

2. Ferraro TN, Buono RJ. The relationship between the pharmacology of antiepileptic drugs and human gene variation: an overview. *Epilepsy Behav* 2005;7:18–36

3. Steinlein OK, Noebels JL. Ion channels and epilepsy in man and mouse. *Curr Opin Genet Dev* 2000;**10**:286–291

4. Yalçın O. Genes and molecular mechanisms involved in the epileptogenesis of idiopathic absence epilepsies. *Seizure* 2012;**21**:79–86

5. Weber YG, Lerche H. Genetic mechanisms in idiopathic epilepsies. *Dev Med Child Neurol* 2008;**50**:648–654

6. Kobow K, El-Osta A, Blümcke I. The methylation hypothesis of pharmacoresistance in epilepsy. *Epilepsia* 2013;**54**(Suppl 2):41–47

7. Vajda FJ, Eadie MJ. The clinical pharmacology of traditional antiepileptic drugs. *Epileptic Disord* 2014;**16**:395–408

8. Desta Z, Zhao X, Shin JG, Flockhart DA. Clinical significance of the cytochrome P450 2C19 genetic polymorphism. *Clin Pharmacokinet* 2002;**41**:913–958

9. Saruwatari J, Ogusu N, Shimomasuda M, et al. Effects of CYP2C19 and P450 oxidoreductase polymorphisms on the population pharmacokinetics of clobazam and N-desmethylclobazam in Japanese patients with epilepsy. *Ther Drug Monit* 2014;**36**:302–309

10. Yamamoto Y, Takahashi Y, Imai K, et al. Influence of CYP2C19 polymorphism and concomitant antiepileptic drugs on serum clobazam and N-desmethylclobazam concentrations in patients with epilepsy. *Ther Drug Monit* 2013;**35**:305–312

11. Yasumori T, Li QH, Yamazoe Y, et al. Lack of low Km diazepam N-demethylase in livers of poor metabolizers for S-mephenytoin 4'-hydroxylation. *Pharmacogenetics* 1994;**4**:323–331

12. Hashi S, Yano I, Shibata M, et al. Effect of CYP2C19 polymorphisms on the clinical outcome of low-dose clobazam therapy in Japanese patients with epilepsy. *Eur J Clin Pharmacol* 2015;**71**:51–58

13. Fohner AE, Ranatunga DK, Thai KK, Lawson BL, Risch N, Oni-Orisan A, Jelalian AT, Rettie AE, Liu VX, Schaefer CA. Assessing the clinical impact of CYP2C9 pharmacogenetic variation on phenytoin prescribing practice and patient response in an integrated health system. *Pharmacogenet Genomics* 2019;29(8):192–199

14. Löscher W, Luna-Tortós C, et al. Do ATP-binding cassette transporters cause pharmacoresistance in epilepsy?: problems and approaches in determining which antiepileptic drugs are affected. *Curr Pharm Des* 2011;**17**:2808–2828

15. Zhang C, Kwan P, Zuo Z, Baum L. The transport of antiepileptic drugs by P-glycoprotein. *Adv Drug Deliv Rev* 2012;**64**:930–942

16. Stępień KM, Tomaszewski M, Tomaszewska J, et al. The multidrug transporter P-glycoprotein in pharmacoresistance to antiepileptic drugs. *Pharmacol Rep* 2012;**64**:1011–1019

17. Bankstahl M, Klein S, Römermann K, Löscher W. Knockout of P-glycoprotein does not alter antiepileptic drug efficacy in the intrahippocampal kainate model of mesial temporal lobe epilepsy in mice. *Neuropharmacology* 2016;**109**:183–195

18. Nakanishi H, Yonezawa A, Matsubara K, Yano I. Impact of P-glycoprotein and breast cancer resistance protein on the brain distribution of antiepileptic drugs in knockout mouse models. *Eur J Pharmacol* 2013;**710**:20–28

19. Chouchi M, Kaabachi W, Klaa H, et al. Relationship between ABCB1 3435TT genotype and antiepileptic drugs resistance in epilepsy: updated systematic review and meta-analysis. *BMC Neurol* 2017;17 (1):32

20. Rogawski MA, Löscher W. The neurobiology of antiepileptic drugs. *Nat Rev Neurosci* 2004;**5**:553–564

21. Tate SK, Depondt C, Sisodiya SM, et al. Genetic predictors of the maximum doses patients receive during clinical use of the anti-epileptic drugs carbamazepine and phenytoin. *Proc Natl Acad Sci USA* 2005;**102**:5507–5512

22. Hung CC, Huang HC, Gao YH, et al. Effects of polymorphisms in six candidate genes on phenytoin maintenance therapy in Han Chinese patients. *Pharmacogenomics* 2012;**13**:1339–1349

23. Abo El Fotoh WM, Abd El Naby SA, Habib MS, ALrefai AA, Kasemy ZA. The potential implication of SCN1A and CYP3A5 genetic variants on antiepileptic drug resistance among Egyptian epileptic children. *Seizure* 2016;41:75–80

24. Thompson CH, Kahlig KM, George AL, Jr. SCN1A splice variants exhibit divergent sensitivity to commonly used antiepileptic drugs. *Epilepsia* 2011;**52**:1000–1009

25. Menzler K, Hermsen A, Balkenhol K, et al. A common SCN1A splice-site polymorphism modifies the effect of carbamazepine on cortical excitability-A pharmacogenetic transcranial magnetic stimulation study. *Epilepsia* 2014;**55**:362–369

26. Lakhan R, Kumari R, Misra UK, et al. Differential role of sodium channels SCN1A and SCN2A gene polymorphisms with epilepsy and multiple drug resistance in the north Indian population. *Br J Clin Pharmacol* 2009;**68**:214–220

27. Jang SY, Kim MK, Lee KR, et al. Gene-to-gene interaction between sodium channel-related genes in determining the risk of antiepileptic drug resistance. *J Korean Med Sci* 2009;**24**:62–68

28. Kumari R, Lakhan R, Garg RK, et al. Pharmacogenomic association study on the role of drug metabolizing, drug transporters and drug target gene polymorphisms in drug-resistant epilepsy in a north Indian population. *Indian J Hum Genet* 2011;**17**(Suppl 1):S32–S40

29. Haerian BS, Baum L, Tan HJ, et al. SCN1A IVS5 N+5 polymorphism and response to sodium valproate: a multicenter study. *Pharmacogenomics* 2012;**13**:1477–1485

30. Kwan P, Poon WS, Ng HK, et al. Multidrug resistance in epilepsy and polymorphisms in the voltage-gated sodium channel genes SCN1A, SCN2A, and SCN3A: correlation among phenotype, genotype, and mRNA expression. *Pharmacogenet Genomics* 2008;**18**:989–998

31. Rogawski MA. The intrinsic severity hypothesis of pharmacoresistance to antiepileptic drugs. *Epilepsia* 2013;**54**(Suppl 2):33–40

32. Escayg A, Goldin AL. Sodium channel SCN1A and epilepsy: mutations and mechanisms. *Epilepsia* 2010;**51**:1650–1658

33. International League Against Epilepsy Consortium on Complex Epilepsies genome-wide mega-analysis identifies 16 loci and highlights diverse biological mechanisms in the common epilepsies. Nat Commun. 2018;9(1):5269

34. Hirose S. Mutant GABA(A) receptor subunits in genetic (idiopathic) epilepsy. *Prog Brain Res* 2014;**213**:55–85

35. Walker LE, Janigro D, Heinemann U, et al. WONOEP appraisal: molecular and cellular biomarkers for epilepsy. *Epilepsia* 2016;**57**:1354–1362

36. Britton J. Autoimmune epilepsy. *Handb Clin Neurol* 2016;**133**:219–245

37. Dixit AB, Banerjee J, Srivastava A, et al. RNA-seq analysis of hippocampal tissues reveals novel

candidate genes for drug refractory epilepsy in patients with MTLE-HS. *Genomics* 2016;**107**:178–188

38. Yan S, Zhang H, Xie W, et al. Altered microRNA profiles in plasma exosomes from mesial temporal lobe epilepsy with hippocampal sclerosis. *Oncotarget* 2017;8(3):4136–4146

39. Lynch BA, Lambeng N, Nocka K, et al. The synaptic vesicle protein SV2A is the binding site for the antiepileptic drug levetiracetam. *Proc Natl Acad Sci USA* 2004;**101**:9861–9866

40. Reddy DS. The utility of cannabidiol in the treatment of refractory epilepsy. *Clin Pharmacol Ther* 2017;**101**:182–184

41. V. R. Yasam, Satya Lavanya Jakki, V. Senthil, N. Jawahar, P et al. An overview of non-drug therapies for the treatment of epilepsy. *Indian J Pharma Sci* 2018;80 (2): 223–234

42. Liao K, Liu Y, Ai CZ, Yu X, Li W. The association between CYP2C9/2C19 polymorphisms and phenytoin maintenance doses in Asian epileptic patients: A systematic review and meta-analysis. *Int J Clin Pharmacol Ther* 2018;56(7):337–346

43. Al-Eitan LN, Al-Dalalah IM, Aljamal HA. Effects of GRM4, SCN2A and SCN3B polymorphisms on antiepileptic drugs responsiveness and epilepsy susceptibility. *Saudi Pharm J* 2019;27 (5):731–737

Malformations of Cortical Development as Causes of Medication-Resistant Epilepsy

Ruben Kuzniecky

Introduction

Malformations of cortical development (MCD) are by now well recognized causes of neurodevelopmental disorders and epilepsy [1]. The precise etiological mechanisms, clinical features and course vary as patients present with a wide range of developmental disorders, associated somatic and cortical malformations, and epilepsy. Specific clinical phenotypes can be recognized in a proportion of patients based on common clinical and imaging features. Furthermore, genetic testing allows for specific phenotype–genotype classification. However, as with many genetic disorders, the phenotypic variability is large, presenting a challenge to the diagnosis and clinical management of these patients.

The availability of in vivo magnetic resonance imaging as a clinical phenotyping tool facilitated the development of a classification of MCDs [2]. More recently, developmental genetic studies have identified many genes that disrupt the main stages of brain formation leading to MCD. Further advances have been possible as our understanding of genetics and basic cellular and metabolic pathways merges.

Aetiology of Malformations of Cortical Development

Hypoxic/ischaemic injury has been recognized as a cause of brain malformations for many years. Congenital cytomegalovirus infection and toxoplasmosis are also well-known causes. Overall, the aetiologies are genetic or presumed genetic in about 50% of cases, whereas early hypoxic/ischaemic injury accounts for 20%, pre-natal infection 10% and 'unknown' (20%). It is likely that the last group is also genetic, making genetic disorders the main cause of MCD.

More than 110 genes are reported to be associated with different types of MCD and the number will continue to increase as molecular genetics improves [3].

Gene and biological pathways affected include mitosis, apoptosis, cell-fate specification, cytoskeletal structure and function, neuronal migration and basement-membrane function. Recent studies have shown that mutations can have variable impacts, not only the pattern of MCD but also on the location of cortical involvement. Byoung-Il et al. reported a mutation in a regulatory element of GPR56 that selectively disrupts human cortex surrounding the Sylvian fissure bilaterally, as seen in patients with bilateral perisylvian polymicrogyria [4]. GPR56 encodes a G-protein-coupled receptor required for normal cortical development. Control of GPR56 expression pattern influences cell proliferation and gyral patterning, affecting certain regions of the cerebral cortex but not others.

Another recent study showed causal post-mitotic mutations in 17% (range 10–30%) of a large sample of patients with MCDs [5]. Mutations were somatic in 30% of the patients, predominantly in double-cortex syndrome (DCX), periventricular nodular heterotopia (PVNH) and pachygyria. Of importance is that, of the detected somatic mutations, the majority were undetectable with common genetic testing as performed with DNA extracted from leukocytes. Instead, it is found through subcloning and subsequent sequencing of the subcloned DNA. Subcortical nodular heterotopia and focal cortical dysplasia (FCD) are frequently focal and unilateral and, thus, it is likely that somatic mutations play a role in their pathogenesis. More recent studies support this by showing several families with focal epilepsy with and without MRI-identified FCD linked to mutations of DEPDC5, NPRL2 and NPRL3 genes, which converge on mTOR pathways [5].

Other causal mutations in candidate genes, such as DYNC1H1, CCND2, PIK3R2 and other genes in patients with pachygyria and PMG with megalencephaly, have been recently identified [6]. It is likely that with improved sequencing techniques we will be able to uncover many more genes involved in the genesis of MCDs.

Mechanism of Epilepsy of Malformations of Cortical Development

The mechanism underlying the genesis of epilepsy in MCD is poorly understood, despite several animal models and many other mechanistic models [7,8]. Studies have suggested a role for GABA or glutamate dysfunction in some malformations [9]. A recent study postulated a hypothesis to explain the mechanism of epileptogenesis in focal cortical dysplasia (FCD), known as the dysmaturity hypothesis [7]. In summary, developmental disorder of cortical formation leads to preservation and malpositioning of a substantial number of subplate and radial glia-like cells. This dysmaturity of neuronal networks and GABA synaptic activity causes depolarizing actions similar to immature developing networks [10,11]. Additionally, spontaneous depolarization and bursting are observed in cytomegalic interneurons, whose function appears to be more like an amplification device instead of a generator of epileptiform activity [11]. It is also postulated that in some MCDs, such as lissencephaly or pachygyria, there is a paucity of GABAergic modulation in the cortex due to failure of tangential radio-glial fibres. Obviously, many factors are involved in the epileptogenic circuitry, and the mechanisms for epilepsy are probably different according to the underlying genetic and pathway abnormalities and/or the structural abnormalities seen in MCDs.

Clinical Classification

The current classification scheme for MCDs is based on the primary developmental steps of cell proliferation, neuronal migration and cortical organization [2]. Although the classification recognizes which process is first disturbed, it is clear that earlier disturbances will affect all steps of brain formation. It is also known that MCD-related genes are implicated in many brain developmental stages that are genetically and functionally inter-dependent giving further support to the above concept of a continuum.

Although the current classification of MCDs has been extremely useful in diagnosing and managing patients during the past decade, it is clear that many patients have distinct enough MCDs or molecular evidence of new gene pathway disturbances deserving re-classification. However, the current classification has its merits and it is still very useful in the grouping and management of patients.

Based on the above main steps of cortical formation, the classification defines four major groups. Group I constitutes malformations secondary to abnormal neuronal and glial proliferation or apoptosis. Group II contains malformations secondary to abnormal neuronal migration. Group III comprises malformations secondary to abnormal migrational and post-migrational development, as the process of cortical organization begins before the termination of neuronal migration. Finally, even though there is no formal classification group that includes those with complex unclassifiable disorders, there are a number of malformations of cortical development that are not yet classified. As our understanding of genes, pathways and the availability of commercially available molecular diagnosis increases, we will be able to implement at a practical level a simpler diagnostic pathway for MCDs.

Guerrini et al. [3] suggested a classification based on pathway disruption and imaging phenotype that merges both clinical and molecular findings. This classification divides MCDs into four different groups: (i) megalencephaly and FCD, (ii) tubulinopathies and lissencephalies, (iii) PMG syndromes and (iv) heterotopia syndromes. This classification scheme is useful as an intermediate step as we move towards a gene pathway classification. Although tuberous sclerosis is an MCD, it is a distinct entity and is not discussed in this chapter.

Group I (Primarily Malformations Secondary to Abnormal Neuronal and Glial Proliferation or Apoptosis)

Megalencephaly, Hemi-Megalencephaly Variants and Focal Cortical Dysplasia

The clinical diagnosis of these patients is based on typical MRI features. In epilepsy, the majority of cases are associated with either polymicrogyria (PMG), bilaterally or diffusely, or with hemi-megalencephaly (HMG). The most severe MCD associated with megalencephaly is HMG and its variants. It is recognized that many cases involve sublobar enlargement rather than hemispheric overgrowth. The pathological changes reported in HMG include a wide range of abnormalities, including changes typically seen in FCD, agyria, PMG and heterotopia. Clinically, most patients present with hemispheric signs, and MRI and EEG are usually concordant. The imaging findings in

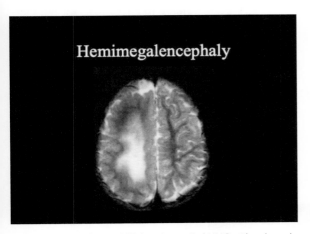

Figure 10.1 Axial T2-W MRI showing typical HMG with enlarged hemisphere, smooth cortex with little sulcation, and abnormal white matter.

HMG and variants are clearly distinct. Enlargement of the entire hemisphere or part of one hemisphere with no consistent preference for a lobe is seen, as well as poor grey and white matter differentiation, hypointense and hyperintense T2-weighted abnormalities in white matter and enlargement of the lateral ventricle, usually on the more dysplastic side (Figure 10.1).

A growing number of syndromes and genes have been associated with HMG, especially with more severe phenotypes. Megalencephaly with polymicrogyria occurs with mutations of PIK3CA and with mutations of PIK3R2 or AKT [6,12]. Isolated HMG most often occurs and has recently been associated with mosaic mutations of PIK3CA, AKT3 and mTOR [13].

The 2011 ILAE classification system for FCD expanded on the original classification to include three main pathologic groups [14]. FCD type I is usually reserved for FCD with abnormal radial (Ia), tangential lamination (Ib) or both (Ic). FCD type II is associated with dysmorphic (IIa) or balloon cells (IIb). Type III includes FCD associated with a number of other pathologies, such as hippocampal sclerosis, glial tumours, vascular malformations, trauma, etc. This classification may have clinical limitations, as in many cases only small samples of brain tissue are available for analysis.

The aetiology of FCD is not known but is likely to be caused in some patients by somatic clonal mutations affecting similar pathways. In fact, studies showed increased mTOR signaling in FCD type IIb, and in HMG and gangliogliomas based on enhanced phosphorylated downstream molecules, such as

protein S6. This is particularly pertinent in FCD type IIb and tubers, in which >80–90% of balloon cells and giant cells, respectively, manifest increased phosphorylation of these proteins [15]. Some cases of FCD type IIb also exhibit activation of the upstream molecules phosphoinositide-3-dependent kinase 1 (PDK1) and AKT, and of the downstream substrates vascular endothelial growth factor (VEGF) and signal transducer and activator of transcription 3. The role of mTOR signaling in the pathophysiology of FCD has been further corroborated in the PTEN knockout mouse model [16]. Furthermore corroboration comes from recent studies in a number of families with focal epilepsy with and without MRI identified FCD due to TSC1, TSC2, DEPDC5 and NPRL2/NPRL3 mutations which involve the same mTOR pathways [17] . The above findings indicate that FCD, HMG and TS share common downstream pathway mechanisms.

The clinical epilepsy presentation is variable and depends on the location and extent of the lesions. However, MRI is the best descriptor and classifier of these lesions. Patients with FCD have focal enlarged smooth gyri and increased cortical/subcortical signal intensity. Transmantle dysplasia and bottom sulcus dysplasia (BSD) are types of FCD characterized by radial white-matter bands that extend from the dysplastic cortex to the periventricular region and can be detected with high-resolution MRI in a large proportion of patients. BSD is restricted to small regions of the gyri or sulcus and often involve the bottom of the sulcus. These lesions are more often seen on the frontal lobes and often give rise to intractable frontal lobe epilepsy (Figure 10.2).

Group 2 (Primarily Malformations Secondary to Abnormal Neuronal Migration)

Tubulinopathies and Lissencephalic/Double Cortex Syndromes

Recent studies have shown that lissencephaly and dysgyria or pachygyria-like malformations are associated with mutations of the same genes and pathways, giving rise to a number of distinct MCDs. The range of these malformations is poorly understood, but they vary from severe lissencephaly with associated malformations to much less severe malformations. Available pathology in the

(A)

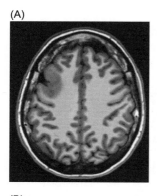

Figure 10.2 Focal cortical dysplasia. (A) Large FCD lateral pre-central region. Thick cortex and abnormal signal of grey matter. (B) Typical bottom of sulcus FCD (arrow). See abnormal signal from bottom of sulcus and abnormal straight frontal gyrus. These lesions are often very small and subtle.

(B)

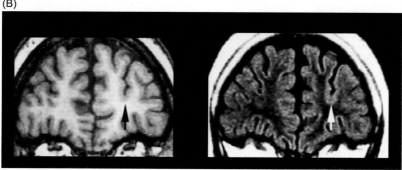

tubulinopathies (TUB) shows absent cortical lamination, radial columnar heterotopia and ectopic neurons in the white matter [18]. In lissencephaly, the cortex is 12–20 mm thick and composed of a normal marginal layer, a superficial cellular layer that corresponds to the cortical plate, a cell-sparse zone and a deep cellular layer composed of heterotopic neurons. Subcortical band heterotopia consists of a normal six-layered cortex and a thin zone of white matter underlying the cortex, and a zone of dense heterotopic neurons [19].

Different patterns of lissencephaly have been reported with mutations of known causative genes. There are about a dozen lissencephalic genes identified so far with LIS1 and DCX mutations being the most common ones [20]. DCX causes X-linked lissencephaly in males and the double cortex syndrome in females. Other genes including LAMB1, NDE1, KATNB1, RELN or VLDLR have been reported with different phenotypes [3].

Imaging features vary from smooth brain surface with completely absent gyri to pebbled or microsulci-like polymicrogyria, and a lack of gyral infolding. Agenesis or dysgenesis of the corpus callosum, with or without cerebellar hypoplasia can be present. Certain imaging patterns are helpful in searching for a genetic cause. Saillour et al. found that 40 of 63 patients with posterior predominant lissencephaly had a LIS1 mutation or deletion, including 1 patient with somatic mosaicism for a nonsense mutation [21]. Most patients with LIS1 mutations had posterior agyria and anterior pachygyria (55.3%). Diffuse agyria was observed in 9 (23.7%) patients and posterior predominant pachygyria was seen in 6 (15.8%). Conversely, with DCX mutations the agyria tends to be mainly anteriorly distributed (Figure 10.3).

The degree of neuromotor impairment was in accordance with the severity of lissencephaly, with a high incidence of tetraplegia (61.1%). However, the severity of epilepsy was less variable, as more than 50% of patients had daily seizures. Mutation type and location does not predict the severity of LIS1-related lissencephaly. In comparison, patients without LIS1 mutation tend to have less severe lissencephaly and no additional brain abnormalities.

Patients with mutations of tubulin genes have severe neurodevelopmental deficits and intractable seizures. Infantile spasms are common. Ocular and ophthalmologic abnormalities are seen in some patients with particular TUB mutations [18].

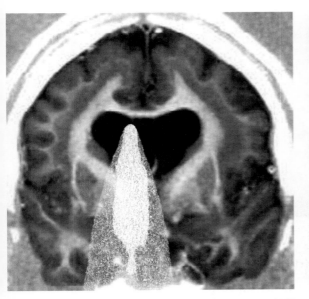

Figure 10.3 DCX mutation. Double cortex syndrome. Coronal MRI shows bilateral symmetric grey matter bands and ventriculomegaly.

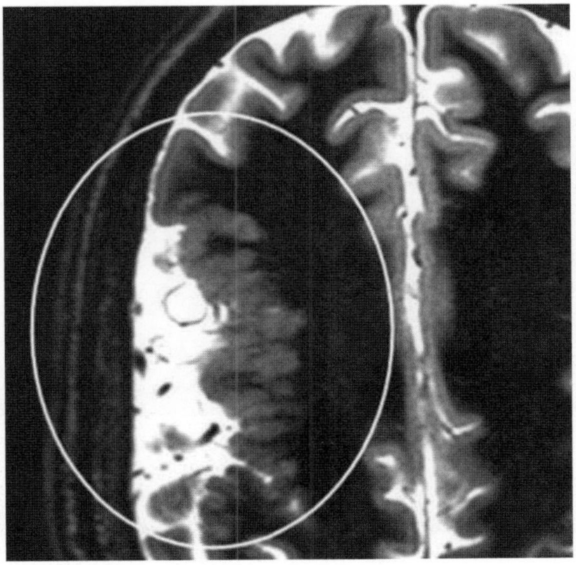

Figure 10.4 Focal PMG. Axial T2W MRI shows abnormal small gyri typical of PMG.

Group 3 (Primarily Malformations Secondary to Abnormal Migrational and Post-Migrational Development)

Polymicrogyria-Associated Disorders

As with other MCDs, PMG is diagnosed on the combination of imaging features and in some cases a syndromic approach with associated abnormalities [22]. PMG is characterized by many excessive cortical small convolutions, which might not be visible on gross inspection of the brain. The aetiology of PMG is highly heterogeneous and there is no correlation between cortical layering patterns and aetiology. PMG is almost always associated with other brain malformations. The distribution of PMG varies greatly from diffuse to bilateral symmetrical to bilateral asymmetrical to unilateral. The perisylvian cortex is the most frequently affected in patients with congenital bilateral perisylvian polymicrogyria (CBPP) or Kuzniecky syndrome [23]. Microscopically, PMG can show several different histologic patterns with two main patterns of unlayered and layered PMG.

The aetiology of PMG is diverse, as it is clear that PMG has genetic as well as acquired causes. A recent study showed that aetiologies found in our patients were genetic or presumed genetic (40%), early

hypoxic/ischaemic injury (21%), pre-natal infection (9%) or 'unknown' (30%) [24].

Although anoxic insult and infectious aetiologies such as cytomegalovirus are well recognized causes of PMG, genetic causes are likely to be more frequent. Deletions of 22q11.2 and 1p36.3 are the only common copy number variations. As reported before, mutations in PIK3R2 can result in CBPP associated with macrocrania, but otherwise it does not seem common to have isolated PMG with mutations. Many complex syndromes with different mutations have been reported. A recent report of an inbred family found a FIG4 mutation associated with temporo-occipital polymicrogyria and epilepsy [25]. The function of FIG4 is related to the Ras GTPases involved in the control of intracellular PI P2 concentration that is crucial for post-migrational development of neurons.

Imaging features are often typical, with cortex that appears thicker (usually 6–8 mm) because of cortical overfolding. However, high resolution often shows the small packed gyri. In young children with PMG, the cortex might not appear thickened because of the immature state of myelination (Figure 10.4).

PMG as stated above is by far more frequent on the perisylvian regions bilaterally or unilaterally. Other patterns have been well-described, such as bilateral frontal PMG and bilateral parietal PMG. Recent studies in selected patients have shown

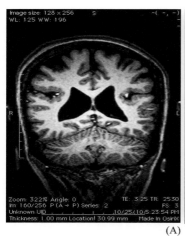
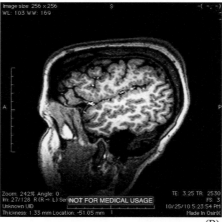

(A)   (B)

Figure 10.5 Congenital bilateral perisylvian polymicrogyria (Kuzniecky syndrome). (A) Coronal T1W image showing typical PMG in insular regions. (B) Saggital T1W image showing small gyri on the sylvian plane.

a clear advantage of high-field MRI at 7 T in mapping PMG areas that otherwise look normal on lower-field MRI [26]. Areas that appear normal at 3 T clearly had PMG cortex underscoring the problem of mapping exactly the extent of PMG or even diagnosing it in some patients (Figure 10.5).

The clinical spectrum is variable, as PMG may be associated with other brain or extra-CNS malformations. Microcephaly is seen in about 35% of patients and macrocephaly in approximately 20%, often associated with other aetiology and genetics. The best clinically defined syndrome is CBPP with oromotor dysfunction, intellectual disability and epilepsy [2]. BPP is likely genetic in some patients, in particular those with macrocrania associated with PIK3R2 mutations. Less frequently, patients have bilateral PMG in other anatomical locations, such as posterior parietal, frontal or occipital. Unilateral perisylvian PMG usually presents with mild hemiparesis and focal seizures. Some patients with unilateral hemispheric PMG develop a transient malignant epileptic syndrome with intractable seizures and epilepsy with continuous spikes and waves during sleep. A recent study showed good long-term outcome for the majority of these patients [27].

Group 4 (Primarily Malformations Secondary to Abnormal Neuronal Migration at Different Stages)

Heterotopia Syndromes

Grey matter heterotopia is defined by the presence of normal neurons in incorrect locations, usually the ventricular wall or in any location along the white matter up to the cortex. Heterotopia are the most frequent MCD seen in the general population. The most common form is periventricular nodular heterotopia or PVNH, but other major types include focal subcortical, laminar or multi-focal heterotopia.

PVNH consists of contiguous or non-contiguous grey matter nodules lining the ventricular walls and protruding into the ventricles. Microscopically, the heterotopic tissue contains neurons and glial cells, and forms clusters of rounded, irregular nodules separated by layers of myelinated fibres. The number of nodules varies, with patients having a single or a few nodules up to a large number of nodules.

Previous genetic studies demonstrated that the most common form of diffuse PVNH is caused by mutations in the X-linked FLNA gene [28]. In familial forms, FLNA1 mutations are extremely common. Overall, FLNA1 mutations are seen in about 50% of individuals with classic PVNH, in both familial and sporadic cases. ARFGEF2 is another gene associated with PVNH and microcephaly. These two genes regulate actin binding, vesicle trafficking, cell adhesion and radial glia function [29]. FLNA1 encodes a large actin-binding phosphoprotein that contributes to formation of adhesions along the ventricular wall. ARFGEF2 encodes a protein that phosphorylates guanine diphosphate, which regulates vesicle trafficking. Other possible candidate genes include CADM1 and DNMT1, as well as SCNA1 mutations. Identified mutations in EML1 (EMAPL) in two families with bilateral giant ribbon-like heterotopia have also been reported. EML1 is a microtubule-associated protein

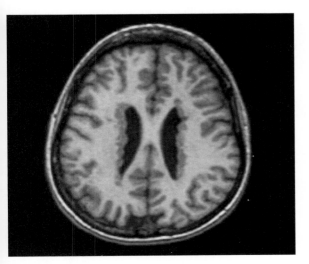

Figure 10.6 Bilateral contiguous periventricular nodular heterotopia.

[30]. Other genetic forms of atypical heterotopia have been mapped to different chromosomes.

Imaging features in patients with FLNA1 mutations are fairly homogeneous. There are bilateral contiguous periventricular nodular masses that spare the temporal horns, and mild cerebellar vermis hypoplasia with mega-cisterna magna. Conversely, a large number of isolated cases have a posterior-predominant pattern, where the heterotopia is limited to the trigone, and temporal and occipital horns, and can be associated with polymicrogyria, hippocampal misrotation, cerebellar hypoplasia, and brainstem and other cortical malformations (Figure 10.6).

The clinical presentation and course in patients with heterotopia varies. In patients with classical PVNH, but no other brain malformations, seizures and normal to moderate neurodevelopmental problems are common. More severe phenotypes are seen in patients with atypical forms, such as those with posterior predominance or those with diffuse heterotopic masses.

Key Points

- Malformations of cortical development (MCDs) are increasingly recognized as causes of epilepsy and neurodevelopmental disorders.
- MCDs are the most common aetiology of intractable epilepsy in children.

- Most MCDs can be classified using high-resolution MRI.
- Recent advances in molecular genetics suggest that several MCDs share similar pathway regulator gene mutations. The clinical variability is likely the result of the developmental stage and location of the lesion.

References

1. Kuzniecky RI. Malformations of cortical development and epilepsy, part 1: diagnosis and classification scheme. *Rev Neurol Dis* 2006;3(4):151–162

2. Barkovich AJ, Guerrini R, Kuzniecky RI, Jackson GD, Dobyns WB. A developmental and genetic classification for malformations of cortical development: update 2012. *Brain* 2012;**135**:1348–1369

3. Guerrini R, Dobyns WB. Malformations of cortical development: clinical features and genetic causes. *Lancet Neurol* 2014;**13**:710–726

4. Bae BI, Tietjen I, Atabay KD, et al. Evolutionarily dynamic alternative splicing of GPR56 regulates regional cerebral cortical patterning. *Science* 2014;**343** (6172):764–768

5. Jamuar SS, Lam AT, Kircher M, et al. Somatic mutations in cerebral cortical malformations. *N Engl J Med* 2014;**371**(8):733–743

6. Lee JH, Huynh M, Silhavy JL, et al. De novo somatic mutations in components of the PI3K-AKT3-mTOR pathway cause hemimegalencephaly. *Nat Genet* 2012;**44**:941–945

7. Marin-Valencia I, Guerrini R, Gleeson JG. Pathogenetic mechanisms of focal cortical dysplasia. *Epilepsia* 2014;**55**(7):970–978

8. Wang VY, Chang EF, Barbaro NM. Focal cortical dysplasia: a review of pathological features, genetics, and surgical outcome. *Neurosurg Focus* 2006;**20**(1):E7

9. Aronica, E., et al. Differential expression patterns of chloride transporters, Na+–K+–2Cl–cotransporter and K+–Cl–cotransporter, in epilepsy-associated malformations of cortical development. *Neuroscience* 2007;**145**(1):185–196

10. Rakhade SN, Jensen FE. Epileptogenesis in the immature brain: emerging mechanisms. *Nat Rev Neurol* 2009;**5**(7):380–391

11. André VM, Wu N, Yamazaki I, et al. Cytomegalic interneurons: a new abnormal cell type in severe pediatric cortical dysplasia. *J Neuropathol Exp Neurol* 2007;**66**:491–504

12. Crino PB. Molecular pathogenesis of focal cortical dysplasia and hemimegalencephaly. *J Child Neurol* 2005;**20**(4):330–336

13. Mirzaa GM, Conway RL, Gripp KW, et al. Megalencephaly-capillary malformation (MCAP) and megalencephaly-polydactyly-polymicrogyria-hydrocephalus (MPPH) syndromes: two closely related disorders of brain overgrowth and abnormal brain and body morphogenesis. *Am J Med Genet A* 2012;**158A**(2):269–291

14. Blumcke I, Thom M, Aronica E, et al. The clinicopathologic spectrum of focal cortical dysplasias: a consensus classification proposed by an ad hoc Task Force of the ILAE Diagnostic Methods Commission. *Epilepsia* 2011;**52**:158–174

15. Hsu PP, Kang SA, Rameseder J, et al. The mTOR-regulated phosphoproteome reveals a mechanism of mTORC1-mediated inhibition of growth factor signaling. *Science* 2011;**332**:1317–1322

16. Zhou J, Blundell J, Ogawa S, et al. Pharmacological inhibition of mTORC1 suppresses anatomical, cellular, and behavioral abnormalities in neural-specific Pten knock-out mice. *J Neurosci* 2009;**29**:1773–1783

17. Epilepsy Electroclinical Study Group, Ricos M Hodgson BL. Pippucci T, et al. Mutations in the mammalian target of rapamycin pathway regulators NPRL2 and NPRL3 cause focal epilepsy. *Ann Neurol* 2016;**79**(1):120–131

18. Romaniello R, Arrigoni F, Bassi MT, Borgatti R. Mutations in a- and b-tubulin encoding genes: implications in brain malformations. *Brain Dev* 2014;**37**(3):273–280

19. Pilz D, Stoodley N, Golden JA. Neuronal migration, cerebral cortical development, and cerebral cortical anomalies. *J Neuropathol Exp Neurol* 2002;**61**(1):1–11

20. Gleeson JG, Allen KM, Fox JW, et al. Doublecortin, a brain-specific gene mutated in human x-linked lissencephaly and double cortex syndrome, encodes a putative signaling protein. *Cell* 1998;**92**:63–72

21. Saillour Y, Carion N, Quelin C, et al. LIS1-related isolated lissencephaly: spectrum of mutations and relationships with malformation severity. *Arch Neurol* 2009;**66**(8):1007–1015

22. Morris EB, 3rd, Parisi JE, Buchhalter JR. Histopathologic findings of malformations of cortical development in an epilepsy surgery cohort. *Arch Pathol Lab Med* 2006;**130**(8):1163–1168

23. Kuzniecky R, Andermann F, Guerrini R. Congenital bilateral perisylvian syndrome: study of 31 patients. The CBPS Multicenter Collaborative Study. *Lancet* 1993;**341**(8845):608–612

24. Jansen AC, Robitaille Y, Honavar M, et al. The histopathology of polymicrogyria: a series of 71 brain autopsy studies. *Dev Med Child Neurol* 2016;**58**:39–48

25. Baulac S, Lenk GM, Dufresnois B, et al. Role of the phosphoinositide phosphatase FIG4 gene in familial epilepsy with polymicrogyria. *Neurology* 2014;**82**(12):1068-1075

26. De Ciantis A, Barkovich AJ, Cosottini M, et al. Ultra-high-field MR imaging in polymicrogyria and epilepsy. *Am J Neuroradiol* 2014;**36**(2):309-316

27. Caraballo RH, Cersósimo RO, Fortini PS, et al. Congenital hemiparesis, unilateral polymicrogyria and epilepsy with or without status epilepticus during sleep: a study of 66 patients with long-term follow-up. *Epileptic Disord* 2013;**15**(4):417–427

28. Fox JW, Lamperti ED, Ekşioğlu YZ, et al. Mutations in filamin 1 prevent migration of cerebral cortical neurons in human periventricular heterotopia. *Neuron* 1998;**21**(6):1315–1325

29. Sheen VL, Topçu M, Berkovic S, et al. Autosomal recessive form of periventricular heterotopia. *Neurology* 2003;**60**(7):1108–1112

30. Kielar M, Tuy FPD, Bizzotto S. Mutations in Eml1 lead to ectopic progenitors and neuronal heterotopia in mouse and human. *Nat Neurosci* 2014;**17**(7):923-933

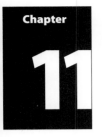

Chapter

11

Hippocampal Sclerosis as a Cause of Medication-Resistant Epilepsy

Fahmida Amin Chowdhury, Beate Diehl and Maria Thom

Introduction

Hippocampal sclerosis (HS) is the most frequent aetiology for medically refractory epilepsy [1]. It was first described by Bouchet and Cazauvielh in 1825 on pathological examination of a patient who had died following seizures [2]. In 1880, Sommer studied pathological samples from over 90 patients with chronic epilepsy, and reported gliosis and pyramidal cell loss in the hippocampus, predominantly in the CA1 region, originally known as Sommer's sector. He proposed that these abnormalities were the cause of the epilepsy. In 1889, Jackson associated focal lesions in the hippocampus with the clinical symptoms of temporal lobe seizures. In addition to the loss of pyramidal cells, the loss of hilar interneurons was recognized as an important feature [3] and is dominant in the type of pathology that came to be described as end-folium sclerosis [4]. Loss of both inhibitory gamma-aminobutyric acid (GABA) neurons and excitatory mossy cells in the hilus reduces their control of the dentate granule cells, and such loss of neurons in the hilus (sometimes included as part of CA4) is one of the most consistent findings in TLE [5,6]. The International League Against Epilepsy has proposed a classification of the distinct patterns of HS to correlate the type of pathological changes to post-surgical outcome [7]. In the 1950s with the development of electroencephalography, HS was linked to electrophysiologic temporal lobe seizures.

The exact prevalence and incidence of HS is unknown, but it is thought to be present in approximately 10% of adults with new-onset focal epilepsy [1]. Furthermore, it often causes medically refractory epilepsy; most epidemiological data on HS comes from surgical series with incidence in large series varying from 34–66% [8]. Many patients referred for surgical management have a long history of epilepsy with seizure onset many years ago and may have benefitted from earlier referral.

Anatomy of the Hippocampus

Structure

The hippocampus forms part of the limbic lobe and is situated in the mesial part of the temporal lobe [9]. It consists of three parts: head, body and tail. It is formed by interlocking bands of dentate gyrus and the hippocampus proper (also known as the cornu ammonis, CA or Ammon's horn). The inner structure of Ammon's horn is made up of four subfields, CA1–4, shown in Figure 11.1, which consist of pyramidal cells. The dentate gyrus consists of three layers: a granule cell layer, an outer molecular layer and a deeper polymorphic layer. The most inferior part of the hippocampal formation is the subiculum, which lies between the CA1 subfield of the hippocampus and the entorhinal cortex, which is part of the parahippocampal gyrus.

Connections

The major excitatory input pathway to the hippocampus comes from the entorhinal cortex to the granule cells of the dentate gyrus and the CA3 pyramidal neurons, via the perforant path. In addition, CA3 pyramidal neurons receive input from the dentate gyrus via mossy fibres. They send axons to CA1 pyramidal cells via the Schaffer collateral pathway; CA1 neurons also receive inputs direct from the perforant path and send axons to the subiculum. The main hippocampal output fibres pass back from the CA1 region to the subiculum, and back to the entorhinal cortex.

Aetiology and Pathogenesis

The aetiology of HS is controversial. It is likely to be multi-factorial due to a combination of acquired and inherited factors. Retrospective studies report 30–50% of patients suffered from an 'initial precipitating injury' before the age of four years [10]. Complex febrile seizures are the most frequently reported

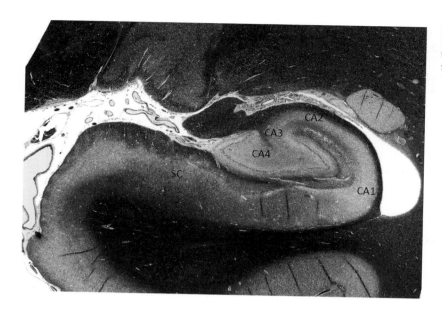

Figure 11.1 Section of normal hippocampus stained with luxol fast blue for myelin and cresyl violet for neurones, showing cornu ammonis (CA) subfields 1–4 and subiculum (SC).

events, followed by birth trauma, head injury and intra-cranial infections.

Acquired Factors

Febrile Convulsions

Patients with HS have a higher incidence of febrile convulsions. There appears to be no increased prevalence after simple febrile seizures compared to the general population, but this rises to 22% after a complicated febrile convulsion, such as febrile convulsions that have focal features or are prolonged.

Status Epilepticus

Animal models of limbic status epilepticus show that this can result in HS. There is also evidence of damage to the hippocampus in humans, detected using magnetic resonance imaging (MRI) following status epilepticus. Longitudinal studies such as FEBSTAT have confirmed that in a minority of cases of febrile status epilepticus, there is subsequent development of HS [11]. In the FEBSTAT study, approximately 10% of children had high T2-weighted signal in the hippocampus with later evolution to HS in most. In the other 90%, there was evidence of decreased hippocampal growth, suggesting subtle hippocampal injury. This study did not allow assessment of whether there were subtle abnormalities of the hippocampus, present prior to the onset of febrile seizures, that may have predisposed to seizures and subsequent HS.

Previous Intracranial Infections

The hippocampus is vulnerable to long-term damage from infections. Viral encephalitis often targets mesial temporal structures with the subsequent evolution to bilateral HS and memory difficulties. Children with a history of meningitis also have higher incidence of HS.

However, about 70% of patients with mesiotemporal sclerosis have no history of febrile convulsions, or status epilepticus, and at least a third have no history of any precipitating injury, suggesting that there are other non-acquired susceptibility factors.

Hippocampal Sclerosis as a Developmental Disorder

The presence of associated subtle cytoarchitectural malformations in the neocortex of patients with HS has led to the suggestions that HS may be part of a wider maldevelopment process. In addition, studies showing pre-existing hippocampal developmental abnormalities have been suggested in neuroimaging studies.

Genetics

HS is generally considered to be a sporadic condition. Though genetic susceptibility determinants have not yet not been clearly elucidated, a few associations have been reported. For example, the Apoε4 genotype has been associated with increased risk of bilateral HS, and more recently, variation around the SCN1A gene was linked with HS and febrile seizures [12]. Rare pedigrees have been identified, with both febrile seizures and HS occurring independently in different family members, providing support for a common genetic basis for these conditions [13]. A number of family-based imaging studies have reported hippocampal atrophy in asymptomatic family members, which may represent that this is an inherited developmental variant that increases risk for HS [14]. Put together, these studies provide support that the genetic background influences the risk of HS.

Immune Mechanisms

Pathological specimens may occasionally show focal infiltrates of microglia, upregulation of interleukin (IL) receptors (IL-1β and IL-1), expression of inter-cellular adhesion molecule 1 (ICAM-1) and expression of kallikrein in glia [15], suggesting that inflammation may play a role. One group reported an increased frequency of a specific interleukin-1beta allele polymorphism in TLE associated with HS and prolonged febrile convulsion [16]. The presence of more widespread inflammation in pathological specimens may indicate the possibility of an underlying or previous autoimmune encephalitis, particularly in adult-onset epilepsy cases. In recent years, specific antibodies, such as voltage-gated potassium channel antibodies have been identified. Usually, these autoantibodies result in acute or subacute encephalitis with MRI showing evidence of enlargement, increased T2-weighted signal and restricted diffusion of the mesial temporal lobe structures. Later, HS can occur, which may be unilateral or bilateral, emphasizing the importance of investigating for autoantibodies and aggressive early immunosuppressive treatment in such patients [1].

Mechanisms of Hippocampal Injury

As described above, the hippocampus is particularly vulnerable to damage by seizures, infection, inflammation and ischaemic/hypoxic injury. Possible mechanisms of neuronal cell loss and selective vulnerability include glutamate neurotoxicity and mitochondrial dysfunction. However, the exact pathways of cell death remain yet to be defined [1].

Mechanisms of Epileptogenicity

In some patients, HS may be progressive, suggesting that seizures arising from the hippocampus can cause further damage to the hippocampus and more widespread structures, including the contralateral hippocampus. The observation that early surgical treatment may result in better outcomes than late surgical intervention, is in support of the hypothesis of the progressive nature of HS [17]. Various theories have been proposed based on animal studies and human pathological studies as to the epileptogenic processes in HS, including: (1) mossy fibre sprouting, resulting in excitatory synaptic contact with apical dendrites, (2) high expression of neuropeptides such as substance P and neuropeptide Y and (3) dysfunction of astroglia and the blood–brain barrier [15].

Clinical Features

Demographics

Onset of seizures is usually between age 4 and 16, typically at the end of the first decade, with equal male and female incidence [18].

Seizure Semiology

Seizure semiology usually consists of characteristic auras, which may evolve to loss of awareness, with or without automatisms. Depending on seizure spread and duration, there may be additional positive ictal motor symptoms. Generalized tonic–clonic seizures are usually infrequent.

There are no semiological features that are specific to medial temporal lobe epilepsy due to HS, and auras usually arise from areas adjacent to the hippocampus [18]. Abdominal auras and early oral automatisms occur more frequently in medial compared to lateral temporal lobe epilepsy [19]. The duration of seizures is usually two to three minutes.

Aura

Abdominal aura (epigastric rising sensation and nausea) is the most commonly reported aura and is probably caused by propagation to the adjacent insular cortex. It is reported to occur in approximately 50% of patients with HS on MRI [20]. Although, abdominal aura may occur in extratemporal epilepsy, when associated with oral and manual automatisms it is reported to have greater than 98% specificity for temporal lobe epilepsy [21].

Other auras may include psychoaffective phenomena such as fear or anxiety in 15–50%, and other psychic auras such as an illusion of familiarity including déjà vu/jamais vu in 20–30%. Autonomic auras can also occur, such as palpitations or feelings of change in temperature. The aura may be non-specific and difficult to describe in words. Rarely, olfactory and gustatory auras that are usually unpleasant are also described.

Clinical Evolution of Seizures

Auras may progress to impaired awareness, the patient may have motor arrest and stare, and there may be associated automatisms. Usually automatisms will involve manual and oral movements, such as fiddling with one or both hands, chewing or lip smacking. However, more complex motor manifestations such as running or pedalling can occur and may indicate propagation to the frontal lobe. Positive motor symptoms can occur with suprasylvian spread and include dystonic posturing, clonic movements or rarely secondary generalization.

Lateralizing Signs

In terms of lateralizing signs, there are none in the above described auras, but unilateral automatisms are usually ipsilateral to the side of HS, although the specificity is relatively low, unless this sign is seen in conjunction with contralateral dystonic posturing. Dystonic limb posturing and clonic limb movements are contralateral signs. Ictal speech is a sign of non-dominant temporal lobe involvement, while postictal dysphasia is a feature of seizures in the dominant temporal lobe. As with other types of seizures, extension of one arm and flexion of the other in a figure of 4 prior to generalization indicates onset contralateral to the extended arm.

Electroencephalogram (EEG)

Scalp EEG

Typical scalp EEG findings can be seen inter-ictally, at seizure onset, as the seizure evolves, and post-ictally (Figure 11.2). Inter-ictal scalp recordings in patients with HS can show non-specific focal slowing in the temporal region. There may also be spikes and sharp waves, maximal in sphenoidal and in anterior and inferior temporal regions (LSph, RSph, F7, F8). This is thought to reflect activity in the parahippocampal gyrus rather than the hippocampus itself. In one study, inter-ictal EEG abnormalities were found in 96% of patients with TLE during prolonged recording, and bilateral independent activity was seen in 42%, predominantly over the side of seizure onset in

half of the patients [22]. An ictal EEG showing lateralized build-up of rhythmic anterior temporal 5–7 Hz activity within 30 seconds of clinical onset is strongly associated with HS [23] and predicts lateralization in 82–94% of cases. Initial attenuation can occur in a unilateral temporal region or more diffusely. Localized EEG onset is reported to occur in 93% of mesiotemporal seizures. Lateralized post-ictal slowing was also a very reliable lateralizing finding. The EEG may be normal in 60% of all auras [24]. In a recent study, the added value of inferior temporal electrodes, computed montages and voltage maps significantly increased the sensitivity for interpreting ictal patterns and identified ictal activity at earlier time-points than visual inspection [25].

Intra-Cranial EEG

Depth recordings show that in patients with mesiotemporal sclerosis as the epileptogenic lesion, ictal onset usually occurs very focally within the hippocampus. Ictal onset patterns usually show high-frequency, low-amplitude spike discharges [18]. However, electrical stimulation and propagation patterns suggest that the symptomatogenic area for most seizures is due to spread to adjacent structures, including insular and temporal neocortex. Compared with other brain areas, propagation is slower, and seizures may also spread to contralateral mesial temporal structures, ipsilateral orbitofrontal and frontal regions.

Imaging

A number of imaging modalities have been applied to investigate patients with HS. Depending on the electroclinical findings, in straightforward situations, structural MRI, ictal and inter-ictal EEG, neuropsychological testing and neuropsychiatric assessment are typically adequate to guide epilepsy surgery. However, if discrepancies in diagnostic test results are noted and it is not clear whether the epilepsy arises from the lesion, or the changes are subtle, further testing may be indicated.

Magnetic Resonance Imaging

MRI is the modality of choice to evaluate the hippocampus; however, a dedicated temporal lobe epilepsy protocol needs to be performed if good sensitivity and specificity are to be achieved. Thin section coronal levels orthogonal to the longitudinal axis of the hippocampus are required, to minimize volume

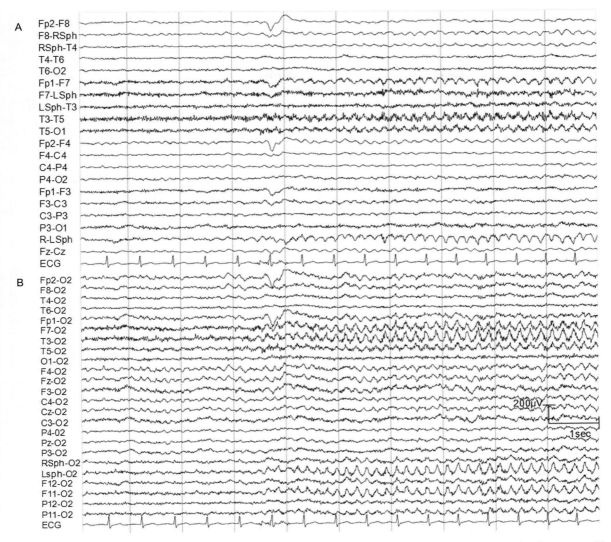

Figure 11.2 EEG example of ictal left temporal theta pattern from a patient with pathologically confirmed left HS on a bipolar montage (A) and referenced to O2 (B), maximal LSph,T3>F7,F11.

averaging. In the last decade, technical improvements have led to increased sensitivity in detecting HS. (Figure 11.3) Coronal volume and coronal high-resolution T2-weighted and FLAIR imaging are the most sensitive sequences to visually detect HS. Findings include: (1) reduced hippocampal volume (detected in 90–95% of pathologically confirmed cases), (2) increased T2 signal (80–85% of surgically treated) and increased FLAIR signal and (3) abnormal morphology, for example loss of internal architecture such as interdigitations of hippocampus (in 60–95%) [18]. Although comparing sides can help with detecting

hippocampal abnormalities, up to 10% of cases are bilateral, and thus if symmetry is the only feature being evaluated, such cases may be misinterpreted as normal. Extrahippocampal abnormalities that may be seen include atrophy of the ipsilateral amygdala, temporal neocortex, fornix and mammillary bodies. Additional quantitative studies such as 3D volumetry and T2 relaxometry may also be useful in detecting subtle HS [26]. In a recent study, HS was identified on T2 values with 100% sensitivity and 100% specificity and was identified using normalized FLAIR signal intensity with 60% sensitivity and 93% specificity

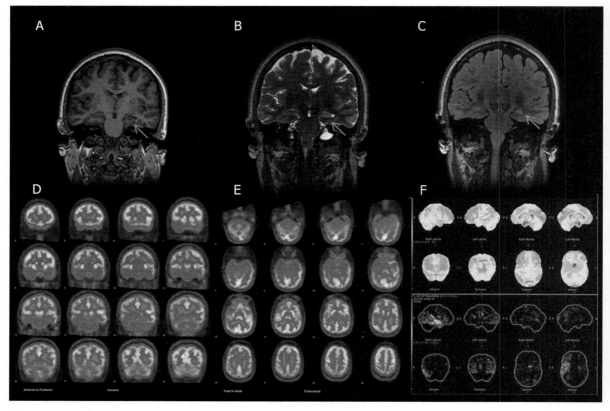

Figure 11.3 MRI from a patient with left HS showing (A) T1 imaging demonstrating a smaller left hippocampus, (B) increased T2 signal and (C) increased fluid-attenuated inversion recovery (FLAIR) signal. PET scan from another patient with right HS showing right temporal hypometabolism on (D) coronal slices, (E) temporal slices and (F) surface rendered imaging.

[27]. This suggests that T2 mapping outperforms normalized FLAIR in identifying HS. However, it must be noted that unilateral HS is found incidentally in 14% of MRI scans, and so the presence of HS does not necessitate that it is the cause of seizures. Further advances may be forthcoming with greater availability of high-field MRI scanners (7 T), although more sophisticated subfield subanalyses using 1.5 or 3 T imaging data already offers insights into patterns of cell loss [28].

Magnetic Resonance Proton Spectroscopy

Magnetic resonance proton spectroscopy (MRS) assesses neuronal integrity by measuring brain metabolites. Due to low signal-to-noise ratio and long acquisition times, only small volumes of brain tissue are sampled. MRS findings may consist of decreased N-acetylaspartate (NAA) and decreased NAA/choline and NAA/creatine (NAA/Cr) ratios in 90% of cases in whom HS is found in resected tissue and is thought to represent neuronal dysfunction. Lactate levels may

rise following a seizure. There is also evidence of reduced NAA in the contralateral hippocampus in 30–40% of patients, which has been reported to be associated with less favourable surgical outcome [29]. Another study that used MRS in patients before and after surgery also found pre-operatively reduced NAA/Cr ratio ipsilaterally in patients who became seizure-free, and bilaterally in those who did not. Furthermore, post-operatively, in patients who became seizure-free, this normalized on the side of surgery and in the one patient who became seizure-free, who had low NAA/Cr prior to surgery, the NAA/Cr ratio on the unoperated contralateral temporal lobe also increased to the normal range. The authors also reported that in patients who did not become seizure-free, NAA/Cr values did not change. This suggests that abnormalities in NAA/Cr reflect altered physiological function of neurons rather than neuronal loss alone, with more remote contralateral changes indicating more severe pathology, and that these changes can be reversible if seizures are controlled [30].

Nuclear Medicine

Single-photon emission computed tomography (SPECT) and positron emission tomography (PET) imaging can be useful adjunctive investigations, particularly in less clear-cut cases. They are, however, not typically needed if structural MRI and electroclinical data are indicative of medial temporal lobe epilepsy with HS. Fluorodeoxyglucose-PET (FDG-PET) measures reductions in regional cerebral glucose metabolism as a surrogate of metabolic dysfunction, while flumazenil-PET (FMZ-PET) is a measure of central benzodiazepine receptors.

FDG-PET shows reduced uptake in the anterior temporal region ipsilateral to the HS, both mesially and laterally in 90% of patients with pathologically confirmed HS. The reduction may also extend to the thalamus, basal ganglia, insula, inferior frontal cortex and lateral parietal cortex. It has high sensitivity, but specificity is limited [31]. ^{11}C-FMZ-PET is a specific antagonist of central benzodiazepine receptors and maps benzodiazepine receptor density, and is decreased in ipsilateral anterior mesiotemporal regions of patients with HS. It has the advantage that reduced FMZ binding correlates with areas of most pronounced neuronal loss and gives more focal results than measures of glucose metabolism. However, its use is limited by cost, availability of tracer and lack of specificity.

Ictal single-photon emission computed tomography (SPECT) scans show hyperperfusion of the anterior temporal region ipsilateral to the HS, in 90% of patients with pathologically proven HS. The abnormal area may also extend to thalamus, insula and basal ganglia [32,33]. Hyperperfusion of the mesial temporal structures is seen for up to two minutes post-ictally, with hypoperfusion of lateral temporal structures, and this is followed by hypoperfusion of the whole temporal lobe. A return to normal perfusion is usually seen within 10–30 minutes. Interictally, hypoperfusion may be seen. The pattern is not specific for HS and may also be seen in other causes of temporal lobe epilepsy, such as low-grade tumours.

A meta-analysis focusing on the FDG-PET in preoperative assessment found that ipsilateral PET hypometabolism had a predictive value of 86% for good outcome [31]. Even in patients with normal MRI the predictive value for good outcome post-operatively was 80% in patients. The added value of ^{11}C- FMZ-PET and MRS is less clear.

Neuropsychology

The dominant hippocampus is involved in anterograde verbal memory, and the non-dominant hippocampus in anterograde non-verbal memory. Studies have shown that degree of deficit correlates with degree of volume loss on MRI. Cross-sectional studies suggest progressive memory decline, but there are no longitudinal studies, and it is difficult to separate duration of epilepsy from cognitive decline due to ageing processes and other factors that may lead to memory impairment, including anti-seizure medication and frequency of seizures.

Post-surgical deficits are most marked in those with least memory dysfunction pre-operatively, limited atrophy on MRI and limited histopathological neuronal loss. In addition, if the contralateral hippocampus is preserved, it can compensate for memory loss.

A recent pathological study found that pathological subtypes are differentially associated with pre-operative cognitive profile, for example CA1 predominant loss was reported to be associated with no declarative memory loss, and dentate gyrus cell density correlated with predictive memory formation. Since odds of seizure freedom post-operatively seem determined in part by pathological subtype, the neuropsychological profile may add to predicting odds of seizure freedom [34].

Psychiatric Co-Morbidity

Psychiatric co-morbidity is found in about 50% of patients with HS, the majority of which are non-psychotic in nature [35]. The most common diagnoses are depression and anxiety, followed by psychosis. A review of this topic found that there was a trend for major psychiatric diagnoses to be more common in patients with right compared to left temporal lobe epilepsy, both before and after surgery [35,36]. Psychiatric dysfunction may improve or worsen after an operation, with post-operative psychiatric conditions usually manifesting within a year of surgery. The two main predictors of psychiatric outcome are seizure freedom and pre-surgical psychiatric history [35]. Therefore, for patients undergoing epilepsy surgery for HS, pre- and post-surgical (within the first six months) psychiatric evaluations are recommended.

Management

Medical vs. Surgical Management

Though medical management should be the first approach, 90% of patients with HS are likely to have medication-resistant epilepsy [37]. Anti-seizure medications tend to control secondary generalization much better than focal seizures. A randomized trial of 80 patients with temporal lobe epilepsy, assigned to surgery or optimal medical treatment with anti-seizure medication for one year, showed that 58% of patients were free of seizures impairing awareness at one year, compared with 8% in the medical group, indicating that surgery is significantly superior to medical management [38]. More recently, another randomized trial, the ERSET trial, reported seizure freedom during two years follow-up; none of the 23 participants in the medical group were seizure-free compared with 11 out of 15 in the surgical group [39].

Surgical Management

A multi-disciplinary team approach is imperative to appraise surgical candidacy and allow for detailed counselling regarding surgical risks, including cognitive, behavioural and psychiatric aspects. These risks need to be balanced against the risks of ongoing intractable epilepsy. In cases with concordant non-invasive tests, such as clear MRI evidence of HS and typical inter-ictal and ictal scalp EEG findings, surgery can be recommended. For MRI-negative cases, if PET is concordant with electroclinical data, then surgery can also be recommended with good expected post-operative outcome, similar to the MRI-positive cases. In patients with contradictory EEG and MRI, further testing, such as intra-cranial recording or functional imaging should be considered.

Surgical Approaches

There are a number of surgical approaches in practice [40]:

1. The 'en bloc' resection, also known as the anterior temporal lobectomy (ATL) was introduced by Falconer in 1967. This resection included mesial as well as lateral structures of the anterior parts of the middle and inferior temporal gyri.
2. The 'Spencer-type' of resection, introduced in 1984, combines a small anterior partial lobectomy (~3 cm) with a more extensive mesial resection.
3. The selective amygdalohippocampectomy (SAH) is a strictly mesial resection with resection of hippocampus, amygdala and parahippocampal gyrus, sparing lateral structures. This can be carried out either as a transcortical approach, through the middle temporal gyrus or as a transylvian approach through the deep sylvian fissure, each with advantages and disadvantages. In the transylvian approach, unnecessary resection of non-epileptogenic temporal neocortex is largely avoided. However, part of the anterior temporal stem of the superior temporal gyrus must be transected. In addition, due to the close proximity of the dissection to major vascular structures in the sylvian fissure, transylvian SAH carries the risk of vascular injury or vasospasm. During the transcortical approach, a portion of the lateral temporal neocortex must be dissected to provide access to the ventricle and the mesiotemporal structures.

Advantages and Risks of Each Approach

The aim of surgical treatment is to give the best chances of seizure freedom, with minimal risk of post-operative deficits. For temporal lobe surgery, the main risks are that of a visual field defect (usually superior quadrantanopia) and neurocognitive deficits (particularly in memory) [41]. The motivation for conservative resection is to try to reduce such deficits. Visual field defect is reported to occur in 17.9% of temporal lobe surgery overall, but is likely to be less for surgery due to HS alone.

A systematic review of studies comparing standard anterior temporal lobectomy with selective amygdalohippocampectomy reported better seizure freedom rates with anterior temporal lobectomy compared to SAH in 11/13 studies. However, several studies have reported a better neuropsychological outcome in SAH [42]. For anterior temporal lobectomy, larger resection seemed to correlate with a better seizure freedom rate in some studies. Cognitive outcome seems to depend on the extent of mesial resection. However, the meta-analysis concluded that overall Class 1 evidence to support that conclusion was rare. The majority of studies were retrospective and did not use post-operative volumetric studies to assess the extent of actual resection; there was also significant variability between intended resection and volumetrically assessed end result. Other limitations were that resections varied across epilepsy surgery centres, and older studies could not differentiate lateral from mesial temporal lobe epilepsy. In terms of seizure outcome, two studies comparing transylvian and transcortical approaches for SAH had similar seizure outcomes for both.

A recent study of a nine-year series with a large number of patients using keyhole corticoamygdalo-hippocampectomy for patients with HS reported a complication rate of 1.76% [34]. Resection was performed through a 2.5-cm keyhole craniotomy at the anterior squamous temporal bone, followed by resection of the anterior-most portions of the middle and inferior temporal gyri and then of the amygdala, uncus and hippocampus-parahippocampal gyrus. The authors reported that 87% of patients had an Engel Class I seizure-free outcome at two years [43].

Post-Operative Outcomes

Seizure Freedom

Positive prognostic factors are concordance of scalp EEG with HS on MRI (predicts seizure freedom in >90%) and shorter duration of epilepsy [44]. Poor prognostic factors include earlier age of onset/longer duration of epilepsy, history of secondarily generalized tonic–clonic seizures, absence of clear lesion on MRI, bilateral PET abnormalities, discordance between functional and anatomical data, and use of intra-cranial recordings [11,17]. Pathological classification is important because it may relate to surgical outcome; type 2 and 3 HS have been shown to have poorer outcome compared with type 1 HS [7,45].

While surgery often improves seizure control, continuation of medications is often necessary. Approximately 75% patients who stop taking medications following successful surgery will have a recurrence of seizures. This finding suggests that in patients who have undergone temporal lobe resections, residual tissue and circuits remain that are capable of generating seizures if medications are discontinued.

Psychological Outcome

Post-operative surgical outcome will depend on pre-operative function and also the degree of function in the contralateral hippocampus [46]. A meta-analysis into post-surgical psychological outcomes reported a 44% risk to verbal memory with left-sided temporal surgery, twice as high as the rate for right-sided surgery (20%). Naming was reduced in 34% of left-sided temporal patients. Variations in surgical techniques did not appear to have a large effect on cognitive outcomes, except for naming outcomes, which appeared better with more conservative resections. For subtemporal vs. transylvian selective amygdalo-hippocampectomy in patients with mesial temporal lobe epilepsy, both surgical approaches caused decline in verbal memory to a similar degree. Differential effects were seen with regard to decline in verbal recognition memory (more affected by left transylvian SAH) as well as in figural memory and verbal fluency (more affected by subtemporal SAH).

Other Techniques

There is evidence that amygdalohippocampal stimulation can improve seizures by more than 50% and in a few cases lead to seizure freedom. Responsive neurostimulation (RNS) may be an option when patients are not suitable candidates for resective surgery, such as those with bilateral HS or when there is a particular concern about memory decline following temporal lobe resection [47]. More studies are required to refine stimulation parameters. A phase 3 randomized clinical trial, radiosurgery or open surgery (ROSE) is currently underway comparing radiosurgery (focused radiation with gamma knife radiosurgery) with temporal lobectomy as a treatment of medial temporal lobe epilepsy. A prior study has shown that focused radiation (radiosurgery) may also reduce or eliminate seizures arising from the temporal lobe [48], although there is a significant delay between intervention and the seizure reduction. It is uncertain whether cognitive outcomes are superior using this technique. Multiple subpial transections of the hippocampus, and stereotactic approaches, including radiofrequency ablation and laser interstitial thermal therapy represent interesting novel strategies. Although numbers are small, those techniques have achieved rates of seizure freedom comparable to open resection, but with fewer neurocognitive adverse effects [49].

Pathology

The pathological diagnosis of HS is based on the identification of pyramidal neuron loss and gliosis affecting specific subfields, primarily CA1, CA4 and CA3. The loss of neurons in these regions may be complete, with only sparse pyramidal and horizontal or interneuronal-type cells remaining (Figure 11.4A).

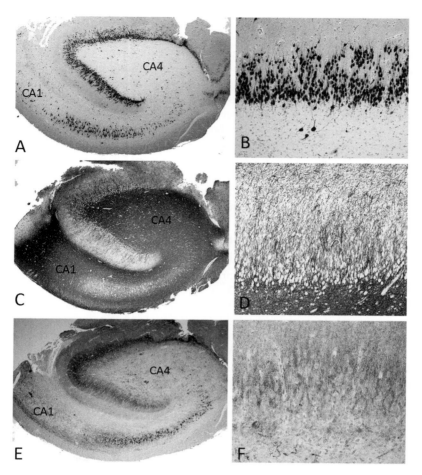

Figure 11.4 (A) Type 1 HS illustrated with NeuN neuronal staining showing loss of neurons in CA1 and CA4 subfield compared to the relative preservation of neurons in CA2 subfield between these regions. (B) The same case at higher magnification of the dentate gyrus, showing dispersion of the granule cell layer. (C) GFAP stain for astrocytes shows dense brown staining in the same regions of neuronal loss and in (D) shows a cellular or isomorphic pattern of gliosis in the dentate gyrus with radially arranged astrocytic fibres. (E) Zinc transporter protein for labelling of the mossy fibres shows patchy residual staining in CA4 and CA3 subfields but a band of staining is seen in the supragranular cell layer (shown in (F) at higher magnification), indicative of mossy fibre sprouting.

Severe neuronal loss is accompanied by the presence of a dense, scar-like fibrous gliosis, particularly in the CA1 subfield (Figure 11.4 C,D). In HS due to epilepsy there is typically a sharp cut-off between the preserved subiculum and the damaged CA1. The granule cell layer and CA2 are regarded as more 'resistant' regions, but patchy neuronal depletion as well as cellular gliosis in these areas is often evident.

There have been many quantitative studies in the last decades aiming to correlate the severity and distribution of hippocampal damage with both clinical and imaging features [50]. In addition, various grading schemes, notably the Wyler score, have been based on regional patterns of neuronal loss and gliosis. The most recent grading system is the International League Against Epilepsy (ILAE) scheme, introduced in 2013, which recognizes three distinct subtypes of HS [42,7]: type 1 pattern (previously known as the 'classical' type of sclerosis) shows significant neuronal loss involving both CA1 and CA4, type 2 (previously termed CA1 predominant sclerosis), shows restricted neuronal loss to the CA1 region, whereas type 3 HS shows significant neuronal loss in the CA4 sector only (previously termed end-folium sclerosis). Early clinico-pathological studies implementing this system suggest that type 1 HS is associated with a better outcome following surgical resection [51] and preserved pre-operative memory function is associated with type 2 HS [52, 53] but requires corroboration from further series. In addition to cell loss and scarring, regenerative changes including axonal sprouting and alteration of interneurons occur in HS in a relatively stereotypical fashion and may be more relevant to the process of epileptogenesis [54]. This includes alteration of interneuronal numbers [55–57] cell hypertrophy, abnormal dendritic projections [58–60] and axonal sprouting. Axonal sprouting in HS is exemplified by the mossy fibre pathway, the axons of the granule cells. Mossy fibre sprouting is relatively specific to epilepsy-related hippocampal damage and readily demonstrated in sections with immunohistochemistry to dynorphin or zinc-transporter 3 (Figure 11.4E,F). Granule cell dispersion is also a common feature in HS [61] defined by increased distances between individual granule cells and overall increased width of the cell layer, which can be up to 400 microns (compared to the normal thickness of around 120 microns) (Figure 11.4B). This 'neo-migration' of dispersed, mature granule cells may relate to a local deficiency in Reelin protein or be a manifestation of aberrant neurogenesis influenced by hippocampal seizures [62].

Bilateral HS and Dual Pathology

Bilateral HS

Bilateral HS can occur in 20% of patients, and they may still benefit from surgery. These patients have generally undergone intra-cranial evaluation, with a recent review reporting 75% Engel Class 1 outcome in patients with unilateral seizure onset on intra-cranial EEG [63]. However, a recent study showed that in bilateral HS with unilateral scalp EEG onset, resection following non-invasive evaluation can result in seizure freedom in 74%. In this study, unilateral inter-ictal discharges were a predictor of good outcome [64]. Cognitive concerns and a risk of memory impairment needs to be carefully assessed and explained to the patient and family in these challenging circumstances.

Dual Pathology

HS may coexist with other pathologies such as focal cortical dysplasia, low-grade neoplasms, periventricular heterotopias and vascular malformations. The most frequently associated pathologies are malformations of cortical development. The prevalence is difficult to assess and is thought to occur in 5–20% of surgical candidates, but this is likely to be an underestimate, as it is based on imaging rather than pathology. The presence of dual pathology results in an increase in resistance to medical treatment, from 11% of patients with HS alone becoming seizure-free with medical treatment to only 3% in those with dual pathology. Individuals with subtle extratemporal abnormalities are also more likely to have seizures post-operatively and removing both the lesion and the abnormal hippocampus has the best outcome in terms of seizure control, emphasizing the role of the hippocampus in temporal lobe seizures, even when there is a second pathology [37,65].

Key Points

- HS is a common pathology in MTLE and is a common cause of medically refractory epilepsy.
- Medication-resistant epilepsy often has a good outcome following resective surgery, and surgery should be considered at an early stage.
- HS has several aetiological factors and pathologic subtypes and is likely to be a heterogeneous condition. New imaging techniques may help us understand these different subtypes better and predict more accurately post-surgical outcome.
- In the future, it will be important to identify distinct patient groups that may need different investigative and surgical approaches to improve seizure outcome.

References

1. Walker MC. Hippocampal sclerosis: causes and prevention. *Semin Neurol* 2015;**35**:193–200

2. Bouchet C, Cazauvielh Y. De l'epilepsie considree dan se rapports avec l'alienation mentale. *Arch Gen Med Par* 1825;**9**:510–542

3. Bruton CJ. *The Neuropathology of Temporal Lobe Epilepsy*. London: Oxford, 1998

4. Margerison JH, Corsellis JA. Epilepsy and the temporal lobes: a clinical encephalographic and neuropathological study of the brain in epilepsy, with particular reference to the temporal lobes. *Brain* 1966;**89**:499–530

5. De Lanerolle NC, Kim JH, Robbins RJ, Spencer DD. Hippocampal interneuron loss and plasticity in human temporal lobe epilepsy. *Brain Res* 1989;**495**:387–395

6. Sloviter RS. Hippocampal pathology and pathophysiology in temporal lobe epilepsy. *Neurologia* 1996;**11**(Suppl 4):29–32

7. Blumcke I, Thom M, Aronica E, et al. International consensus classification of hippocampal sclerosis in temporal epilepsy: a Task Force Report from the ILAE Commission on Diagnostic Methods. *Epilepsia* 2013;**54**:1315–1329

8. De Tisi J, Bell GS, Peacock JL, et al. The long-term outcome of adult epilepsy surgery, patterns of seizure remission, and relapse: a cohort study. *Lancet* 2011;**378** (9800):1388–1395

9. lmgren K, Thom M. Hippocampal sclerosis – origins and imaging. *Epilepsia* 2012;**53**(S4):19–33

10. Blumke I, Thom M, Wiestler OD. Ammon's horn sclerosis; a maldevelopment disorder associated with temporal lobe epilepsy. *Brain Pathol* 2002;**12**(2):199–121

11. Lewis DV, Shinnar S, Hesdorffer DC, et al. Hippocampal sclerosis after febrile status epilepticus: the FEBSTAT study. *Ann Neurol* 2014;**75**:178–185

12. Kasperaviciute D, Catarino CB, Matarin M, et al. Epilepsy, hippocampal sclerosis and febrile seizures linked by common genetic variation around SCN1A. *Brain* 2013;**136**:3140–3150

13. Baulac S, Gourfinkel-An I, Nabbout R, et al. Fever, genes, and epilepsy. *Lancet Neurol* 2004;**3**:421–430

14. Tsai MH, Pardoe HR, Perchyonok Y, et al. Etiology of hippocampal sclerosis: evidence for a predisposing familial morphologic anomaly. *Neurology* 2013;**81**:144–149

15. Thom M. Review. Hippocampal sclerosis in epilepsy: a neuropathology review. *Neuropathol Appl Neurobiol* 2014;**40**:520–554

16. Kanemoto K, Kawasaki J, Yuasa S, et al. Increased frequency of interleukin-1beta-511 T allele in patients with temporal lobe epilepsy, hippocampal sclerosis, and prolonged febrile convulsion. *Epilepsia* 2003;**44**:796–799

17. Janszky J, Janszky I, Schulz R, et al. Temporal lobe epilepsy with hippocampal sclerosis: predictors for long-term surgical outcome. *Brain* 2005;**128**(2):395–404

18. Wieser HG et al. ILAE Comission report: mesial temporal lobe epilepsy with hippocampal sclerosis. *Epilepsia* 2004;**45**:695–714

19. Gil-Nagel A, Risinger MW. Ictal semiology in hippocampal versus extrahippocampal temporal lobe epilepsy. *Brain* 1997;**120**(1):183–192

20. Dupont S, Samson Y, Nguyen-Michel VH, et al. Are auras a reliable indicator in medial temporal lobe epilepsy with hippocampal sclerosis? *Eur J Neur* 2015;**22**:1310–1316

21. Henkel A, Noachtar S, Pfandel M, et al. The localising value of abdominal aura and its evolution: a study in focal epilepsies. *Neurology* 2002;**58**:271–276

22. Williamson PD, French JA, Thadani VM, et al. Characteristics of medial temporal lobe epilepsy: II. Interictal and ictal scalp electroencephalography, neuropsychological testing, neuroimaging, surgical results, and pathology. *Ann Neurol* 1993;**34**(6):781–787

23. Risinger MW, Engel J, Jr, Van Ness PC, et al. Ictal localisation of temporal lobe seizures with scalp/ sphenoidal recordings. *Neurology* 1989;**39**:1288–1293

24. Foldvary N, Klem G, Hammel J, et al. The localizing value of ictal EEG in focal epilepsy. *Neurology* 2001;**57**(11):2022–2028

25. Rosenzweig I, Fogarasi A, Johnsen B, et al. Beyond the double banana: improved recognition of temporal lobe seizures in long-term EEG. *J Clin Neurophysiol* 2014;**31**(1):1–9

26. Jackson GD, Berkovic SF, Duncan JS, et al. Optimizing the diagnosis of hippocampal sclerosis using MR imaging. *Am J Neuroradiol* 1993;**14**:753–762

27. Rodionov R, Bartlett PA, He C, et al. T2 mapping outperforms normalised FLAIR in identifying hippocampal sclerosis. *Neuroimage Clin* 2015;**7**:788–791

28. Kim H, Bernhardt BC, Kulaga-Yoskovitz J, et al. Multivariate hippocampal subfield analysis of local MRI intensity and volume: application to temporal lobe epilepsy. *Med Image Comput Comput Assist Interv* 2014;**17**(2):170–178

29. Duc CO, Trabesinger AH, Weber OM, et al. Quantitative 1H MRS in the evaluation of mesial temporal lobe epilepsy in vivo. *Mag Reson Imaging* 1998;**16**(8):969–979

30. Cendes F, Andermann F, Dubeau F, et al. Normalisation of neuronal metabolic dysfunction after surgery for temporal lobe epilepsy: evidence from proton MR spectroscopic imaging. *Neurology* 1997;**49**:1525–1533

31. Willmann O, Wennberg R, May T, et al. The contribution of 18 F-FDG-PET in pre-operative epilepsy surgery evaluation for patients with temporal lobe epilepsy: a meta-analysis. *Seizure* 2007;**16**:509–520

32. Sequeira KM, Tabesh A, Sainju RK, et al. Perfusion network shift during seizures in medial temporal lobe epilepsy. *PLoS One.* 2013;**8**(1):e53204

33. Duncan R, Patterson J, Roberts R, et al. Ictal/postictal SPECT in the pre-surgical localisation of complex partial seizures. *J Neurol Neurosurg Psychiatry* 1993;**56**:141–148

34. Coras R, Blümcke I. Clinicopathological subtypes of hippocampal sclerosis in temporal lobe epilepsy and their differential impact on memory impairment. *Neuroscience* 2015;**309**:153–161

35. Foong J, Flugel D. Psychiatric outcome of surgery for temporal lobe epilepsy and pre-surgical considerations. *Epilepsy Res* 2007;**75**:84–96

36. Macrodimitris S, Elisabeth MS, Sherman EMS, et al. Psychiatric outcomes of epilepsy surgery: a systematic review. *Epilepsia* 2011;**52**(5):880–890

37. Semah F, Picot MC, Adam C, et al. Is the underlying cause of epilepsy a major prognostic factor for recurrence. *Neurology* 1998;**51**(5):1256–1262

38. Wiebe S, Blume WT, Girvin JP, et al. A randomised control trial of surgery for temporal lobe epilepsy. *N Eng J Med* 2001;**345**(5):311–318

39. Early Randomized Surgical Epilepsy Trial (ERSET) Study Group, Engel J, Jr, McDermott MP, Wiebe S, et al. Early surgical therapy for drug-resistant temporal lobe epilepsy: a randomized trial. *J Am Med Assoc* 2012;**307**(9):922–930

40. Schramm J. Temporal lobe epilepsy surgery and the quest for optimal extent of resection: a review. *Epilepsia* 2008;**49**(8):1296–1307

41. Hader WJ, Tellez-Zenteno J, Metcalfe A, et al. Complications of epilepsy surgery: a systematic review of focal surgical resections and invasive EEG monitoring. *Epilepsia* 2013;**54**(5):840–847.

42. Josephson CB, Dykeman J, Fiest KM. Systematic review and meta-analysis of standard vs selective temporal lobe epilepsy surgery. *Neurology* 2013;**80**(18):1669–1676

43. Yang PF, Zhang HJ, Pei JS, et al. Keyhole epilepsy surgery: corticoamygdalohippocampectomy for mesial temporal sclerosis. *Neurosurg Rev* 2016;**39**(1):99–108

44. Tonini C, Beghi H, Berg AT. Predictors of epilepsy surgery outcome: a meta-analysis. *Epilepsy Res* 2004;**62**:75–87

45. Thom M, Liagkouras I, Elliot KJ, et al. Reliability of patterns of hippocampal sclerosis as predictors of postsurgical outcome. *Epilepsia* 2010;**51**(9):1801–1808

46. Sherman EMS, Wiebe S, Fay-McClymont TB. Neuropsychological outcomes after epilepsy surgery: systematic review and pooled estimates. *Epilepsia* 2011;**52**(5): 857–869

47. Thomas GP, Jobst BC. Critical review of the responsive neurostimulator system for epilepsy. *Med Devices* 2015;**1**(8):405–411

48. www.clinicaltrials.gov/ct2/show/NCT00860145 (Accessed March 2020)

49. Gross RE, Mahmoudi B, Riley JP. Less is more: novel less-invasive surgical techniques for mesial temporal lobe epilepsy that minimize cognitive impairment. *Curr Opin Neurol* 2015;**28**(2) 182–191

50. Steve TA, Jirsch JD, Gross DW, et al. Quantification of subfield pathology in hippocampal sclerosis: a systematic review and meta-analysis. *Epilepsy Res* 2014;**108**(8):1279–1285

51. Na M, Ge H, Shi C, et al. Long-term seizure outcome for international consensus classification of hippocampal sclerosis: a survival analysis. *Seizure* 2015;**25**:141–146

52. Coras RE, Pauli E, Li J, et al. Differential influence of hippocampal subfields to memory formation: insights from patients with temporal lobe epilepsy. *Brain* 2014;**137**(7):1945–1957

53. Deleo F, Garbelli R, Milesi G, et al. Short- and long-term surgical outcomes of temporal lobe epilepsy associated with hippocampal sclerosis: relationships with neuropathology. *Epilepsia* 2016;**57**(2):306–315

54. Thom M. Review. Hippocampal sclerosis in epilepsy: a neuropathology review. *Neuropathol Appl Neurobio* 2014;**40**(5):520–543

55. Sloviter RS, Sollas AL, Barbaro NM, et al. Calcium-binding protein (calbindin-D28 K) and parvalbumin immunocytochemistry in the normal and epileptic human hippocampus. *J Comp Neurol* 1991;**308**(3):381–396

56. Arellano JI, Muñoz A, Ballesteros-Yáñez I, et al. Histopathology and reorganization of chandelier cells in the human epileptic sclerotic hippocampus. *Brain* 2004;**127**(1):45–64

57. Toth K, Eross L, Vajda J, et al. Loss and reorganization of calretinin-containing interneurons in the epileptic human hippocampus. *Brain* 2010;**133**(9): 2763–2777

58. Maglóczky Z, Wittner L, Borhegyi Z, et al. Changes in the distribution and connectivity of interneurons in the epileptic human dentate gyrus. *Neuroscience* 2000;**96**(1):7–25

59. Wittner L, Eross L, Szabo Z, et al. Synaptic reorganization of calbindin-positive neurons in the human hippocampal CA1 region in temporal lobe epilepsy. *Neuroscience* 2002;**115**(3):961–978

60. Wittner L, Eross L, Czirjak S, et al. Surviving CA1 pyramidal cells receive intact perisomatic inhibitory input in the human epileptic hippocampus. *Brain* 2005;**128**(1):138–152

61. Houser CR. Granule cell dispersion in the dentate gyrus of humans with temporal lobe epilepsy. *Brain Res* 1990;**535**:195–204

62. Hester MS, Danzer SC. Hippocampal granule cell pathology in epilepsy – a possible structural basis for comorbidities of epilepsy? *Epilepsy Behav* 2014;**38**:105–116

63. Aghakhani Y, Liu X, Jette N, et al. Epilepsy surgery in patients with bilateral temporal lobe seizures: a systematic review. *Epilepsia* 2014;**55**(12):1892–1901

64. Ravat S, Rao P, Iyer V, et al. Surgical outcomes with non-invasive presurgical evaluation in MRI determined bilateral mesial temporal sclerosis: a retrospective cohort study. *Int J Surg* 2016;**36**(Pt B):429–435

65. Li LM, Cendes F, Andermann F, et al. Surgical Outcome in patients with epilepsy and dual pathology. *Brain* 1999;**122**(5):799–805

Chapter 12

Autoimmune Causes of Medication-Resistant Epilepsy

Anteneh M. Feyissa and Jeffrey W. Britton

Introduction

Epilepsy affects approximately 65 million people worldwide. Despite expanding treatment options, up to one-third of patients remain medically intractable [1]. With the exception of surgery in a subset of these patients, epilepsy treatment is usually limited to suppression of seizures with anti-seizure medications (ASMs). Accumulating data support an autoimmune aetiology in some patients [2,3]. Identification of neural antibodies allows a direct means of establishing an autoimmune cause in many of these cases [3–6]. Table 12.1 shows the best-known currently identified autoimmune epilepsy syndromes.

The role of immunity and inflammation in epilepsy is increasingly recognized [7–9] (see Figure 12.1). Paraneoplastic encephalitis has been recognized as a potential cause of seizures for many years [5]. Non-paraneoplastic encephalitides associated with neural antibodies responsive to immunotherapy have been discovered more recently [10–13]. The observation that seizures often complicate systemic autoimmune disorders suggests a broader role for immune mechanisms in seizure pathogenesis [14,15]. In this chapter, we review the clinical characteristics of several autoimmune epilepsy syndromes, and discuss current diagnosis and therapy.

Approach to Patients with Suspected Autoimmune Epilepsy

Clinical Features

Clinical features suggesting an autoimmune epilepsy syndrome are summarized in Table 12.2. The onset is often subacute. A history of preceding febrile illness is not uncommon. Unlike epilepsies due to other causes, seizures often occur up to several times a day at their inception. Focal seizures are the most common seizure type, usually of temporal origin. The seizures may be brief and may not be associated with loss of awareness. Affected patients are often refractory to standard ASMs; however, some will respond, so intractability should not be considered a sole criterion.

Diagnostic Evaluation

The detection of neural autoantibodies is important in establishing the diagnosis. The clinical features between different neural antibodies can overlap. Therefore, it is important to order a comprehensive neuroimmunology panel in suspected cases instead of targeting a specific antibody [5]. CSF examination should also be considered. It should be appreciated that several of the current neural antibodies were not discovered until recently, commensurate with technologic advances. Therefore, a negative comprehensive panel does exclude the possibility of an autoimmune aetiology. Autoimmune epilepsies may arise as a paraneoplastic phenomenon; therefore, evaluation with FDG-PET/CT, colonoscopy and mammography may need to be considered. In addition, for NMDA receptor (NMDAR) encephalitis, transvaginal ultrasound and gynaecologic evaluation is warranted to screen for ovarian teratoma. In men, urological examination and ultrasound for testicular and prostate cancer should be considered [5].

CSF investigation is important for several reasons: (a) in some cases, like NMDAR encephalitis, antibodies may be present in CSF only; (b) for some disorders, the concentration of CSF antibodies correlates better with clinical course; (c) as some neural antibodies are found in serum in the general population, the presence of antibodies in CSF helps provide evidence of relevance and (d) the antibodies in CSF and serum may differ in the same patient, and in such cases, the CSF antibodies usually correlate best with the clinical picture [5]. Other CSF findings indicative of inflammation include pleocytosis, elevated CSF protein and presence of oligoclonal bands.

Table 12.1 Autoimmune epilepsy syndromes grouped according to antigen location, seizure prevalence, clinical and laboratory features, association with cancer and response to immunotherapy

	Prominent seizure type and clinical features	Seizure prevalence	Frequency of cancer, main cancer type	Unique findings (serum, EEG and CSF)	Imaging findings	Response to immunotherapy
Antibodies targeting cell-surface antigens						
VGKC-complex Ab LGI1 +ve LE	Faciobrachial dystonic and temporal lobe seizures	Up to 100%	<20%, thymoma	hyponatraemia; acellular CSF with oligoclonal bands; temporal lobe IEDs and seizures (EEG)	Temporal lobe T2 signal abnormality in 50%; striatal T1 and/or T2 hyperintensity	Good
CASPR2+ve Morvan syndrome LGI1-ve/CASPR2-ve LE	Focal seizures	Less than LGI1 LE	20–50%, thymoma	Similar to LGI1+ve LE	Temporal lobe T2 signal abnormality in few cases	Good
	Mesial temporal lobe seizures	50–90%	<20%, thymoma	Similar to LGI1 +ve LE	Temporal lobe T2 and striatal T1/T2 signal abnormalities, hippocampal and striatal PET hypermetabolism	Moderate
NMDA receptor encephalitis	Focal and generalized seizures, psychosis, hypoventilation, autonomic instability, catatonia, orofacial dyskinesia	70–80%	30–40%, ovarian teratoma	Abs found in the serum and CSF; generalized rhythmic delta or delta brush pattern (EEG)	Often normal	Good
GABA-AR Ab encephalitis	Refractory status epilepticus or epilepsia partialis continua (EPC)	Major feature	<5%, thymoma	High Ab titer in CSF and serum; focal and generalized IEDs (EEG)	Multifocal or diffuse cortical and basal ganglia T2 signal changes	Good
GABA-BR Ab LE	Seizure is a prominent feature, complex partial	Up to 100%	70% SCLC	Lymphocytic pleocytosis in CSF; temporal seizures and IEDs (EEG)	Often with T2 signal changes in the mesial temporal region	Good
AMPAR-associated encephalitis	Temporal lobe seizures, opsoclonus	Minor feature	70%, thymoma and SCLC	Elevated CSF protein and pleocystosis in the majority : temporal IEDs	PET and MRI abnormalities mesial and neocortical temporal	Good
mGluR5 Ab LE	Seizure infrequent; myoclonic jerks; Ophelia syndrome	Minor feature	>90%, Hodgkin's lymphoma	Abs found in serum and CSF	Temporal lobe and parieto-occipital T2 hyperintensity	Good
GlyR Ab PERM	EPC and refractory status epilepticus; myoclonus; stiff-person syndrome	10–50%	10–20%, thymoma	Abs found in serum and CSF; focal IEDs and seizures; generalized seizures and IEDs (EEG)	+/- T2 signal change in the temporal lobe	Good

Table 12.1 (cont.)

	Prominent seizure type and clinical features	Seizure prevalence	Frequency of cancer, main cancer type	Unique findings (serum, EEG and CSF)	Imaging findings	Response to immunotherapy
Antibodies targeting intra-cellular antigens						
ANNA-1-associated LE	TLE; cerebellar degeneration, peripheral neuropathy, radiculopathy, sensory neuronopathy, autonomic dysfunction	Major feature	95%, SCLC	Pleocytosis and elevated protein in majority of cases (CSF); EEG with temporal lobe IEDs (33%), extratemporal IED (25%), both (42%)	Mesial temporal or extratemporal T2 signal hyperintensity	Poor
Ma 2-associated LE	TLE; cerebellar degeneration and hypothalamic dysfunction	Fairly common	>95%, testicular germ cell tumours	Pleocytosis and elevated protein in majority; temporal lobe IEDs and seizures	Mesial temporal or diffuse T2 signal changes	Poor
GAD65 Ab-associated LE	TLE; ataxia; brainstem; diabetes mellitus; stiff-person syndrome	Common feature	25%, thymoma and SCLC	High titer serum GAD65 (low titre non-specific); CSF often normal; temporal IEDs (EEG)	Mesial temporal T2/FLAIR hyperintensity	Mixed

AMPA = alpha amino-3-hydroxy-5-methyl-4-isoxazolepropionic acid, ANNA-1= Type 1 anti-neuronal nuclear antibody, GAD = glutamic acid decarboxylase, LGI1 = leucine-rich glioma inactivated 1, CASPR2 = contactin-associated protein 2, GABA-B = gamma-aminobutyric acid B, NMDA = N-methyl- D-aspartate, IED = inter-ictal epileptiform discharges, VGKC = voltage-gated potassium channel complex, SCLC = small cell lung cancer, mGluR5= metabotropic glutamate receptor 5

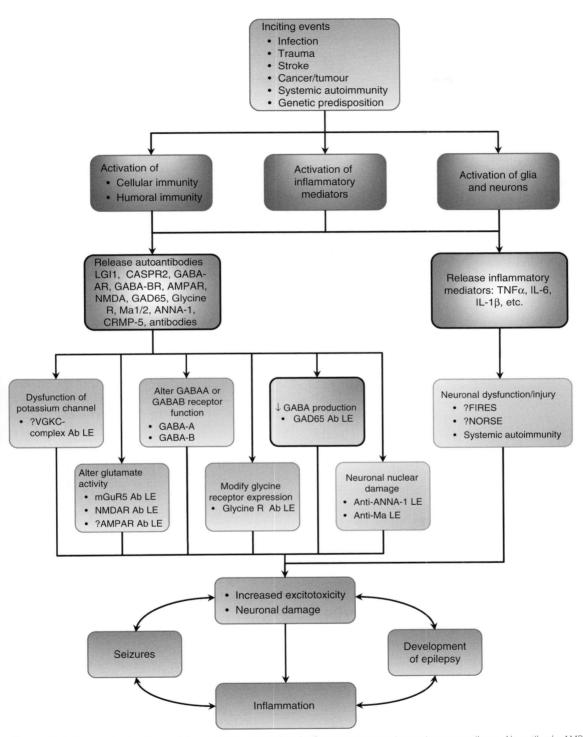

Figure 12.1 Hypothesized pathophysiology of immunological and inflammatory events in autoimmune epilepsy. Ab, antibody; AMPA,α-amino-3-hydroxy-5-methyl-4-isoxazolepropionic acid; ANNA-1, anti-neuronal nuclear antibody type 1; CRMP-5, collapsin response mediator protein 5; FIRES, febrile infection-related epilepsy syndrome; GABA-A, gamma-aminobutyric acid A; GABA-B, gamma-aminobutyric acid B; GAD65, glutamic acid decarboxylase 65; IL, interleukin; LE, limbic encephalitis; mGluR5, metabotropic glutamate receptor 5; NMDA, N-methyl-D-aspartate; NORSE, new-onset refractory status epilepticus; TNF, tumour necrosis factor; VGKC, voltage-gated potassium channel.

Table 12.2 Features suggestive of autoimmune epilepsy

Clinical features

- Acute/subacute onset
- Personal or family history of autoimmunity
- Risk factors for cancer
- Preceding infection, febrile syndrome
- Coexisting encephalopathy, movement disorders, neuropsychiatric impairment

Seizure types or patterns

- Frequent, recurrent temporal seizures
- Onset with status epilepticus or flurry of seizures
- Multi-focal seizures, epilepsia partialis continua
- Faciobrachial dystonic seizures

Imaging and other investigations

- MRI: Inflammatory changes (high T2/FLAIR signal/ contrast enhancement) medial temporal; increased T1/T2 or enhancement basal ganglia
- FDG PET: Hypermetabolic mesial temporal abnormalities; diffuse hypometabolism
- EEG: Frequent bilateral temporal lobe seizures; generalized rhythmic delta activity and extreme delta brush
- CSF: Mild to moderate mononuclear pleocystosis and protein elevation, abnormal synthesis rate, oligoclonal bands
- Positive cell surface or intracellular neural antibodies (serum and/or CSF)
- Histopathological findings compatible with inflammation on biopsy (chronic encephalitis)

EEG is usually abnormal, typically showing slowing, inter-ictal epileptiform discharges (IEDs) and occasionally seizures. Patients with limbic encephalitis (LE) often show unilateral or bilateral temporal abnormalities; however, multi-focal and extratemporal discharges may also be present. Ictal discharges may be lacking during recorded focal aware seizures, which can lead to misdiagnosis of a functional aetiology. Multi-focal discharges and seizures may be present in status epilepticus (SE) cases [3]. Examples of EEG patterns seen in different types of autoimmune epilepsy syndromes are provided in Figure 12.2. Radiological evidence of LE such as FLAIR signal hyperintensity in the mesial temporal regions may be present in up to 25–50% of cases. Signal abnormalities may also be present in other cortical and subcortical regions, including the basal ganglia [16]. However, conventional MRI may be normal, and does not exclude the diagnosis. FDG-PET may show limbic hypermetabolism in LE due either to inflammation or seizure activity. Conversely, FDG-PET in anti-NMDAR encephalitis may show striatal hypermetabolism and cortical (particularly posterior) hypometabolism [5]. Examples of imaging abnormalities noted in different autoimmune epilepsy syndromes are provided in Figures 12.3, 12.4 and 12.5. Brain biopsy is of limited value. An immunohistopathological study of 17 adult cases showed inflammatory infiltrates and perivenular cuffing resulting in mild to severe degrees of neuronal loss [9].

Treatment of Suspected or Confirmed Autoimmune Epilepsy

There is no Class I evidence establishing optimal therapy, and current treatment is based on open-label single- and multi-centre experience [10–13]. First-line treatment typically includes immunotherapy with corticosteroids, intravenous immunoglobulin (IVIg) or plasma exchange (PLEX). Second-line therapies when first-line treatment fails include cyclophosphamide or rituximab. Early diagnosis is important as efficacy is correlated with duration of illness at treatment inception. A detailed therapeutic approach is provided in the 'Treatment' section below.

Autoimmune Epilepsy Syndromes

A list of currently identified autoimmune epilepsy syndromes is shown in Table 12.1. A more detailed discussion of these syndromes follows.

Autoimmune Encephalitis with Seizures

Neuronal Cell-Surface Antibody Syndromes
LGI/CASPR2 Antibody-Associated Encephalitis

VGKC-complex antibodies, particularly those targeting leucine-rich glioma inactivated 1 (LGI1) protein, can lead to LE and seizures [17]. Patients typically present with subacute onset of seizures and encephalopathy. Seizures arising from the temporal region are common, some presenting with autonomic features such as unilateral piloerection or palpitations, and others with an aura often described as a 'wave' coursing through their body. Faciobrachial dystonic seizures (FBDS), manifested by paroxysmal contractions of the face and ipsilateral

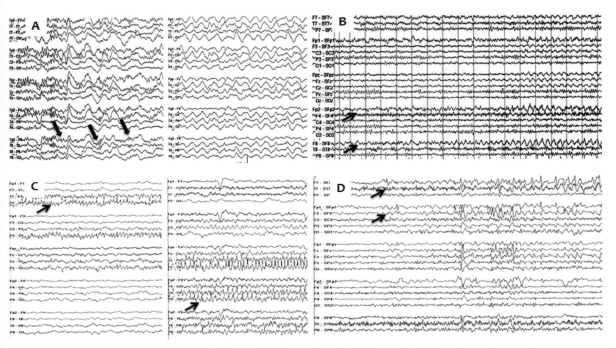

Figure 12.2 EEG findings in autoimmune epilepsy. (A) Extreme delta brushes (arrows, left) and generalized rhythmic delta activity (right) in a patient with anti-NMDAR encephalitis and seizures. (B) Right frontotemporal (arrows) seizure discharge in a patient with limbic encephalitis and temporal lobe seizures associated with GAD-65 antibodies. (C) Rhythmic seizure discharges independently arising from the left posterior (arrow, left) and right centroparietal regions (arrow, right) in a two-year-old girl with FIRES. (D) Left frontotemporal seizure discharge (arrows) in a patient with ANNA-1 antibody encephalitis and seizures.

upper extremity lasting a few seconds, recurring multiple times a day, are characteristic and unique to this antibody syndrome [16–18]. FBDS may affect both sides at different times, and sometimes a contraction on one side is followed immediately by another on the opposite side. FBDS often lack an ictal EEG discharge and can be misdiagnosed as functional [16].

Certain specific antigenic targets of VGKC-complex antibodies have been identified, including LGI1, contactin-associated protein-like 2 (CASPR2), and Contactin-2 [16–20]. In some VGKC patients, the precise antigenic target remains unknown. Seizures are most common with LGI1 antibodies, however they also can occur in CASPR2 patients, and in those without a specific antigenic target. The majority of patients with LGI1 antibodies do not have an associated tumour [17–19]. The mechanism of seizures is not definitively known. Some have suggested that VGKC-complex antibodies arise as a secondary response to neuronal damage and are not ictogenic. Others have proposed that the

antibodies lead to dysfunction of potassium channels, resulting in impaired repolarization, favouring excitation [19]. The good clinical response to immunotherapy coinciding with a fall in serum antibody titre suggests a pathogenic role for VGKC-complex antibodies[18].

The CSF may be acellular. A mild protein elevation is present in 47%. Oligoclonal bands may be present. VGKC-complex antibodies are not consistently present in CSF [17–20]. MRI FLAIR signal hyperintensity, gadolinium enhancement and restricted diffusion may be present in the hippocampus. A unique MRI finding is T1 and/or T2 hyperintensity involving the striatum [16]. FDG-PET hypermetabolic abnormalities may be present in the hippocampi and striatum as well (see Figure 12.3 and 12.4A).

Most respond favourably to corticosteroid therapy [10–13]. When corticosteroids are inadvisable, IVIg can be considered. The responder rate to either treatment is generally excellent, ranging from 60–100%. Failure to respond in the first six weeks of immunotherapy should prompt consideration of another

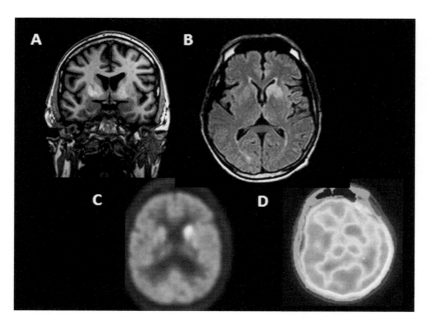

Figure 12.3 MRI and FDG-PET imaging in patients with LGI1 antibodies presenting with faciobrachial dystonic seizures. (A) Increased T1 signal right putamen on MRI. (B) Increased FLAIR signal right caudate and putamen. (C) Increased uptake left caudate on FDG-PET. (D) Increased uptake left striatum and right putamen on FDG-PET.

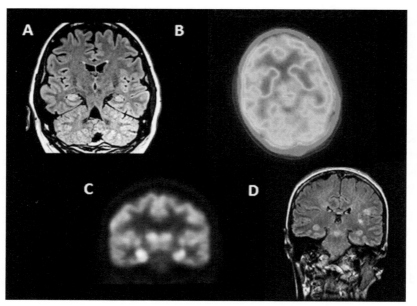

Figure 12.4 Neuroimaging findings in autoimmune epilepsy. (A) Enlarged right hippocampus with increased FLAIR signal in patient with LGI1 antibody-related epilepsy. (B) Diffuse cerebral hypometabolism on FDG-PET in patient with NMDAR encephalitis (cortex is hypometabolic relative to basal ganglia). (C) Increased uptake involving both hippocampi on FDG-PET in patient with epilepsy associated with GAD65 antibody. (D) Increased FLAIR signal involving left peri-insular and external capsule region in patient with focal encephalitis and right hemi-clonic seizures associated with ANNA-1 antibodies.

first-line treatment. Second-line treatment should be considered in the absence of response to first-line therapies, options of which include PLEX, cyclophosphamide or rituximab [11–13]. It is controversial whether chronic maintenance therapy should be initiated, as the clinical course may be monophasic and relapses occur in the minority. Mycophenolate or azathioprine are used by some to prevent relapse, but the benefits of this practice are not definitively established.

NMDA Receptor Antibody-Associated Encephalitis

NMDA receptor (NMDAR) encephalitis is an immune-mediated disorder associated with IgG antibodies to the GluN1 subunit of the NMDA receptor [2,3,21]. Although initially identified in young women in association with ovarian teratoma, NMDAR encephalitis has been reported in all ages and genders, and often occurs without teratoma. Epidemiological studies suggest that this disorder is the most common autoimmune encephalitis after acute demyelinating encephalomyelitis [21,22]. The initial symptoms are usually acute behavioural change, psychosis and catatonia, followed by seizures, memory deficit, dyskinesias, speech problems, autonomic instability and central hypoventilation, often requiring ICU and ventilatory care [22]. The neuropsychiatric presentation is heralded by emotional and behavioural disturbances, fear, depression, cognitive impairment, psychosis, ataxia and choreiform movements. Seizures are usually focal and may be subtle clinically, with EEG monitoring often required to detect them. Children are more likely to have seizures as the presenting symptom [4,22].

NMDAR antibodies form cross-links with the NMDA receptors, followed by intra-cellular internalization. This internalization leads to cerebral hypofunction. These antibodies lead to elevated extracellular glutamate concentration in the brain, and NMDAR antibodies from CSF suppress induction of long-term potentiation (LTP) in murine hippocampal slices. These findings suggest a direct pathogenic role for NMDAR antibodies in glutamatergic signalling [21].

NMDAR antibodies are sometimes only present in CSF. They may persist long after clinical resolution, and have also been identified in patients relapsing after initial recovery from herpes simplex virus encephalitis [5]. A characteristic EEG finding in NMDAR encephalitis is generalized rhythmic delta, which is sometimes associated with superimposed intermittent bursts of low-amplitude high-frequency activity, termed the 'excess delta brush' pattern (see Figure 12.2A). Structural MRI is unremarkable in 50% of patients, the remainder showing non-specific abnormalities. However, FDG-PET may show patchy cerebral hypometabolism (see Figure 12.4B). In addition, functional MRI has been reported to show reduced functional connectivity of the hippocampi with the anterior default-mode network, and diffusion tensor imaging (DTI) shows impairment of white matter integrity in the cingulum [5,22].

Although the presentation is often severe, the potential for recovery wth immunotherapy is reasonably high. In a cohort of 360 patients, 75% experienced complete or near complete recovery [22]. Relapses occur in 20–25%, presenting most commonly with speech dysfunction, psychiatric symptoms, seizures or disturbances of consciousness or attention [21,22]. Relapse rates are higher in patients not treated with immunotherapy, and in those without a removable teratoma. Chronic immunosuppression with mycophenolate mofetil or azathioprine has been suggested by some to prevent relapse [22].

GABA-A Receptor Antibodies

GABA-A receptor (GABA-AR) antibodies lead to a selective reduction of synaptic GABA-A receptors, and have been identified in patients with encephalitis, seizures and refractory SE. Most patients respond to immunotherapy [23,24].

GABA-B Receptor Antibodies

Antibodies against GABA-B receptors (GABA-BR) have been identified in adults with LE [25]. Although these antibodies target the cell surface, they are often paraneoplastic, associated with small-cell lung carcinoma. Seizures are common and typically drug resistant. Patients may present in SE. Seizures are thought to result from GABA-BR impairment. However, many affected patients also have GAD65, anti-thyroid peroxidase (TPO) and N-type calcium channel antibodies, which may also contribute to seizure propensity [24,25]. Corticosteroids, IVIg, and other immunotherapies are all effective, with 75–90% responding [25].

AMPA Receptor Antibodies

Autoantibodies directed at the GluR1/GluR2 subunits of the AMPA receptors (AMPAR), may lead to LE and seizures [26]. AMPAR antibodies cause a reduction in receptor number, especially at synapses. Patients typically present with symptoms of LE, including memory loss, behavioural changes, agitation/aggression or hypersomnolence. Most have a favourable response to immunotherapy [26].

Glycine Receptor Antibodies

Glycine receptor antibodies are typically associated with a syndrome known as progressive encephalomyelitis with rigidity and myoclonus (PERM) and stiff-person syndrome [27]. However, they may also present with encephalitis and focal seizures. In the largest published series, 73% presented with PERM and seizures were present in 13% [27]. Most respond to immunotherapy [27].

Metabotropic Glutamate Receptor 5 Antibodies

Metabotropic glutamate receptor 5 (mGluR5) antibodies have been reported in two patients with autoimmune encephalitis in the setting of Hodgkin's lymphoma, termed Ophelia syndrome. In published reports, patients respond favourably to Hodgkin's treatment [28].

Neuronal Intra-Cellular Antibody Syndromes

GAD65 Antibody-Associated Encephalitis and Seizures

The enzyme glutamic acid decarboxylase (GAD) catalyzes the conversion of L-glutamic acid to GABA [23]. GAD65 antibodies are associated with a variety of neurologic symptoms, including ataxia, vertigo, brainstem dysfunction, limbic encephalopathy, extrapyramidal signs, myelopathy and seizures [23,29]. Seizures and epilepsy may be the primary presentation, wth patients typically experiencing temporal lobe seizures (see Figure 12.2B). Patients may also present in non-convulsive SE (NCSE). It is unknown whether GAD65 antibodies are pathogenic, or represent a biomarker of immune-mediated neuronal injury [23,29]. MRI and PET may show temporal abnormalities (see Figure 12.4B), and EEG typically shows epileptiform discharges primarily involving the temporal region [29].

An immunotherapy trial is warranted in GAD65 patients with medically unresponsive seizures. However, the results are relatively disappointing compared to patients with cell-surface antibody-associated syndromes. In patients with diabetes, glucose monitoring is necessary when using corticosteroids. IVIg may be considered. In patients who do not respond to first-line therapy, rituximab, mycophenolate, PLEX and azathioprine can be tried, but evidence of efficacy is limited [12,13,29].

Onconeuronal Antibody-Associated Encephalitis and Seizures

Some antibodies are nearly always associated with an underlying tumour and are considered paraneoplastic. Paraneoplastic antibodies include anti-Yo, Hu (ANNA-1), Ma1/2, CRMP-5 and amphiphysin antibodies. Of these, ANNA-1 antibodies are those most frequently associated with seizures [3,4]. These patients may also present with epilepsia partialis continua (EPC) and NCSE. EEG and imaging abnormalities in ANNA-1 encephalitis commonly involve limbic structures, but may also affect extratemporal regions (see Figure 12.2D and Figure 12.4D). Ma1/2 antibodies were initially recognized in cases of brainstem encephalitis characterized by gaze palsies, ptosis, opsoclonus, dysarthria and facial weakness. Later studies of Ma1/2 antibody syndromes confirmed that LE and seizures can also occur. Immunotherapy is not consistently effective in these patients, and treatment of the underlying neoplasm is typically prioritized [4,5].

Rasmussen's Encephalitis

Rasmussen's encephalitis (RE) is an uncommon disorder characterized by unilateral encephalitis, medication-resistant epilepsy, and progressive neurological and cognitive deterioration. Inflammatory changes are prominent on pathologic evaluation; however, it is still unknown whether RE represents an autoimmune disease or is infectious in origin [30]. RE primarily affects children and young adults, with a median age of onset of six years. The acute stage is marked by frequent seizures arising from one cerebral hemisphere, manifested as EPC. Progression typically occurs over months but can 'burn itself out' after a period of time, leaving the patient with a static hemiplegia, residual focal motor seizures and other lateralized neurologic deficits [30].

Most evidence suggests that that the immunopathogenesis in RE is mediated by T-cells and microglia. Initially, GluR3 receptor antibodies were thought to play a pathogenic role in RE. However, subsequent studies found that GluR3 antibodies were absent in many RE patients, and were present in other chronic epilepsies. The histopathological hallmarks of RE are cortical inflammation, microglial nodules, perivascular cuffing, neuronal loss and gliosis, all predominantly involving one hemisphere [31].

MRI of the brain has become a mainstay for diagnosis and follow-up in RE. Within months of onset of the acute stage, most patients show unilateral hemispheric atrophy. Any area of the brain can be affected, but there is a predilection for the fronto-insular region [30,31] (see Figure 12.5A). Ipsilateral atrophy of the head of the caudate is a typical but not invariable feature, and can be an early sign. The EEG typically shows focal and multifocal IEDs, asymmetric background slowing and may show lateralized seizure discharges [31]. However, EPC is not always accompanied by an EEG correlate. Independent IEDs over the non-affected hemisphere occur in 62% within three to five years from seizure onset [30].

The seizures in Rasmussen's encephalitis are notoriously unresponsive to ASMs. Despite the prominent inflammation, immunotherapy with steroid pulses, PLEX and rituximab generally shows temporary benefit. Surgery, either functional hemispherectomy or hemispherotomy, remains the most effective treatment [31].

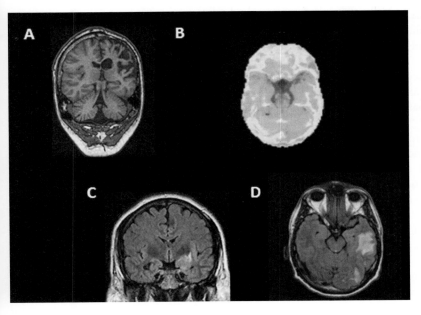

Figure 12.5 Neuroimaging in autoimmune epilepsies not associated with specific neural autoantibodies. (A) T1-weighted MRI showing marked left hemispheric atrophy in patient with Rasmussen's encephalitis. (B) FDG-PET showing asymmetric bitemporal hypometabolism maximal on the right in patient with CNS lupus and temporal lobe seizures. (C) FLAIR hyperintensity involving left amygdala and inferior putamen in a patient with temporal lobe seizures and neurosarcoidosis. (D) FLAIR hyperintensity involving left temporal-occipital parenchyma in a patient with SNALE.

Epilepsy Associated with Systemic Autoimmune Diseases

Seizures complicate a number of systemic autoimmune disorders [15]. A recent population-based retrospective cohort study using insurance claims data found a two- to ninefold risk of seizures among patients with 12 common autoimmune diseases [14]. Mechanisms underlying CNS manifestations in these disorders include vascular lesions (secondary to prothrombotic state, anti-cardiolipin antibodies, cardioemboli and vasculitis), anti-neural antibodies, immune complex deposition, cytokines and opportunistic infection [15].

Systemic Lupus Erythematosus

Seizures occur in approximately 15% of systemic lupus erythematosus (SLE) cases [32]. Seizures are a symptom at initial diagnosis in a third of cases. SLE patients with seizures have a higher frequency of other neuropsychiatric symptoms compared to those without seizures. Anti-cardiolipin and anti-Smith antibodies are more common in SLE patients with seizures. The main pathologic findings in CNS lupus is progression of a small vessel, inflammatory vasculopathy, leading to the accumulation of ischemic lesions which are thought to predispose to seizures [15]. MRI may show cerebral atrophy and subcortical white matter hyperintensities on FLAIR sequences, but these findings are not specific [32].

Some SLE patients who present with a first seizure will not have another. However, ASMs should be considered if high-risk features are present, such as the occurrence of a second seizure, the presence of serious brain injury, structural abnormalities on MRI, focal neurological signs, partial seizure as the first seizure and IEDs. Corticosteroids are commonly used in more severe cases of CNS lupus. High-dose (2 g/kg) IVIg therapy has been proposed as an option in CNS lupus. Non-myeloablative hematopoietic stem cell transplant following administration of high-dose cyclophosphamide has also been used in severe cases [15,32].

Hashimoto's Encephalopathy

Hashimoto's encephalopathy (HE), also known as steroid-responsive encephalopathy associated with autoimmune thyroiditis (SREAT), is an immunotherapy-responsive condition, manifested by subacute encephalopathy, myoclonus, ataxia, tremor and stroke-like episodes. Seizures occur in two-thirds of cases, including generalized tonic–clonic, partial, absence, myoclonic seizures and SE [33].

The pathogenesis underlying the seizures in HE is uncertain. A direct role of anti-thyroid antibodies has not been established, and the TPO antibodies are largely considered an epiphenomenon serving as a biomarker indicating the presence of an underlying autoimmune state [15]. Other neural autoantibodies, such as antibodies targeting a 36 kD antigen derived from the cerebral cortex, another directed against the NH_2-terminal of alpha-enolase and GAD-65 antibodies have been identified in these patients. Autoimmune vasculitis has also been proposed as a mechanism. However, autopsy and biopsy cases usually show perivenular inflammatory changes and not vasculitis [15,33].

HE patients are typically euthyroid. The serologic hallmark of HE is the presence of anti-TPO or thyroglobulin antibodies and these should be obtained in suspicious cases. Low titres are common in the general population; HE patients typically have very high titres. Patients may also be ANA positive, potentially causing confusion with CNS lupus. CSF is abnormal in 80%, showing elevated protein, oligoclonal bands occasionally and lymphocytic pleocytosis. EEG is usually abnormal, showing focal or diffuse slowing, frontal intermittent rhythmic delta activity, triphasic waves or IEDs [15]. The degree of abnormality on EEG correlates with the severity of the encephalopathy, and usually improves in parallel with treatment response. MRI is often normal, but may show focal or diffuse atrophy, subcortical white matter changes, or oedema. FDG-PET may show multifocal hypometabolism during active encephalopathy, with normalization following treatment [33].

Corticosteroids are the mainstay of therapy for HE. The response is relatively prompt, with improvement typically occurring within a few weeks or months. For corticosteroid-resistant or dependent cases, IVIg, other immunosuppressant medications or PLEX may be effective. HE may relapse, especially after tapering corticosteroids, prompting some authorities to recommend chronic immunosuppression in some cases, with rituximab, IVIg, azathioprine or mycophenolate [15,33].

Other Systemic Autoimmune Diseases Associated with Seizures

Seizures may also occur in other autoimmune diseases including coeliac disease, Sjögren's, neurosarcoidosis (see Figure 12.5C), Behçet disease, Perry–Romberg syndrome and Crohn's disease [15]. Clinical features and potential response to therapy are provided in Table 12.3.

Table 12.3 Prevalence, features and response to immunotherapy with systemic autoimmune disorders

	Seizure prevalence	Associated neuropsychiatric signs and symptoms	Treatment type and response
CNS lupus	7–40%	Encephalopathy; depression; psychosis; headaches; stroke; pseudotumour cerebri; myelitis; peripheral neuropathy	Corticosteroids or IVIg + ASMs; cyclophosphamide; ?rituximab for refractory cases
Hashimoto's encephalopathy	>50%	Encephalopathy; delirium; depression; psychosis; stroke like; dementia; ataxia; chorea; myoclonus; tremor	Corticosteroids – prompt and excellent response, may relapse
Neurosarcoidosis	10% (adult) 35% (paediatric)	Cranial neuropathy; leptomeningeal disease; headache; hydrocephalus; pituitary dysfunction; SIADH; parenchymal lesions (see Figure 12.5C); myelopathy; polyneuropathy; myopathy	Corticosteroids + ASM (transient); variable response, may relapse; cytotoxic therapy in intractable cases
Behçet's disease	2–27%	Parenchymal lesions; dural venous sinus thrombosis; intracranial hypertension	Corticosteroids and cytotoxic agents; variable response
Crohn's disease	3.5–6%	Central demyelination; stroke; peripheral neuropathy; myelitis	Immunosuppressive agents and monoclonal antibodies; variable response
Coeliac disease	1–5%	Ataxia; headache; cognitive dysfunction; mood disorder; vestibular dysfunction; cerebral (occipital) calcification; peripheral neuropathy	Gluten free diet, folic acid supplement; good response
Perry–Romberg syndrome	1–3%	Localized sclerodermal lesion affecting face and brain, characterized by meningo-cortical dysmorphism and central atrophy localized to region underlying facial lesion	Corticosteroid or IVIg; poor response; seizures often refractory

ASM = anti-seizure medications, IVIg = intravenous immunoglobulin, SLE = systemic lupus erythematosus

Acute Epilepsy Syndromes of Possible Autoimmune Origin: AERRPS/FIRES/DESC/NORSE

Several syndromes of acute encephalitis manifested by the onset of SE in the context of a recent or current febrile illness, have been reported in adults and children. This syndrome has been reported under several names, including: acute encephalitis with refractory repetitive partial seizures (AERRPS), febrile infection-related epilepsy syndrome (FIRES), devastating epileptic encephalopathy in school-aged children (DESC) and new-onset refractory status epilepticus (NORSE) [34,35]. These syndromes have in common the acute onset of recurrent focal or generalized seizures and encephalopathy following or during a febrile illness, culminating in super-refractory SE. Affected patients typically require anaesthetic dosages of benzodiazepines, barbiturates, propofol or ketamine, often for weeks in duration [35].

As the syndrome is preceded by a febrile illness, an inflammatory pathogenesis has been suspected. In fact in the largest series of NORSE cases, an autoimmune aetiology was eventually identified in roughly 37% of cases (18% paraneoplastic, 19% non-paraneoplastic) [35]. Nonetheless, in many cases, firm support for an autoimmune pathogenesis is lacking. Furthermore, empiric trials of immunotherapy are often unsuccessful. Other hypotheses have been considered, including the possibility that affected patients potentially could harbour a channelopathy or metabolic or mitochondrial defect, the manifestations of which only becoming symptomatic under times of physiologic stress imposed by fever [7,9,34,35]. Alternatively, an ictogenic role for inflammatory mediators such as interleukin-1B (IL-1B), IL-6, and tumour necrosis factor (TNF) have been proposed as precipitating factors [2,7,9].

CSF typically shows a mild pleocytosis or slight increase in protein, and may show upregulation of inflammatory markers such as IL-6 or neopterin [34,35]. EEG typically shows diffuse background slowing and multi-focal spikes and seizures (see Figure 12.2C). Neuroimaging may show temporal lobe signal abnormalities; however, whether these represent peri-ictal phenomena or active inflammation is unclear. Other reported findings include leptomeningeal enhancement, T2 signal hyperintensity in the peri-insular region and pulvinar. Over time, marked diffuse cerebral atrophy frequently develops [34,35].

Both the acute and post-encephalitic seizure phases in these cases are ASM resistant. A ketogenic diet has been reported to be successful in a few cases [34]. At our centre we successfully treated a two-year-old girl with FIRES using anakinra, an IL-1 receptor antagonist (unpublished report). Attempts to wean her off resulted in seizure recurrence, with seizure remission resulting again following reinstitution. Interestingly, activation of IL-1R1/TLR4 signaling occurs after epileptogenic injuries in animal models, and IL-1 receptor blockade has been demonstrated to inhibit seizures. Response to immunotherapy with high-dose steroids, IVIg and PLEX has been reported in NORSE [35].

Chronic or New-Onset Epilepsy with Autoantibodies in the Absence of Encephalitis

Anti-neural antibodies may be present in patients with chronic epilepsy outside of the context of an encephalitic presentation [3,6,14]. While this raises important questions as to pathogenesis, the therapeutic implications may be different. For example, GAD65 antibodies are present at low titre in 1–3% of patients with focal epilepsy, a rate significantly higher than in idiopathic generalized epilepsy and non-epilepsy populations [3]. Brenner et al. [6] found the following autoantibodies in 416 chronic epilepsy patients: VGKC-complex (5%), glycine receptor (3%), GAD65 (1.7%) and NMDAR (1.7%). Antibody titre is often low in these cases, and immunotherapy is often ineffective. Most patients responding to immunotherapy present with acute onset of seizures with high seizure frequency.

Seronegative Autoimmune Limbic Encephalitis

Seronegative autoimmune limbic encephalitis (SNALE) is a term reserved for a non-paraneoplastic, non-infectious subgroup of LE, in which immunological mechanisms are suspected, but the targeted neural autoantigens are unknown [36]. Patients typically present with acute or subacute onset of encephalopathy, temporal lobe seizures and neuropsychiatric disorders. SNALE may masquerade as glioma, resulting in unnecessary and ineffective lesionectomy. CSF and serum autoimmune testing is often unremarkable. EEG typically shows temporal slowing and

IEDs. In the majority of the reported cases, MRI reveals unilateral or bilateral hyperintense signal changes in the temporal lobe or hippocampus (see Figure 12.5D) Pathology usually shows intense peri-vascular and parenchymal mixed lymphocytic inflammatory infiltrates, microglial nodules and entrapped lymphocytes in neurons. The response to immune therapy is variable, and spontaneous resolution may occur without immunotherapy [36].

Treatment

There currently are no randomized controlled trials on immunotherapy in autoimmune epilepsy syndromes [10–13]. However, an immunotherapy trial is generally considered justified in the aforementioned autoimmune epilepsy syndromes, given their gravity and the multiple reports of success published by several centres. It is important to establish a baseline assessment before commencing treatment in all cases, so that efficacy can be clearly gauged at future intervals. One metric for autoimmune epilepsy is seizure rate pre- and post-treatment. This can be measured in terms of number of seizures per week, in some cases seizures per day, and seizure-days per month. Other clinical metrics include mental status scores. Serial EEG is also helpful if baseline is abnormal. Serial MRIs may demonstrate resolution or progression of radiologic changes, including development of changes involving the contralateral side and frequent development of mesial temporal sclerosis (MTS).

The following observations have been made in the treatment of autoimmune epilepsy syndromes: (a) early initiation of treatment is correlated with more favourable outcome; (b) responders tend to improve within four to six weeks, so reassessment should occur in that time frame and (c) certain antibodies and autoimmune epilepsy syndromes have a better prognosis than others [10–13]. For example, prognosis is relatively optimistic for epilepsies resulting from Hashimoto's and LGI1/CASPR2 and NMDAR antibody encephalitis, but is guarded for patients with seizures related to GAD 65, onconeural antibodies and seronegative autoimmune encephalitis [2,3]. Figure 12.6 summarizes the therapeutic approach used at our institution.

A search for occult neoplasm is clearly justified in the presence of onconeural antibodies and other antibodies with a high association with underlying tumours (see Table 12.1). Treatment of an underlying tumour is usually recommended prior to immunotherapy. For example, in NMDAR encephalitis, removal of the teratoma is associated with neurologic improvement, as is treatment for Hodgkin's in patients with anti-mGluR5 and Ophelia syndrome [5,20]. Some autoimmune epilepsy syndromes have a significantly lower association with underlying neoplasm, rendering the yield of investigation correspondingly lower (see Table 12.1).

Acute Treatment

First-Line Therapy Trial

Corticosteroids are the most commonly used first-line therapy. Intravenous methylprednisolone is often used; however, oral therapy has been advocated by some. The typical initial dose is 1 g methylprednisolone IV daily for three to five days, then weekly for six weeks, and every other week for six weeks. Patients are typically seen in follow-up at six weeks to evaluate efficacy [10–13]. Methylprednisolone inhibits phospholipase A2 activity and prostaglandin synthesis, leading to dampening of the inflammatory cytokine cascade, inhibition of T cell activity and reduction of immune cell extravasation into the CNS. Methylprednisolone also facilitates apoptosis of activated immune cells and indirectly decreases cytotoxic effects mediated by nitric oxide and TNFα. The potential side effects of corticosteroid therapy include weight gain, hypertension, hyperglycaemia, insomnia and increased susceptibility to opportunistic infections. For this reason, sulfamethoxazole with trimethoprim is usually recommended to prevent *Pneumocystis* pneumonia. With long-term corticosteroid use, osteopaenia can develop, hence calcium and vitamin D supplementation are commonly recommended.

IVIg is also commonly used as first-line treatment. However, cost and insurance approval requirements are barriers to its use. Dosing is variable and has not been defined by clinical trials. The protocol for IVIg at our institution is 0.4 g/kg IV daily for three to five days, then weekly for six weeks, then every other week for six weeks [12,13]. As with corticosteroid treatment, patients should be seen in follow-up after six weeks of treatment. IVIg is a purified blood product, composed mainly of immunoglobulin G (IgG) (95%) with the remainder consisting of IgA and negligible concentrations of IgM. IgA-depleted IVIg dosage forms should be considered in IgA-deficient patients. IVIg side effects include headache, hives, low-grade fever, aseptic meningitis, haemolytic anaemia, venous thrombosis and acute renal injury.

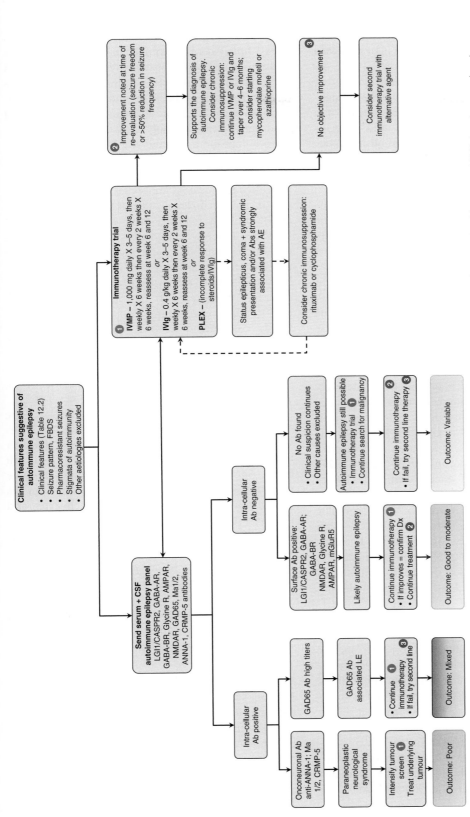

Figure 12.6 Diagnostic and therapeutic approach to autoimmune epilepsy. AMPA, alpha-amino-3-hydroxy-5-methyl-4-isoxazolepropionic acid receptor; ANNA-1, anti-neuronal nuclear antibody type 1; CRMP-5, collapsin response mediator protein 5; CASPR2, contactin-associated protein-like 2; GABA-A, gamma-aminobutyric acid-A; GABA-B gamma-aminobutyric acid-B; GAD65, glutamic acid decarboxylase 65; IVIg, intravenous immunoglobulin; IVMP, intravenous methylprednisolone; LE, limbic encephalitis; mGluR5, metabotropic glutamate receptor 5; NMDA, N-methyl-D-aspartate; PLEX, plasma exchange; VGKC, voltage-gated potassium channel.

PLEX is sometimes used as first-line treatment in critically ill patients in which the goal is to achieve a rapid reduction in circulating antibodies. While the concept of this is compelling, its superiority to other treatments in this clinical context has not been established. PLEX usually necessitates placement of a special intravenous cannula into the subclavian or internal jugular vein, which risks embolism, pneumothorax and infection [11–13].

Second-Line Therapy

When first line therapies fail, second-line treatments are usually considered. Typically, if an initial first-line therapy is found to have failed at six week follow-up, the other is tried for 6–12 weeks before a second-line treatment is used, at least in less severe clinical situations. Progression between first-line therapies and initiation of second-line therapies may be more rapid in critical situations. Second-line treatments include cyclophosphamide, and monoclonal antibody therapies, most commonly rituximab [10–13].

Immunosuppressive Agents

Immunosuppressant agents may be used in acute treatment, but are more commonly used as maintenance therapy following a response to first-line treatment. Cyclophosphamide is a cytotoxic agent affecting lymphocytes and myeloid cells. It has been used successfully in refractory SE, secondary to anti-GAD65 antibodies, and in NMDAR encephalitis, and is sometimes used as maintenance treatment. Mycophenolate mofetil is used to prevent relapse in VGKC-complex and NMDAR encephalitis. However, clinical trials establishing the risks and benefits of its use in maintenance therapy are lacking. Mycopholate mofetil is teratogenic and must be used with caution in females of child-bearing potential. Azathioprine is an alternative option [2,3,10–13].

Monoclonal Antibody Therapies

Monoclonal antibodies engineered to target specific components of the immune response have been established as effective in a number of inflammatory disorders. Rituximab is an anti-CD20 monoclonal antibody that results in B-cell depletion [19]. Open-label studies have reported benefit in NMDAR encephalitis [22]. There are anecdotal reports regarding the use of rituximab and other monoclonal antibodies in other autoimmune epilepsy syndromes, including LE associated with anti-GAD and LGI1/CASPR2 autoantibodies, and

in a case of FIRES with multi-focal super-refractory SE [3,34]. Initial doses of rituximab are associated with infusion-related hypersensitivity reactions in 50%, and 10% experience more serious reactions, including hypotension, rigors, bronchospasm and angioedema. Other reactions include cardiac arrhythmia, acute coronary syndrome, interstitial lung disease, bowel perforation, Stevens–Johnson syndrome and infection. Progressive multi-focal leukoencephalopathy has also been reported.

Other monoclonal antibodies with anecdotal efficacy include tocilizumab, an anti-IL-6 receptor monoclonal antibody reported to be effective in a case of CASPR2 antibody encephalitis [19]. Bortezomib, a monoclonal antibody targeting antibody-producing plasma cells, and alemtuzumab, a monoclonal antibody targeting CD52 antigens on memory B and T cells, have been reported as efficacious in refractory anti-NMDAR encephalitis [20]. While one cannot widely recommend these therapies at the present time, they deserve careful evaluation as to their potential future role in these disorders, particularly those unresponsive to first-line treatment.

ASM Therapy

Although intractability is a common feature in autoimmune epilepsy, some respond to ASMs, and they remain an important aspect of therapy in these cases. Some ASMs affect cellular and humoral immune responses [37]. For example, vigabatrin increases the proportion of CD8 T-suppressor lymphocytes and increases the activity of natural killer cells [37]. Whether these effects are relevant to the clinical management is unclear. In our experience, carbamazepine has been efficacious in some patients refractory to other ASMs. If carbamazepine is used, however, monitoring for hyponatraemia should be performed, as this can complicate autoimmune encephalitis itself. At this time, no single ASM stands out as superior to others in autoimmune epilepsy.

Epilepsy Surgery

Epilepsy surgery has been attempted in some cases of autoimmune epilepsy, but the results outside of hemispherectomy for Rasmussen's encephalitis are largely disappointing [32]. There are also cases where the diagnosis of autoimmune epilepsy was identified after surgical pathologic inspection in failed epilepsy surgery cases. The lack of efficacy of surgery in autoimmune epilepsy is not surprising, given the multi-focal nature of seizures in these patients and likely diffuse distribution of inflammation.

Potential Future Therapies

Drugs that influence the inflammatory response, such as interleukin-1-converting enzyme/caspase-1 inhibitors and interleukin-1 beta receptor antagonists are currently being evaluated as potential treatments for epilepsy [38]. While the use of such agents in autoimmune epilepsy syndromes is compelling, clinical data is lacking. IL-1 receptor antagonists (IL-1Ra) have been shown to confer protection and seizure termination in animal models of epilepsy. Anakinra, a recombinant version of the naturally occurring IL-1Ra, is one such available agent that may be worth study [38]. Two neurosteroid agents, ganalaxone and allopregnanolone are currently in clinical trials for epilepsy and refractory SE respectively. Given their dual GABAergic and potential anti-inflammatory effects, it is tempting to speculate whether they will have a unique role in the management of autoimmune epilepsy.

Prognosis

Prognosis is highly dependent on the type of autoimmune epilepsy syndrome. The prognosis in patients with onconeural antibody encephalitis is generally less favourable than that due to cell-surface antibodies. In paraneoplastic cases, treatment of the underlying tumour is essential where feasible, and patients receiving only immunotherapy do not generally improve. Treatment outcomes in epilepsy associated with intra-cellular GAD65 antibody is likewise generally unfavourable, although responders to immunotherapy are reported [2,4,29]. In contrast, the prognosis of immunotherapy in seizures associated with LGI1/CASPR2, NMDAR, AMPAR, GABA-BA, GABA-BR and mGluR5 antibodies is generally favourable [2,4,29]. Early diagnosis and initiation of immunotherapy is an important determinant of prognosis, as unfettered inflammation may lead to continued seizures and neuronal injury, which negatively influences outcome.

Conclusions

The finding of inflammatory markers and especially neural autoantibodies in new-onset seizures of unknown aetiology has opened up a new treatment paradigm for some patients. Seizures occur as an early and prominent feature in autoimmune epilepsy syndromes, and are characteristically refractory to conventional ASM therapy. The earliest reports of autoimmune epilepsy syndromes focused on paraneoplastic LE due to onconeural antibodies, such as anti-Ma2 and ANNA-1, and those due to GAD65 antibodies, in which immunotherapy is largely unsuccessful. The recent discovery of antibodies directed at cell-surface antigens, however, has identified syndromes which have proven to be highly responsive to immunotherapy. Outcome studies in the latter group show responder rates of 60–100%, justifying an immunotherapy trial in these cases.

The scope of autoimmune epilepsy also includes seizures complicating other systemic autoimmune conditions such as SLE. Therefore evaluation in suspected autoimmune epilepsy cases includes testing for ANA and extractable nuclear antibodies, as well as a neuroimmunology panel. In addition, CSF examination is highly recommended in suspected cases in order to help establish the presence of CNS inflammation and to allow for neuroimmunology antibody testing. Because of the efficacy of immunotherapy, it is essential that an autoimmune aetiology be considered early in such patients.

Key Points

- Autoimmune epilepsy (AE) is an immunologically mediated disorder in which recurrent seizures are a primary and persistent clinical feature.
- It is estimated that up to 20% of patients with epilepsy of unknown aetiology may be due to AE.
- The most commonly identified antibodies are those targeting NMDA receptor (NMDAR), leucine-rich glioma-inactivated protein 1 (LGI1) and glutamic acid decarboxylase 65 (GAD65).
- When AE is suspected on clinical grounds consideration of early immunotherapy is indicated.
- Immunotherapies have demonstrated higher efficacy in patients with cell-surface antibody-associated AEs (e.g. LGI1) than those with intra-cellular antigen-associated AEs (e.g. GAD65).

References

1. Kwan P, Brodie MJ. Early identification of refractory epilepsy. *N Engl J Med* 2000;**342**:314–319
2. Greco A, Rizzo MI, De Virgilio A, et al. *Autoimmun Rev* 2016;**15**:221–225

3. Irani SR, Bien CG, Lang B. Autoimmune epilepsies. *Curr Opin Neurol* 2011;**24**:146–153

4. Suleiman J, Dale RC. The recognition and treatment of autoimmune epilepsy in children. *Dev Med Child Neurol* 2015;**57**: 431–440

5. Graus F, Titulaer MJ, Balu R, et al. Clinical approach to diagnosis of autoimmune encephalitis. *Lancet Neurol* 2016;**15**:391–404

6. Brenner T, Sills GJ, Hart Y, et al. Prevalence of neurologic autoantibodies in cohorts of patients with new and established epilepsy. *Epilepsia* 2013;**54**:1028–1035

7. De Vries EE, van den Munckhof B, Braun KP, et al. Inflammatory mediators in human epilepsy: a systematic review and meta-analysis. *Neurosci Biobehav Rev* 2016;**63**:177–190

8. Johnson MR, Behmoaras J, Bottolo L, et al. Systems genetics identifies Sestrin 3 as a regulator of a proconvulsant gene network in human epileptic hippocampus. *Nat Commun* 2015;**6**:6031

9. Bien CG, Vincent A, Barnett MH, et al. Immunopathology of autoantibody-associated encephalitides: clues for pathogenesis. *Brain* 2012;**135**: 1622–1638

10. Byun JI, Lee ST, Jung KH, et al. Effect of immunotherapy on seizure outcome in patients with autoimmune encephalitis: a prospective observational registry study. *PLoS One* 2016;**11**:e0146455

11. Bello-Espinosa LE, Rajapakse T, Rho JM, Buchhalter J. Efficacy of intravenous immunoglobulin in a cohort of children with drug-resistant epilepsy. *Pediatr Neurol* 2015;**52**:509–516

12. Toledano M, Britton JW, McKeon A, et al. Utility of an immunotherapy trial in evaluating patients with presumed autoimmune epilepsy. *Neurology* 2014;**82**: 1578–1586

13. Quek AM, Britton JW, McKeon A, et al. Autoimmune epilepsy: clinical characteristics and response to immunotherapy. *Arch Neurol* 2012;**69**:582–593

14. Ong M, Kohane IS, Cai T, et al. Population-level evidence for an autoimmune etiology of epilepsy. *J Am Med Assoc Neurol* 2014;**71**:569–574

15. Devinsky O, Schein A, Najjar S. Epilepsy associated with systemic autoimmune disorders. *Epilepsy Curr* 2013;**13**:62–68

16. Flanagan EP, Kotsenas AL, Britton JW, et al. Basal ganglia T1 hyperintensity in LGI1-autoantibody faciobrachial dystonic seizures. *Neurol Neuroimmunol Neuroinflamm* 2015;**2**:e161

17. Lai M, Huijbers MGM, Lancaster E, et al. Investigation of LGI1 as the antigen in limbic encephalitis previously attributed to potassium channels: a case series. *Lancet Neurol* 2010;**9**:776–785

18. Irani SR, Michell AW, Lang B, et al. Faciobrachial dystonic seizures precede Lgi1 antibody limbic encephalitis. *Ann Neurol* 2011;**69**:892–900

19. Irani SR, Gelfand JM, Bettcher BM, et al. Effect of rituximab in patients with leucine rich, glioma-inactivated antibody-associated encephalopathy. *J Am Med Assoc Neurol* 2014;**71**:896–900

20. Krogias C, Hoepner R, Müller A, et al. Successful treatment of anti-Caspr2 syndrome by interleukin 6 receptor blockade through tocilizumab. *J Am Med Assoc Neurol* 2013;**70**:1056–1059

21. Peery HE, Day GS, Dunn S, et al. Anti-NMDA receptor encephalitis: the disorder, the diagnosis and the immunobiology. *Autoimmun Rev* 2012;**11**:863–872

22. Titulaer MJ, McCracken L, Gabilondo I, et al. Treatment and prognostic factors for long-term outcome in patients with anti-NMDA receptor encephalitis: an observational cohort study. *Lancet Neurol* 2013;**12**:157–165

23. Prud'homme GJ, Glinka Y, Wang Q. Immunological GABAergic interactions and therapeutic applications in autoimmune diseases. *Autoimmun Rev* 2015;**14**:1048–1056

24. Petit-Pedrol M, Armangue T, Peng X, et al. Encephalitis with refractory seizures, status epilepticus, and antibodies to the GABAA receptor: a case series, characterization of the antigen, and analysis of the effects of antibodies. *Lancet Neurol* 2014;**13**:276–286

25. Lancaster E, Lai M, Peng X, et al. Antibodies to the GABA(B) receptor in limbic encephalitis with seizures case series and characterization of the antigen. *Lancet Neurol* 2010;**9**:67–76

26. Lai M, Hughes EG, Peng X, et al. AMPA receptor antibodies in limbic encephalitis alter synaptic receptor location. *Ann Neurol* 2009;**65**:424–434

27. Carvajal-González A, Leite MI, Waters P, et al. Glycine receptor antibodies in PERM and related syndromes: characteristics, clinical features and outcomes. *Brain* 2014;**137**:2178–2192

28. Lancaster E, Martinez-Hernandez E, Titulaer MJ, et al. Antibodies to metabotropic glutamate receptor 5 in the Ophelia syndrome. *Neurology* 2011;**77**:1698–1701

29. Malter MP, Helmstaedter C, Urbach H, et al. Antibodies to glutamic acid decarboxylase define a form of limbic encephalitis. *Ann Neurol* 2010;**67**:470–478

30. Pradeep K, Sinha S, Mahadevan A, et al. Clinical, electrophysiological, imaging, pathological and therapeutic observations among 18 patients with Rasmussen's encephalitis. *J Clin Neurosci* 2016;**25**:96–104

31. Marras CE, Granata T, Franzini A, et al. Hemispherectomy and functional hemispherectomy: indications and outcome. *Epilepsy Res* 2010;**89**:104–112

32. Hanly JG, Urowitz MB, Su L, et al. Seizure disorders in systemic lupus erythematosus results from an international, prospective, inception cohort study. *Ann Rheum* 2012;**71**:1502–1509

33. Olmez I, Moses H, Sriram S, et al. Diagnostic and therapeutic aspects of Hashimoto's encephalopathy. *J Neurol Sci* 2013;**331**: 67–71

34. Howell KB, Katanyuwong K, Mackay MT, et al. Long-term follow-up of febrile infection-related epilepsy syndrome. *Epilepsia* 2012;**53**:101–110

35. Gaspard N, Foreman BP, Alvarez V, et al. Critical Care EEG Monitoring Research Consortium (CCEMRC). New-onset refractory status epilepticus: etiology, clinical features, and outcome. *Neurology* 2015;**85**:1604–1613

36. Najjar S, Pearlman D, Zagzag D, Devinsky O. Spontaneously resolving seronegative autoimmune limbic encephalitis. *Cogn Behav Neurol* 2011;**24**:99–105

37. Beghi E, Shorvon S. Antiepileptic drugs and the immune system. *Epilepsia* 2011;**52**(Suppl 3):40–44

38. Dinarello CA, Simon A, van der Meer JW. Treating inflammation by blocking interleukin-1 in a broad spectrum of diseases. *Nat Rev Drug Discov* 2012;**11**:633–652

Chapter 13

Medication-Resistant Epilepsy Syndromes in Children

Elia M. Pestana Knight and Elaine Wyllie

Introduction

Medically refractory epilepsies account for 20–30% of the patients evaluated in an epilepsy centre. With more than 50% of paediatric epilepsies persisting into adulthood, it is very important for the epileptologist to have an updated understanding of the current advances in the field of medically refractory paediatric epileptic syndromes.

Refractory epilepsies are common in children. Medical intractability becomes quickly apparent after seizure onset in children with developmental epileptic encephalopathies [1].

Refractory epilepsies with onset at paediatric age have some features in common. They typically involve more than one seizure type, they are resistant to treatment and they are often associated with cognitive, emotional and behavioural problems. Neurological morbidity is high and early mortality is not uncommon, especially when associated with other systemic problems or metabolic aetiology.

Considering that medically refractory paediatric phenotypes are age-related, this chapter addresses the most relevant syndromes by age group.

Neonatal Syndromes

Ohtahara Syndrome or Early Infantile Epileptic Encephalopathy and Early Myoclonic Epileptic Encephalopathy

Ohtahara syndrome or early infantile epileptic encephalopathy (EIEE) with suppression burst and early myoclonic epileptic encephalopathy (EMEE) are rare forms of early infantile encephalopathy that typically present with refractory epilepsy in the first week of life, but presentation within the first month of life is also possible [2,3]. There are reports of presentation even during the pre-natal period with abnormal fetal movements perceived by the mother.

Tonic seizures can be isolated or in clusters and involve the whole body, but often are asymmetrical or segmental. Other symptoms are hiccups or partial seizures.

Myoclonic seizures occur in clusters or as isolated events. Often they are segmental and affect one limb, but subsequent jerks can be in other locations and often on the opposite side of the body.

The frequent tonic and segmental myoclonic seizures usually correlate well with the EEG findings. EEG shows periods of suppression that alternate with bursts of irregular and disorganized high-voltage spikes and polyspikes. This is known as a suppression burst pattern (Figure 13.1A and B). It is important to clarify that this EEG pattern is not exclusively seen in these early epilepsies and it is more commonly seen in severe hypoxic ischaemic encephalopathy.

It has been suggested that a predominance of tonic seizures and grossly abnormal MRI defines Ohtahara syndrome or EIEE with suppression burst, while a predominance of myoclonic seizures with a normal brain MRI indicates a diagnosis of EMEE. The clinical reality indicates that myoclonic and tonic seizures overlap in both group of patients with or without partial seizures. Furthermore, recent developments in the field of genetics indicate that multiple gene disorders with no associated visible abnormality in the brain MRI are seen in both clinical phenotypes. There is abundant clinical, aetiological and outcome data to consider EIEE and EMEE phenotypical variations of a severe neonatal-onset epileptic encephalopathy that affects extensive areas of the newborn brain, whether or not an abnormality is visible on brain MRI.

In children with EIEE/EMEE, brain MRI findings range from normal to extensive brain malformations, such as hemimegalencephaly, megalencephaly, lissencephaly, polymicrogyria, focal or multi-focal cortical dysplasia, porencephaly, agenesis of the corpus callosum or the mamillary bodies, posterior fossa abnormalities, etc. Findings of severe and diffuse forms of

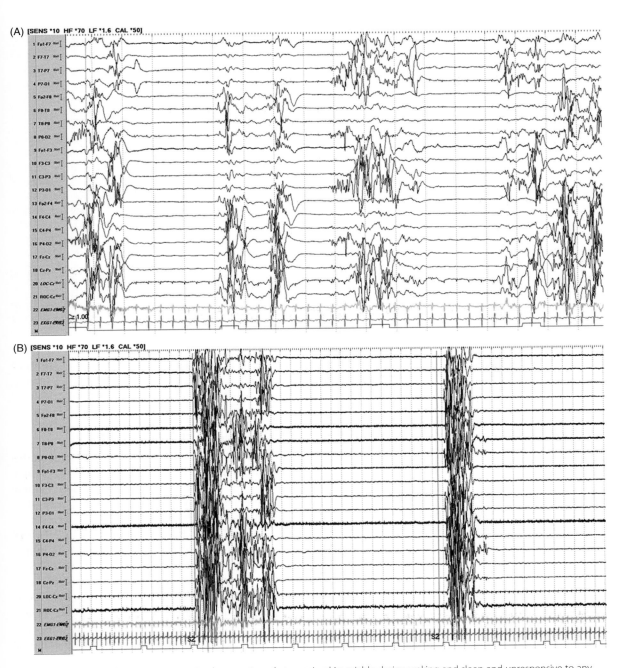

Figure 13.1 (A) EEG showing a suppression burst pattern that remained invariable during waking and sleep and unresponsive to any treatment. The burst lasted 2–3 seconds. (B) EEG compressed to 60 seconds showing the effect of treatment with dextromethorphan.

hypoxic ischaemic encephalopathy may also be seen on the brain MRI. Genetic metabolic work up is important and recommended in these cases. Diagnoses include specific genetic defects such as ARX, AARS, CDKL5, CACNA2D2, GNAO1, SLC25A22 and STXBP1, KCNQ2, KCNT1, NECAP1, PIGA, PIGQ, SCN2A, SCN8A, SIK1, and ALDH7A1, mitochondrial diseases, inborn error of the metabolism such as non-ketotic hyperglycinaemia or glycine encephalopathy, propionic or methylmalonic acidaemia, molybdenum cofactor deficiency, and other more rare inborn errors of the metabolism. Study of the CSF is important to rule out neonatal infectious disease and other neurotransmitter-related conditions [3–5].

Seizures become quickly refractory to phenytoin, barbiturate and benzodiazepines. Treatment of these patients should include a trial of pyridoxine and folinic acid, as well as drugs such as topiramate, vigabatrin, zonisamide, acetazolamide, ACTH and dextromethorphan, once it becomes clear that seizures are refractory. A ketogenic diet and epilepsy surgery are other treatment alternatives for selected, very refractory cases [6,7].

Even in cases in which seizures are reduced or minimized with the aid of some ASMs, the pattern of suppression burst remains. Along with a persistent suppression burst pattern, a lag in neurodevelopment in children who survive this catastrophic epilepsy shows that these early-onset encephalopathies carry high neurological and systemic morbidity and mortality. For a long time, outcome data has provided evidence of a continuum or evolution from EIEE or Ohtahara syndrome to other age-dependent epileptic encephalopathies, in particular to West syndrome, and later to Lennox–Gastaut syndrome. This evolution is now supported by the recent medical findings of shared genetic mutations between these phenotypes. It also indicates that earlier seizure development may represent a more severe phenotype of the underlying genetic abnormality [4]. Evolution from EIEE to migrating partial epilepsy phenotype has also been reported [6].

In the case of EMEE, even when considered an independent neonatal disease, the current medical literature recognizes it as a rare phenotype of the neonatal epileptic encephalopathies, with only around 30 cases reported in the literature up to 2006 [2]. The EMEE phenotype has a higher mortality within the first two years of life than the EIEE phenotype. Patients who survive EMEE remain in a persistent vegetative state [4].

The differential diagnosis of these neonatal epileptic encephalopathies include early-onset infantile spasms, which will be associated with an electrographic pattern of hypsarrhythmia. Benign infantile myoclonus and benign neonatal familial convulsions are also in the differential diagnosis, but all have neonatal EEGs with a normal background for age.

Infants who survive the neonatal encephalopathies in general will develop infantile spasms or migrating partial epilepsy phenotypes as they approach the first six months of life.

Case 13.1 Early Myoclonic Epileptic Encephalopathy

A three-month-old girl was born at 37 weeks gestational age after an uncomplicated pregnancy. She presented on day 5 of life with three different seizure types: (1) multiple segmental myoclonus in clusters or not (predominant type), (2) tonic seizures and (3) bilateral eye clonic seizures mixed with episodic, hiccups and staring. Brain MRI showed a very small left periventricular cyst. Whole-gene exon and chromosome microarray, and basic metabolic work up and CSF studies were all negative. Seizures were refractory to phenobarbital, phenytoin and levetiracetam, pyridoxine and folinic acid. Intensity and duration of the seizures were reduced to six per minute on a combination of clonazepam and topiramate. Treatment with dextromethorphan reduced the seizures and burst periods to two per minute with some bursts no longer correlating with the seizures, but this medication prolonged the burst to 5–6 seconds.

Case 13.1 illustrates the clinical features and EEG findings of a patient with early myoclonic epileptic encephalopathy.

Other Neonatal Encephalopathies

Advances in the field of genetics have shed light on the genetic mutations behind two well-described benign epilepsies with onset in the neonatal period: benign familial neonatal seizures (BFNS) and benign familial neonatal-infantile seizures (BFNIS). Both autosomal dominant epilepsies have a remitting course in the first year of life. BFNS has been associated with mutations in the KCNQ2 and KCNQ3 genes; BFNIS is caused by a mutation in KCNQ2. Nevertheless, studies of neonates with severe encephalopathies have also linked these genetic defects to a more severe neonatal encephalopathy phenotype in this age group [8]. Retigabine (also known as ezogabine), a neuronal potassium channel enhancer was investigated as a specific therapy for neonates with these epilepsies [9,10]. Results from a small series indicated improvement of seizures and development in patients treated before the age of six months [11]. However, retigabine was withdrawn from the market in 2017. Interestingly, these infants respond very favourably to therapy with carbamazepine or phenytoin [12,13]. This observation is understandable based on the colocalization of the KCNQ channels and sodium channels in the axon initial segment of the principal neurons in the network [14].

Infant and Early Onset Epileptic Syndromes

Infantile Spasms and Hypsarrhythmia

Infantile spasm (IS) is an age-specific epilepsy of early infancy and the most common encephalopathy in this age group. The incidence has been estimated as 0.25–0.60 per 1000 live births [15–17]. A recently published population-based study on the incidence and outcome of the epilepsy syndromes with onset in the first year of life in Finland documented that the incidence of epilepsy in the first year of life was 124/100000, with West syndrome being the most common (41/100000) [18]. Boys are more often affected than girls.

This epileptic syndrome was initially described by Dr James West in 1841 when he described the seizures his infant son was experiencing [19]. The epilepsy was named West syndrome in his honour and includes an epilepsy with onset in infancy with the main seizure type described as axial spasms in clusters, and abnormal neurodevelopment that ranges from lack of progression to frank regression on developmental milestones.

In 1952, the Gibbs' described the classical EEG pattern of hypsarrhythmia [20]. This finding completed the West syndrome triad along with the infantile spasms and psychomotor retardation.

The most common age of onset is between four and seven months of age, but earlier onset is also seen. Onset beyond age 18 months is rare, but some children who presented with this epilepsy phenotype during infancy continue to have epileptic spasms combined with other seizure types well into school age and adolescence. There are reports of late-onset epileptic spasms during adolescence in patients with malformation of cortical development [21].

The typical description of IS includes flexion or extension of all limbs in a symmetrical or asymmetrical or asynchronous fashion, but asymmetries and a mixture of flexion and extension are commonly seen. Detailed study of the movements documents that the infant will have a brief phasic contraction of the muscles followed by a gradually relaxing tonic phase. Spasms can also be focal associated with atonia or mixed with partial seizures, with spasms either preceding or leading to the partial seizures or presenting at the end of the partial seizures [22]. Most commonly the spasms present in clusters when the patient is falling asleep or when awakening. Asymmetric IS are a common feature in children with focal brain pathology, in particular focal cortical dysplasia [23]. The coexistence of IS and partial seizures has been recognized for many years [24].

The classic clinical presentation of IS can be easily diagnosed by observing the patient, but subtle spasms often are missed by parents and physicians. Episodes of yawning, facial grimacing, abnormal eye movements such as nystagmus, ocular flutter or ocular gyration, transient focal motor activity, sighing and other behaviours can occur in clusters coinciding with typical ictal EEG changes of IS [24,25]. Subclinical IS has also been noted. Subtle spasms can be seen at the presentation of the IS or early in the clusters before the more typical movements are seen. Subtle IS can also be seen in patients with partial response to treatment of IS.

Once there is clinical suspicion for IS, the EEG will add the third component of the triad: hypsarrhythmia. Classic hypsarrhythmia as described by Gibbs includes irregular high voltage (more than 200 μV) inter-mixed with polymorphic spikes and sharp waves with multi-focal location [20]. Figure 13.2A shows the EEG of an infant with classic hypsarrhythmia. Hrachovy et al., in their classic 1984 report, offered a detailed description of variants of hypsarrhythmia or modified hypsarrhythmia which may also be seen in patients with IS. These variants include: hypsarrhythmia with increased inter-hemispheric synchronization (Figure 13.2B), asymmetrical hypsarrhythmia (Figure 13.2C), hypsarrhythmia with a consistent focus of abnormal discharges (Figure 13.2D), hypsarrhythmia with episodes of attenuation (Figure 13.2E) and hypsarrhythmia with primary high-voltage slow activity with little sharp wave or spike activity (Figure 13.2F) [26]. It is important to know that in some cases, IS can present without hypsarrhythmia [27] and hypsarrhythmia can be seen without a history or video documentation of IS. Despite the detailed description by Hrachovy and collaborators, the identification of hypsarrhythmia by paediatric electroencephalographers still has a lower inter-rater reliability than is needed to increase the identification of infants who could benefit from adequate treatment [28].

The ictal patterns associated with epileptic spasms also have electrographic variability. There are three main patterns described that include

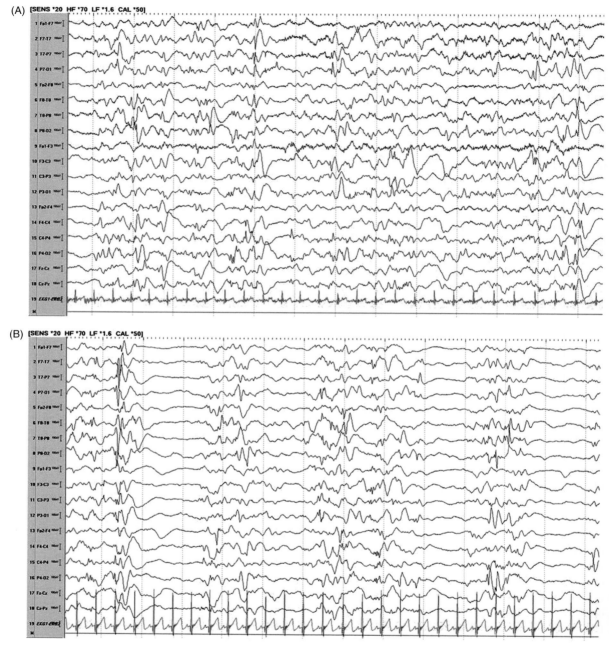

Figure 13.2 (A) and (B) These interictal EEGs were recorded in an infant who presented with extensor infantile spasms at the age of six months. Treatment with ACTH began five days after the diagnosis of IS. Two weeks later EEG showed complete resolution of the hypsarrhythmia and IS. (A) EEG with classic hypsarrhythmia of high-voltage delta and multi-focal spikes and sharp waves (as seen in (B)), but during sleep, episodes of generalized attenuation were seen alternating with episodes of hypsarrhythmia. This second pattern was seen in 20–30% of the sleep. (C) Hypsarrhythmia with bifrontal inter-hemispheric synchronization in a four-year-old male with medically refractory CDKL5 epileptic encephalopathy. (D) Asymmetrical hypsarrhythmia with a predominance in the left hemisphere, mainly in the posterior quadrant. Notice attenuation of the background rhythms in the left parasagittal fronto-central region. This EEG was recorded in a seven-month-old with known left perinatal MCA stroke and right hemiparesis, presented with a two-week history of asymmetrical IS. IS resolved with ACTH treatment. (E) Hypsarrhythmia with a consistent focus of abnormal discharges in the left posterior temporal region. This child is a 15-month-old with onset of IS at seven and a half months. Brain MRI showed a left temporal low-grade grail/glioneuronal tumour that was resected surgically two months after the onset of the IS. Her seizures had partial response to vigabatrin and ACTH. (F) This EEG shows hypsarrhythmia with primary high-voltage slow activity with little sharp wave or spike activity in a nine-year-old female with CDKL5. Her seizures began at age two months with IS. Currently she has a mixture of seizures that include isolated epileptic spasms, myoclonic seizures and prolonged seizures with multiple phases that include tonic–clonic, hypomotor and autonomic features.

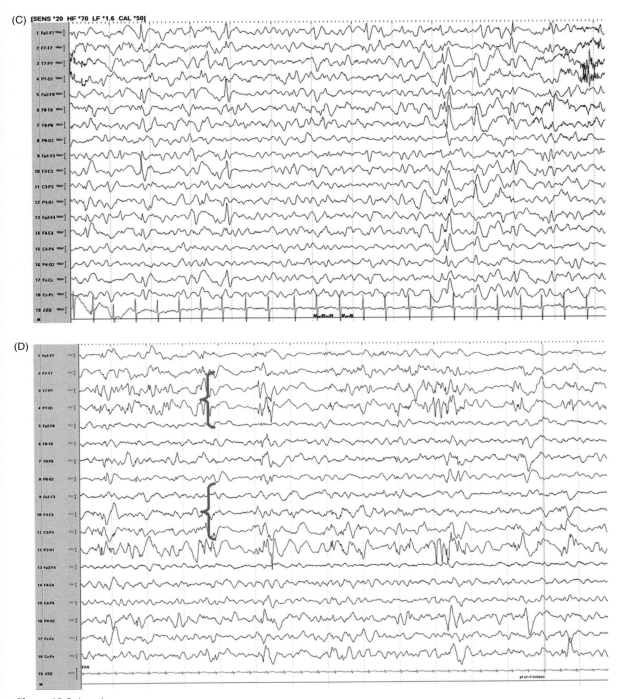

Figure 13.2 (cont.)

diffuse slow waves with maximum positivity in the vertex (Figure 13.3A), generalized or diffuse fast activity (Figure 13.3B) and diffuse electrodecrement (Figure 13.3C) [29]. It is not uncommon to find different types of ictal patterns intermixed in a single patient or during the same cluster of IS.

More than 200 aetiologies can lead to a phenotype of IS. Recently, the Commission of Pediatric Epilepsy

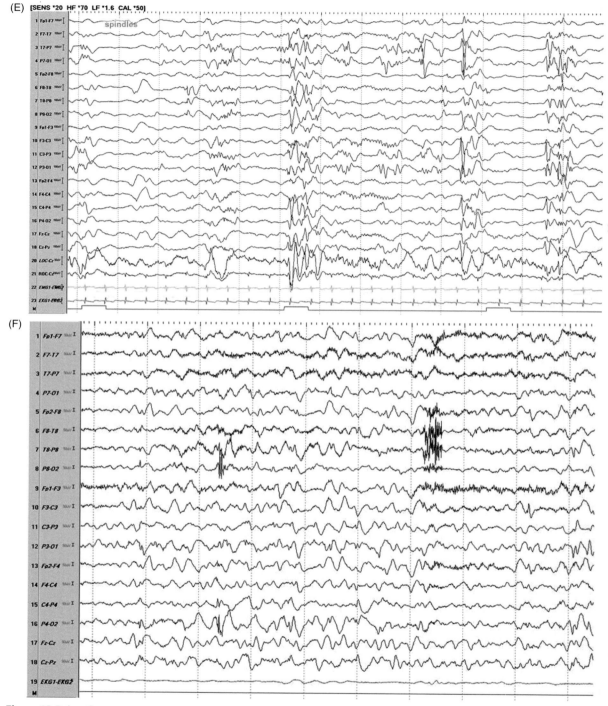

Figure 13.2 (cont.)

(A)

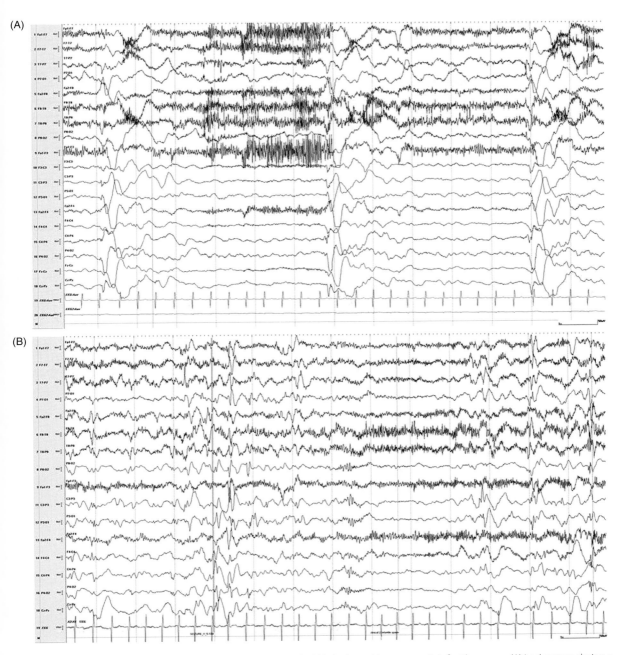

(B)

Figure 13.3 EEG samples (A) and (B) correspond to an eight-month old baby boy with cryptogenic infantile spasms. (A) Ictal pattern during a cluster of infantile spasms with characteristic diffuse delta waves with maximum positivity in the midline region. (B) Another ictal pattern recorded during a cluster of IS and showing diffuse fast activity. (C) This EEG shows an ictal pattern of relative electrodecrement recorded during a cluster of IS at age eight months in a child with migrating partial epilepsy of infancy phenotype.

of the ILAE provided recommendations for the evaluation and management of infantile seizures based on the current medical evidence [30]. The recommendations emphasize the standard of care for suspected infantile spasms at all levels of care and specify the expected evaluation at the tertiary and quaternary levels of epilepsy care.

Figure 13.4 shows the diagnostic algorithm for the diagnostic evaluation of an infant with suspected infantile spasms.

(C)

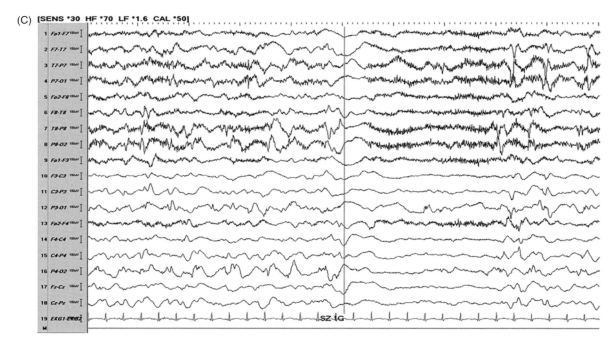

Figure 13.3 (cont.)

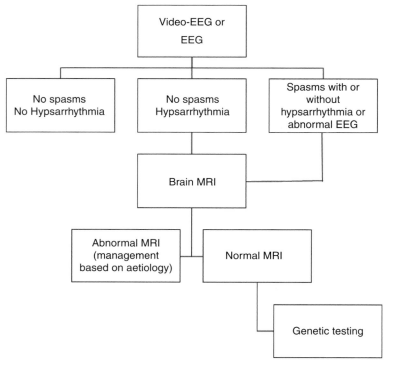

Figure 13.4 Algorithm for the evaluation of infants with suspected spasms.

Brain MRI is the initial test to be performed in children with any age-related epileptic encephalopathy. Results from the Pediatric Epilepsy Research Consortium showed that the brain MRI provided a diagnosis in 55% of children with IS. Along with the brain MRI, currently available genetic metabolic testing can clarify the aetiology of IS in 64.4% of the cases [31]. The ILAE Commission on Pediatrics recommended serum glucose, basic haematologic screening, liver function tests, ammonia, urine analysis, pH, arterial gases, plasma electrolytes (sodium, potassium and chloride), CSF and plasma lactate, and CSF glucose as the standard of care work-up for children with suspected metabolic conditions. The evaluation in tertiary and quaternary centres should be expanded to include amino acids, organic acids, enzyme studies, genetic testing and even tissue biopsy. The extended genetic screen should include array comparative genomic hybridization, targeted single nucleotide polymorphism array, specific genetic testing, epilepsy gene panel, whole exome/genome sequencing, mitochondrial single nucleotide polymorphism array and mitochondrial panel [30].

The yield of the metabolic testing is low for many of the tests recommended for standard of care according to results from the National Infantile Spasms Consortium [31]. Blood and serum studies were normal in 77.6% of the children, urine studies were normal in 88.6%, and CSF studies were normal in 78.2% and non-specific in 18.2%. In 2 cases out of 55 children, CSF studies were abnormal (3.6%). In one of these two cases, diagnosis was possible by epilepsy gene panel. Karyotype provided information about abnormalities in 85% of the children tested and often the test was done due to developmental concerns and before the onset of IS. Array comparative genomic hybridization showed abnormalities in 15% who were tested after the onset of IS. Targeted chromosomal single nucleotide polymorphism revealed the aetiology in 50%. Targeted single gene testing showed abnormalities in 83.3% (five cases) tested before the onset of IS and 33.3% (six cases) tested after IS. Epilepsy gene panels showed abnormalities in 32.4% (11 cases).

Another study on the diagnostic yield of genetic testing in epileptic encephalopathy of childhood examined a sample of patients referred to an epilepsy genetic clinic over a period of two years. Results showed identification of genetic causes in 28% of the patients, and 7% of the patients had inherited metabolic disorders of

which 4.5% had available treatment opportunities. Targeted next-generation sequencing epileptic encephalopathy panels provided genetic diagnosis in 45% of the patients [32]. Taking into account these results, modern genetic testing should be done expeditiously in children with infant-onset epileptic encephalopathies because the diagnostic yield is much higher than the formerly recommended metabolic tests [33].

Treatment in children with epileptic spasms should be started as soon as possible. There is Class B evidence that both low and high doses of ACTH are probably effective for the treatment of epileptic spasms, resulting in a strong recommendation for its use in this condition. There is Class C evidence that prednisone and vigabatrin are possibly effective in the treatment of IS with a weak level of recommendation. The exception is tuberous sclerosis complex, in which vigabatrin offers a favourable treatment option for IS in the setting of this specific genetic disease [30].

Treatment response of IS according to the 2004 AAN practice parameters is considered when there is complete cessation of spasms confirmed by video-EEG and abolition of hypsarrhythmia on prolonged EEG [34].

Recently, a report from the National Infantile Spasms Cohort that included 230 infants with IS documented a higher response rate in children who received standard therapy for IS (46%) vs. children who received non-standard therapy (9%). Response to initial treatment was 56% with ACTH, 39% with oral corticosteroids and 9% with vigabatrin; 14% of the children received non-standard therapy with levetiracetam, topiramate, clobazam, valproic acid, zonisamide, oxcarbazepine, phenobarbital, clonazepam and ketogenic diet [35]. Children with IS and a focal brain lesion should be referred to a tertiary/quaternary epilepsy centre for epilepsy surgery evaluation.

Factors associated with best prognosis in children with IS are short treatment lag between the onset of spasms and adequate treatment, cryptogenic aetiology, normal neurodevelopment at the onset of the spasms, age of onset under four months, absence of atypical spasms or focal seizures, absence of asymmetries in the EEG and quick and sustained response to treatment [36].

Almost a third of the patients will progress to the Lennox–Gastaut phenotype, another age-related epileptic encephalopathy [37]. Therefore, when considering the long-term prognosis into adulthood of these patients, some of the outcome data of children who suffered from infantile spasms will be lumped together with other symptomatic generalized epilepsies of childhood onset. One study from Finland reported on the 20–35-year follow-up of 214 patients who were diagnosed with West syndrome and received treatment with ACTH [38,39]. One-third of the patients had died by age three years, one-third were seizure-free and the final third remained with daily to monthly seizures. IQ was below 68 in two-thirds of the patients. More than half of the patients were unable to receive education, around a quarter completed special education and a little less than a quarter completed primary or secondary education. Only 10 of 147 patients married, 11 were able to drive, 23 had an independent life and 9 had some dependency. As many as 113/147 had total dependency with 30 of them living in institutions. Of the 36 patients who achieved independent life, some were able to gain some form of occupation, including professional, manual labour, sales and office work, and some were able to do house work. A quarter of the patients in this series had psychiatric problems that included hyperactivity and autism.

Migrating Partial Epilepsy of Infancy

Malignant migrating partial seizures of infancy (MMPSI) is a rare epileptic encephalopathy syndrome described by Coppola et al. in 1995 [40]. Clear knowledge about this syndrome is needed when evaluating infants for epilepsy surgery because initially seizures can be unilateral and later become multi-focal or migrate to other regions of the brain.

Seizures typically start in the first six to seven months of life, but more commonly around age two to three months. Typically, infants have a mixture of epileptic spasms, tonic seizures, myoclonic seizures and partial seizures with ictal onsets independently in the right and left hemispheres. Along with frequent seizures, there is progressive neurodevelopmental retardation or lack of progression. The infants can also have gastrointestinal dysmotility, movement disorders and abnormalities in muscle tone [41].

Initially, the seizures may be sporadic, weekly or monthly, but soon become refractory to medical treatment. Focal motor seizures can be one-sided or involve a single limb or alternate from one limb to another. Secondary generalization and status epilepticus can occur. Autonomic symptoms such apnoeas, drooling, facial flushing, cyanosis or pupillary changes are common. Between seizure onset and first year of life, seizures become multiple per day or can occur in clusters or continuously. Other focal ictal symptoms develop, including eye or head deviation to one side, eyelid clonic activity, or clonic or tonic activity involving one limb, or one or both sides of the body. Autonomic symptoms with or without oral automatism may also be present. Seizures can evolve into generalized clonic seizures. Duration can be variable, but seizures lasting over two minutes are not uncommon. Sometimes between the first and fifth year of life, seizures become milder and more prominent during intercurrent illnesses. Status epilepticus may occur [42].

The changes on EEG evolve along with the different periods of this epileptic syndrome. At the onset of the seizures, the EEG can show diffuse slow background for age and multi-focal spikes or sharp waves when the child is awake or asleep, and unilateral focal seizures can be seen. As the syndrome progresses to a more florid phase, sleep spindles begin to fade, multi-focal spikes become more frequent and ictal patterns with onset in any region of the brain can be recorded. Hypsarrhythmia with epileptic spasms and a burst suppression pattern can also occur [41]. The ictal patterns during focal seizures have very distinctive characteristics (Figure 13.5A and B). Typically, at the onset of an ictal pattern there is high-voltage, sharply contoured activity within the alpha to theta range of frequencies that can be located in the occipital, temporal, rolandic or frontal regions, and quickly spreads to other regions of the brain. Seizures can be seen independently in the right or left hemispheres. Often the ictal patterns are localized to the posterior quadrants of the brain. As seizures begin to subside, the inter-ictal epileptiform discharges can become more frontal and exhibit inter-hemispheric synchronization [40,42].

Brain MRI is normal in the majority of the cases, but brain atrophy can occur as the disease progresses, with delayed myelination and putamen atrophy. There have been reports of mesial temporal sclerosis and dual pathology. Decreased N-acetyl aspartate can be seen on magnetic resonance spectroscopy [40–42].

Multiple genes have been described as causative, including SCN1A [43]; PLCB1 [44]; QARS, TBC1D24 [45]; SLC25A22 [46]; SLC12A5, SCN2A [47]; KCNT1 [41,48]; SCN8A [48,49] and CLCN2 [50]; multiple

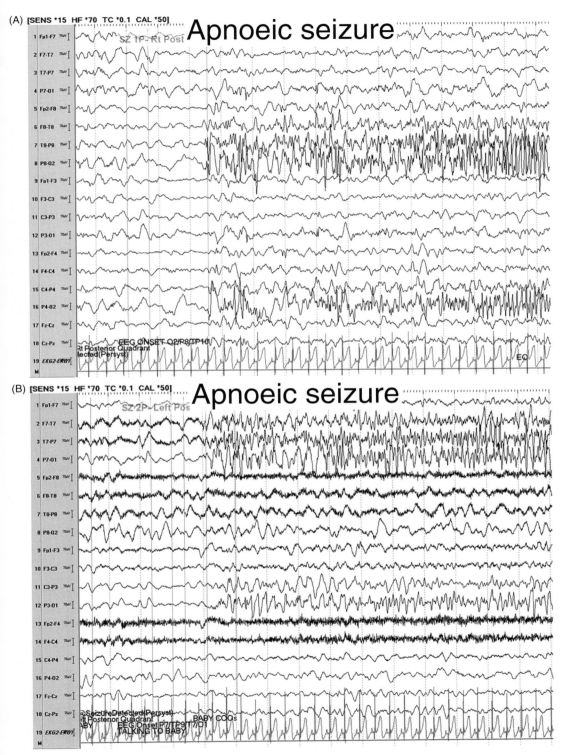

Figure 13.5 Figures showed focal seizures arising from the right (A) and left (B) posterior quadrant that clinically correlated with apnoeic seizures in a 10-month-old infant with MPEI. This child died aged 12 months.

sodium channel gene deletions, including SCN1A, SCN2A, SCN3A, SCN7A and SCN9A [51], and chromosomal abnormalities such as 47XYY [52] and WWOX tumour gene autosomal recessive defect in chromosome 16q23.1 (a case encountered in our practice). In a subset of patients, the aetiology remains unknown [53].

Seizures in MMPSI are refractory to conventional anti-seizure medications. There are reports of successful treatment when using a combination of stiripentol and clobazam [54] or of stiripentol, levetiracetam and bromides [55]. Seizure reduction of 50% has been reported with rufinamide [56] and a ketogenic diet [57,58]. Levetiracetam has been useful for the treatment of status epilepticus in patients with MMPSI [59]. Acetazolamine [60] can be useful for seizure control. Seizure reduction from daily to weekly has been reported with treatment with potassium bromide or cannabidiol. Potassium bromide initial dose was 50 mg/kg/day with subsequent titration by 10 mg/kg/day each week to a goal of 80 mg/kg/day [61]. Cannabidiol was used at an initial dose of 10 mg/kg/day divided into twice-daily doses and increased to 25 mg/kg/day over 15 days [62]. Quinidine can be a treatment choice for children with KCNT1 mutations. Quinidine was administered at an initial dose of 2 mg/kg/day divided every six hours and then titrated to 33 mg/kg/day with monitoring of the serum levels. The maximal dose reported was 42 mg/kg/day [63]. Another patient with MMPSI also had a reduction in seizures of 80% when receiving quinidine [64]. Despite the initial enthusiasm for the potential of quinidine to mitigate the gain in potassium currents mediated by KCNT1 in infants with MPEI attributable to such mutations, results have not been consistent [63,65].

Treatment with dextromethorphan in an infant with early myoclonic encephalopathy suppressed the myoclonic seizures and aided in the transition to MMPSI phenotype, but did not provide a treatment benefit for MMPSI seizures [6].

Worsening of seizures in patients with MMPSI has been reported with vigabatrin and carbamazepine [40,42].

Prognosis is poor for seizure control and neurodevelopment. All children have developmental delay or intellectual disabilities. Children with milder symptoms can walk, but there is no language development. Microcephaly develops over time and mortality is high [40–42].

Dravet Syndrome

Dravet syndrome was initially described by Charlotte Dravet in 1978. This epilepsy phenotype was initially named severe myoclonic epilepsy of infancy, but after the association of the genetic defect with other epilepsy phenotypes, such as borderline severe myoclonic epilepsy of infancy, intractable epilepsy of infancy with tonic–clinic seizures and genetic epilepsies with febrile seizure plus (GEFS+), the ILAE name was changed to Dravet syndrome [66,67].

Dravet syndrome is one of the epileptic encephalopathies with fever susceptibility. The typical presentation is around the age of six months with a convulsion or hemiconvulsion in the setting of fever either triggered by infectious disease, typically viral, or due to fever secondary to vaccination [68]. Seizures can be prolonged. Febrile convulsions become frequent and recurrent. Hemiconvulsions can occur on either side of the body. Febrile and afebrile status epilepticus are common. Following the initial febrile seizures, other afebrile seizure types can appear at the end or beginning of the first year of life. These seizure types include myoclonic seizures, absence seizures, generalized tonic–clonic (GTC) seizures, tonic seizures, focal partial seizures and atonic seizures. Nevertheless, when considering the diagnosis of Dravet syndrome, it is important to take into account that not all patients will have myoclonic or absence seizures and not all patients will present with febrile seizures. Dravet syndrome has a variable phenotype with different degrees of severity and milder forms are encountered in clinical practice.

Other neurological symptoms include pyramidal and extrapyramidal motor signs, moderate to severe cognitive impairment and ataxia [69]. Some studies clarify that instead of cognitive regression, there is lack of progression or cognitive stagnation [70].

A family history of epilepsy is common and can be better seen in large families, in particular in those families with SCN1A mutations leading to GEFS+. A negative family history does not exclude the diagnosis of Dravet syndrome. Nevertheless, most of the cases with Dravet syndrome have a de novo mutation in the SCN1A gene that encodes for the neuronal voltage-gated sodium channel alpha 1 subunit (Nav1.1). This mutation is present in 70–80% of the Dravet cases. Mutations in other genes such as SCN1B and GABARG2 also can produce a Dravet syndrome phenotype. X-linked protocadherin PCDH19 mutation can produce a similar phenotype in girls, with variable cognitive function from normal to intellectual disability, with or without autistic features [71]. Other genetic defects have been reported in children with Dravet phenotype and negative for SCN1A mutation. They include GABRA1, GABRG2, HCN1 and STXBP1.

A mutation of SCN1A can be also found in other well-recognized epileptic phenotypes, such as migrating partial epilepsy of infancy, myoclonic astatic epilepsy, and early infantile epileptic encephalopathy.

In Dravet syndrome, the EEG findings are not specific to the syndrome and are more related to the patient's seizure types. EEG can be normal early in the disease. The presence of posterior dominant rhythms is variable, and a diffuse slow background can be found in more severe cases. Focal slowing can be seen. Focal, multi-focal or generalized spikes, and polyspikes or spike and wave complexes of variable frequency can be seen, along with other generalized or focal ictal patterns. Photic stimulation can elicit photoparoxysmal response, but this is not specific.

Brain MRI is Non-Revealing

Seizures in Dravet syndrome are refractory to medical treatment. There is Class A evidence and therefore a strong recommendation for the use of stiripentol in patients with Dravet syndrome. Class C evidence for topiramate, zonisamide, valproate, bromide and ketogenic diet indicate that these medications are possibly effective with weak efficacy. There is Class A evidence that lamotrigine, carbamazepine and phenytoin can exacerbate the seizures in patients with Dravet and should be avoided [30]. More recently, cannabidiol has been approved by the US FDA for the treatment of children with Dravet syndrome and provides a seizure reduction of 38–50% [72]. Fenfluramine is another medication being investigated for Dravet syndrome [73].

The long-term prognosis of Dravet syndrome includes high mortality (16–20.8%); patients with Dravet have increased susceptibility to SUDEP. Studies of adults with Dravet syndrome document that seizure control is achieved in less than 16% of cases. Sensitivity to fevers and high temperature remains in 30–50% of the patients. Almost all patients will experience generalized convulsions during sleep, but status epilepticus becomes less frequent over time [74,75]. Most adults with Dravet syndrome will have moderate to severe cognitive problems [69] and almost a quarter of the patients will continue to have serious behavioural problems [74]. Communication

Case 13.2 SCN1A Mutation

A 13-year-old male presented with a febrile prolonged convulsion at age 11 months. Some of the initial febrile seizures were described as having head deviation to the right followed by right side body shaking. Afebrile seizures began at age 18 months and had persisted since then with intermittent periods of seizure freedom lasting up to two years. He only has one type of seizure, described as generalized tonic–clonic. His seizures increase during hot summers, which led the family to relocate to the Midwest of the USA from the south. His seizures have worsened with carbamazepine, oxcarbazepine, lamotrigine, levetiracetam and lacosamide. Valproate provided a period of seizure freedom but caused pancreatitis and hepatic dysfunction. Seizures have been better controlled with clobazam, phenobarbital and rufinamide. A vagus nerve stimulator was recently implanted.

He has an uncle with infancy-onset epilepsy who currently is an adult with severe intellectual and physical disability and occasional 'grand mal seizures'.

Recent genetic testing showed a pathogenic variant in the SCN1A gene.

limitations range from no language or few words in almost half of the patients to poorly structured language or simple conversational language in some [74,75]. Only 3–14% of the patients can achieve an independent life, 14–34% are partially independent and 54–71% are totally dependent [69,74,75]. These data are important when arranging transition of care and succession of care in adults with Dravet syndrome and aging primary caregivers [76].

Case 13.2 illustrates the clinical features and EEG findings (Figure 13.6) of a patient with an SCN1A mutation who has EEG markers for SUDEP.

Epilepsy with Myoclonic Absences

Epilepsy with myoclonic absences is a genetic generalized epilepsy syndrome recognized by the ILAE [77,78]. This rare epilepsy has received less attention in the medical literature than other equally rare syndromes. This syndrome is probably more commonly encountered in tertiary and quaternary centres that provide care for children with medically refractory epilepsies.

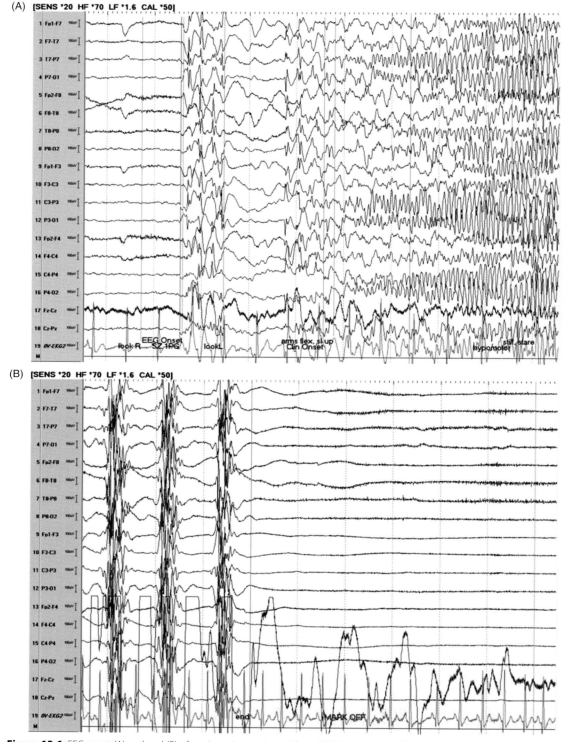

Figure 13.6 EEG onset (A) and end (B) of a seizure in a patient with an SCN1A mutation. Diffuse electrodecrement on the EEG is a well-recognized marker for SUDEP.

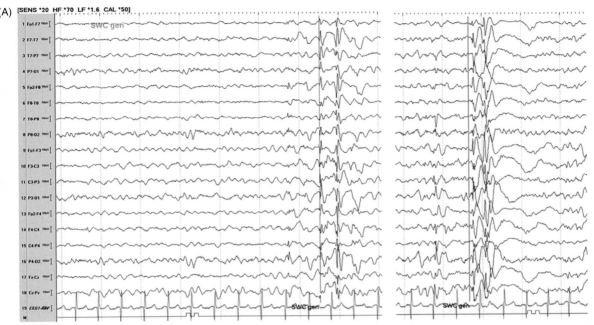

Figure 13.7 (A) Inter-ictal EEG of a four-year-old girl with epilepsy with myoclonic absence, showing a high-voltage burst of 3 Hz spike and wave complexes, and polyspike and wave complexes. (B) A typical myoclonic absence seizure with interruption of activity and rhythmic jerking of the shoulders and arms. (C) A myoclonic clonic seizure that occurred during sleep. Seizures in this patient are controlled on a combination of ethosuximide, valproate and topiramate. Seizures were refractory to monotherapy with each drug independently and also a ketogenic diet.

The age at onset is variable, from the first year of life until the pre-teenage years, but most commonly is seen in early-school-age children. In our experience, a pre-school-age onset (around three years) is common.

As its name describes, there is a combination of absence seizures with superimposed myoclonic seizures. During the seizures, the children can exhibit sudden interruption of activity or staring. Myoclonic seizures are bilateral, rhythmic or irregular and can affect the chin, the neck muscles, the shoulders or less commonly the whole body. Sometimes, isolated myoclonus without absences can occur, producing falls. At times, myoclonic seizures can progress into a generalized clonic seizure, but in general convulsions are infrequent. The frequency of the seizures is high. Seizures can occur when awake or asleep.

At the onset of the epilepsy, the neurological exam and development are normal. As the epilepsy progresses, some cognitive decline can occur. In some children with this epileptic syndrome, evolution to Lennox–Gastaut phenotype has been reported [79] (Case 13.3).

The background rhythms are typically normal for age. EEG shows inter-ictal bursts of high-voltage generalized spike and wave complexes and polyspikes that at times can be seen bifrontally (Figure 13.7A). The frequency of the spike and wave complexes is typically around 3 Hz, but faster and slower frequencies can be seen. Polyspike and wave discharges are more common than the typical 3 Hz spike and wave complexes seen in childhood absence epilepsy. Myoclonic seizures typically follow the frequency of the spike and wave complexes. Multi-focal spikes are not uncommon. During seizures, a mixture of polyspikes and spike and wave complexes is typically seen (Figure 13.7B,C).

Brain MRI Does Not Reveal Any Abnormalities

The evidence for the treatment of this type of epilepsy is at the expert level (Level D evidence). It can be refractory to monotherapy, with some anti-myoclonic seizure drugs. In our experience, children often need combination treatment with ethosuximide, valproate, topiramate or levetiracetam. Worsening of seizures with phenobarbital or carbamazepine has been reported. Lamotrigine can be ineffective in many cases [79,80] .

(B) [SENS *20 HF *70 LF *1.6 CAL *50]

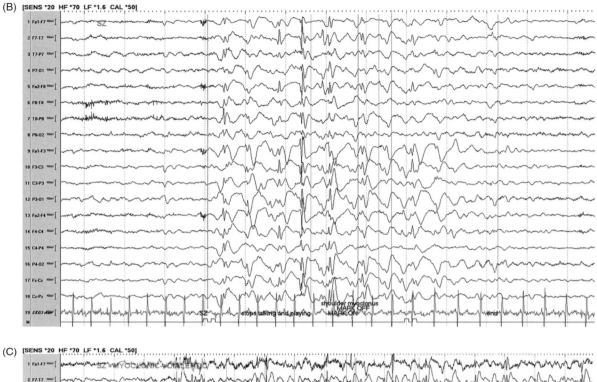

(C) [SENS *20 HF *70 LF *1.6 CAL *50]

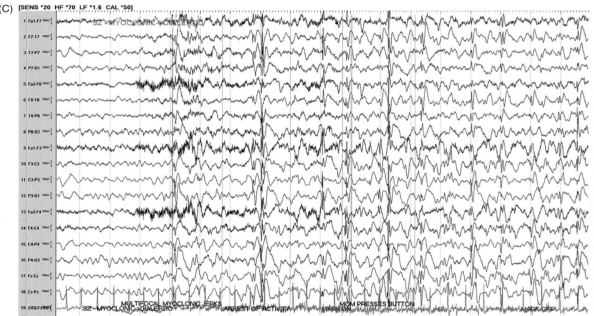

Figure 13.7 (cont.)

Table 13.1 Progressive myoclonic epilepsy, relevant clinical features and genetic testing

Disease	Relevant clinical features	Genetic testing
Unverricht–Lundborg disease (EPM1)	Prevalance in Finland (1/20 000) Refractory myoclonus More progression in adolescence and slowing down of progression in adulthood Preserved cognition MRI: mild atrophy of brain, cerebellum and brainstem ASMs: VPA, ZON, LEV, high-dose piracetam AVOID: phenytoin (can worsen ataxia)	Gene test: EPM1 (CSTB) mutation analysis
Lafora body disease (EPM2)	Autosomal recessive Onset: 8-18 years Occipital seizures Profound dementia Death by aspiration in less than 10 years from onset	Skin biopsy: Lafora bodies Gene tests: EPM2A or EPMP2B(NHLRC1) mutation analysis
Neuronal ceroid lipofuscinoses (NCL)	Currently 14 forms described (CLN1 to CLN14) Main symptoms: seizures, cognitive and motor decline, and retinal pathology and visual loss, in particular macular degeneration Myoclonic seizures May be infrequent during the disease course of some forms except in late stages when myoclonus, tremor or involuntary movements occur Length of survival is related to the specific type, but they all lead to early death	Skin biopsy: Granular osmophilic deposit Leukocyte enzyme analyses: PPT1,TPP1, CTSD Gene tests: CLN1/PPT1, CLN2/TPP1, CLN3, CLN4/ DNAJC5, CLN5, CLN6, CLN7/ MFSD8, CLN8, CLN10/CTSD, CLN11/GRN, CLN12/ATP13A2, CLN13/CTSF, CLN14/ KCTD7 mutation analysis
Sialidosis	Type 1: Juvenile onset Action and intention myoclonus with axial involvement is disabling Progressive visual failure (cherry red spot) Normal cognition No dysmorphic features No visceromegaly Type 2: Onset birth to second decade Dysmorphism: coarse face, cornel clouding, skeletal dysplasia Cognitive problems, mainly learning	Urine: Sialo-oligosaccharides Leukocyte enzyme analysis: Neuraminidase Gene test: NEU1 mutation analysis

The prognosis is for resolution around two to five years after epilepsy onset, but in about 50% of the cases, treatment with anti-seizure medications must continue long term.

Progressive Myoclonus Epilepsy

Progressive myoclonus epilepsy (PME) represents a group of diseases in which there is a clinical combination of myoclonus, GTC seizures, cognitive decline and ataxia [81]. While age of onset for PME is variable and extends beyond infancy, it is an important diagnostic consideration for infant-onset disease, particularly when myoclonus is present.

Common conditions that cause PME are listed in Table 13.1, along with other relevant clinical features and currently available genetic testing. In the early stages, PME can mimic other epilepsies in which myoclonus is a prominent feature, in particular juvenile myoclonic epilepsy (JME), so this epilepsy should be considered in cases of JME with associated neurological symptoms or cognitive decline.

EEG in PME cases shows inter-ictal generalized spikes and polyspikes with a variable frequency from 2.5–6 Hz. Focal spikes can be present in some conditions as well. Photoparoxysmal response and photoconvulsion are common (Figure 13.8).

The understanding of these diseases has been expanded as the field of genetics has developed (see Table 13.1). Although treatment remains symptomatic for most, patients with Gaucher disease can benefit from enzyme replacement [82].

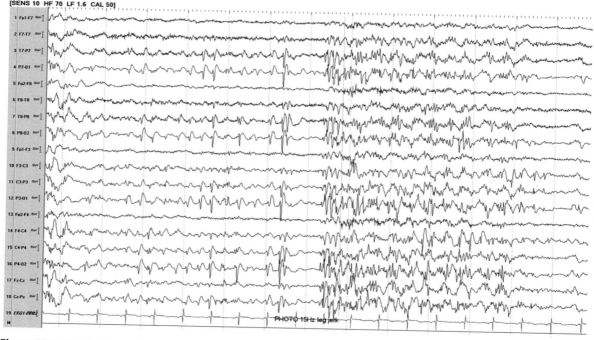

[SENS 10 HF 70 LF 1.6 CAL 50]

Figure 13.8 EEG of a 17-year-old male diagnosed with Gaucher disease at age seven years, showing a segmental myoclonus of the legs elicited by photic stimulation at 15 Hz. In the sample, photoparoxysmal response is seen, as well as multi-focal sharp waves over the posterior head regions, as has been typically described for this condition.

Childhood Syndromes

Lennox–Gastaut Syndrome

Lennox–Gastaut Syndrome (LGS) is a severe epileptic encephalopathy in children [83]. LGS syndrome has an incidence of 1.9–2.1 per 100 000 and represents 6–7% of the medically refractory paediatric epilepsies.

The onset of LGS is in childhood during the first two to four years of life. It can present de novo or in children with a history of infantile focal seizures or infantile spasms (one-third of the patients). There is male predominance for this epilepsy phenotype.

The class triad of LGS includes multiple seizure types that are refractory to medication, cognitive dysfunction/developmental delay and typical EEG with diffuse slow spike and wave, polyspikes and slow background.

Seizure types include tonic seizures, atonic seizures, atypical absences, myoclonic seizures, GTC seizures and partial seizures.

Tonic seizures typically involve the axial muscles, producing elevation or extension of the arms. Tonic seizures seem to increase during sleep, causing a very

Case 13.3 Lennox–Gastaut Syndrome

A 10-year-old female had the diagnosis of Lennox–Gastaut syndrome secondary to HSV encephalitis infection at age six weeks. Her seizures presented at five months of age with infantile spasms that improved but did not resolve with treatment with ACTH and vigabatrin. The brain MRI showed right temporal lobe encephalomalacia that was resected at age two years. Nevertheless, seizures relapsed at age three years with daily tonic seizures, atypical absence seizures and GTC seizures. A vagus nerve stimulator was implanted at age five years. Her seizures have been refractory to phenobarbital, oxcarbazepine, lamotrigine, clobazam and valproate. Seizures are now weekly on a combination of topiramate, clorazepate and ethosuximide.

fragmented and non-restful sleep that can add to the increased seizure burden.

Atonic seizures can produce sudden falls to the floor due to loss of muscle tone. Along with tonic and myoclonic seizures, atonic seizures are a major cause of injuries in these patients. As all these seizures produce falls, use of a helmet with face cover is recommended. It can be difficult for the caregiver to distinguish between atonic and tonic seizures, and for this reason they are often lumped together as 'drop attacks' in studies of drug efficacy in LGS [84,85].

Atypical absence seizures are very common. They may be less obvious than typical absences. When reviewing the video-EEG records of these patients, atypical absence seizures have a gradual onset from an activity level that can be increased or reduced. In a child with a baseline reduced level of activity, it is difficult to identify the clinical onset of the atypical absence seizures. Atypical absence seizures are usually longer than typical absences. Clinically the patient can have prolonged staring episodes, arrest or diminution of behaviour, or act confused, for example when eating trying to continue to eat from outside the food plate. The end of the atypical absence seizures is often unclear as well, with some children returning to their baseline level of activity.

In patients with early focal or hemispheric brain lesions on MRI, the possibility of epilepsy surgery must be considered, despite the presence of generalized inter-ictal and ictal patterns [86,87].

Status epilepticus, convulsive or non-convulsive, is frequent. Some children with an incomplete phenotype are assigned a diagnosis of symptomatic generalized epilepsy rather than LGS.

The degree of developmental delay and cognitive impairment is variable from mild to severe, with some patients being completely dependent on caregivers for activities of daily living. Language impairment is variable. In some patients, the cognitive impairment worsens as epileptic encephalopathy develops over time and more ASMs are added to the treatment. Neuro-motor comorbidities like spasticity, cerebral palsy, dystonia, dyskinesia, choreoathetosis and hypotonia are not uncommon, but some children can walk, putting them at risk of accidents during the seizures. Neuropsychiatric comorbidities such as ADHD, autism, explosive behaviour and anxiety are frequent in affected children, as is depression in the caregivers.

EEG shows a posterior dominant rhythm background that is slow for age or completely absent, with only diffuse delta inter-mixed with intermittent rhythmic slow activity. Slow spike and wave at a frequency of less than 2.5 Hz, typically around 1 Hz, is common (Figure 13.9A). This pattern correlates with atypical absences. During sleep, there is a predominance of generalized polyspikes or paroxysmal fast activity that is often followed by periods of relative electrodecrement (Figure 13.8B). This pattern correlates with tonic seizures and can be seen at the onset of the convulsions as well (Figure 13.9C). Multifocal spikes are seen often. Seizures occur when awake or sleep and have a variable duration.

Aetiology is symptomatic in two-thirds of patients and varies from genetic to structural lesions, acquired or congenital. Brain MRI can be normal or reveal a variety of structural lesions. Recent advances in genetics support the notion of a continuous age-related phenotype with shared aetiology for IS and LGS. Among the genes found in patients with both epileptic encephalopathy phenotypes are CDKL5, KCNQ2, KCNT1, SCN1A, SCN2A, SCN8A and STXBP1, GABRB3, ALG13, CHD2, GRIN2A and SYNGAP1 [8,88,89].

Treatment of patients with LGS often requires polytherapy with more than three ASMs.

There is FDA approval for adjunctive treatment of LGS with topiramate, felbamate, lamotrigine, rufinamide, clonazepam and clobazam. Valproate can be very effective, particularly in combination with lamotrigine. Zonisamide and levetiracetam have also shown some efficacy. Ethosuximide is useful when atypical absence seizures are present. Vigabatrin, which is indicated for the treatment of IS and partial seizures, can also be used in children with LGS with some efficacy. Phenobarbital, often excluded from the treatment choices in patients with LGS given the cognitive side effects, may be an efficacious drug for these patients. Steroids [90–92] and IVIg [93,94] can temporarily reduce the seizure burden in selected cases, but the level of evidence is low and based on case series. Carbamazepine and oxcarbazepine can worsen the seizures overall, but improve the generalized tonic–clonic type. The aetiology of LGS needs to be considered when clarifying why these medications worsen the seizures in some patients.

Diets, neurostimulation and surgeries become necessary treatment in LGS patients with poor response to medical treatment.

A ketogenic diet is commonly used in young children, but diet alternatives such as the Atkins diet and the modified Atkins diet can be attractive alternatives for older children and adults [89,95–97].

Vagus nerve stimulation is another commonly used therapy for patients with LGS, producing a

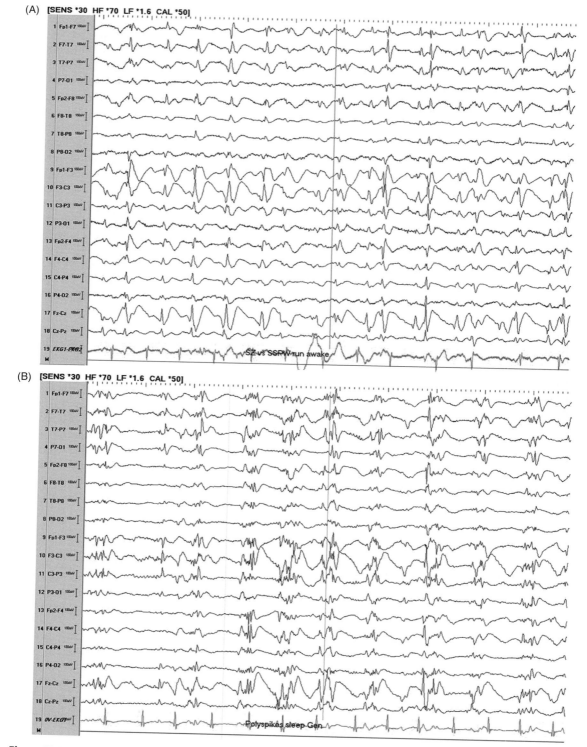

Figure 13.9 (A) A classic slow wave spike at 1.5 Hz recorded in this case. (B) Runs of generalized polyspikes recorded during sleep. Notice the asymmetry of the grapho-elements in the right hemisphere due to surgical resection of the right temporal lobe. (C) A tonic seizure occurring during sleep with the corresponding EEG electrodecrement followed by fast activity.

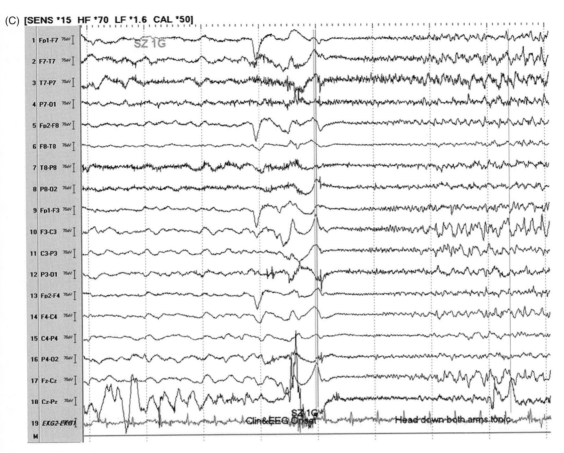

(C) [SENS *15 HF *70 LF *1.6 CAL *50]

1 Fp1-F7
2 F7-T7
3 T7-P7
4 P7-O1
5 Fp2-F8
6 F8-T8
7 T8-P8
8 P8-O2
9 Fp1-F3
10 F3-C3
11 C3-P3
12 P3-O1
13 Fp2-F4
14 F4-C4
15 C4-P4
16 P4-O2
17 Fz-Cz
18 Cz-Pz
19 EKG2-EKG1

SZ 1G

S4 1G
Clin&EEG Onset
Head down both arms tonic

Figure 13.9 (cont.)

seizure reduction of around 50% after six months of treatment [98].

Corpus callosotomy reduces injuries from atonic seizures in LGS [99–101]. Advances in epilepsy surgery have made it possible for these patients to have focal or multi-focal resection or hemispherectomy with resolution of the seizures in 50–60% of the cases.

Premature mortality is high in patients with LGS compared to other seizure phenotypes.

The long-term prognosis into adulthood for children who have LGS is refractory seizures in 62%, with 20.4% having focal seizures and neuropsychiatric problems [102] and cognitive deficit with autism being very common [103]. Patients often live in home groups or institutions when their caregivers are no longer able to care for them.

Despite the advances on the epilepsy field, the long-term prognosis of these patients remains the same. It is important to keep in mind that when not all the clinical features of LGS are present, patients are lumped into a broader category of refractory epilepsy known as generalized symptomatic epilepsies. A more recent long-term outcome study by Carol and Peter Camfield that included adults with generalized symptomatic epilepsies of childhood onset showed mortality of 11.4% of the patients, remission without anti-seizure medications in a quarter of the patients and refractory epilepsy in almost half of the patients [37]. Ambulation was limited in 48% of the patients. Mental retardation/intellectual disability was seen in 90% of the patients, being severe or profound in 71% of the adults. Neuropsychology testing was completed in 39 patients and showed normal intelligence without limitations in 9% of the cases [37,104]. The authors reported limitations in the activities of daily living in 63% of the patients, 60% required total care, 38% were unable to feed themselves or required feeding tubes, 57% lived in home groups or institutions

139

and 86% were dependent on their primary caregivers or society.

Myoclonic Astatic Epilepsy

Myoclonic astatic epilepsy (MAE) or Doose syndrome was first described in 1970 [105]. It accounts for 1–2% of childhood epilepsies. Age of onset for this epilepsy ranges from seven months to six years with a peak between two and five years. There is a male predominance for this epilepsy and a susceptibility to seizures with fever.

Most of the children have normal neurodevelopment at the time of seizure onset, but cognitive deterioration can be seen in children with evolution to a refractory phenotype.

Seizures are myoclonic, atonic or a combination. Typically, children have a brief jerk of the limbs that can be follow by a loss of tone. Atonic seizures with falls can occur without a preceding myoclonus and can range from a loss of neck muscle tone with a head drop to full loss of tone. Some children develop tonic seizures and absence seizures mixed with myoclonus and clonic features. In some cases this epilepsy can evolve into an LGS phenotype with tonic seizures, GTC seizures and poor response to ASMs [106]. A family history of epilepsy is present in some cases.

EEG shows bursts of irregular polyspikes and spike and wave at a frequency of 2–4 Hz. Multi-focal spikes in the fronto-central regions can also be seen. (Figure 13.10A). The seizures are associated with high-voltage generalized spikes or polyspikes that can also be bilateral fronto-central (Figure 13.10B). The background of the EEG when awake and asleep can be normal and remains so in patients with better controlled seizures. When the phenotype evolves into LGS, slowing of the background is seen.

Brain MRI is Normal

MAE has a shared genetic susceptibility with patients with Dravet syndrome and GEFS+. An SCN1A mutation is reported in around 2% of patients with epileptic encephalopathy and an MAE phenotype [107]. When cognitive deterioration is present, work-up should be expanded to rule out neurometabolic conditions, in particular PME.

Treatment recommendations for MAE are at the level of evidence of expert opinion. Valproate, ethosuximide, topiramate, levetiracetam and lamotrigine are useful drugs either alone or combined with benzodiazepines. More refractory cases may require polytherapy and other drugs such as zonisamide, felbamate, vigabatrin, steroids and IVIg [108]. A ketogenic diet has been reported to be very beneficial for these patients, especially in those with a mutation in the SLC2A1 gene, which codes for the glucose transporter GLUT1 [109].

The prognosis of MAE is variable. Between 50% and 70% of children become seizure-free.

Most children can achieve complete seizure remission with anti-seizure medications and some have remission without ASMs. Unfortunately, there is a small subset that develops severe and frequent seizures that are at times indistinguishable from LGS syndrome [110].

Epilepsy with Continuous Spike Wave of Sleep and Landau–Kleffner Syndrome: The Most Severe Forms of the Epilepsy–Aphasia Spectrum

Epilepsy with continuous spike wave of sleep (CSWS) and Landau–Kleffner syndrome (LKS) are rare epileptic encephalopathies that affect school-aged children and adolescents. Both syndromes are characterized by seizures, cognitive regression or deterioration of school performance, and electrographic status epilepticus of sleep (ESES) on EEG. In the case of LKS, there is also language regression as a predominant clinical symptom, with EEG spiking typically maximal in the left posterior temporal or centrotemporal regions.

CSWS and LKS present in children with a history of normal development in the first three to five years of life. Seizures start and in the case of LKS this is followed by language regression.

In CSWS, various seizure types can occur particularly during sleep. Seizures can be partial or generalized atypical absence seizures, and begin around the age of two to four years. Most commonly partial seizures are rolandic.

Seizures are typically easier to control with conventional ASMs than the cognitive dysfunction caused by the abundant spikes seen when the child falls asleep. In a subset of patients, a more severe phenotype with absence, clonic and GTC seizures can develop, along with poor response to treatment.

More troublesome than the seizures are the behavioural and cognitive problems associated with CSWS. Problems include inattention, poor impulse

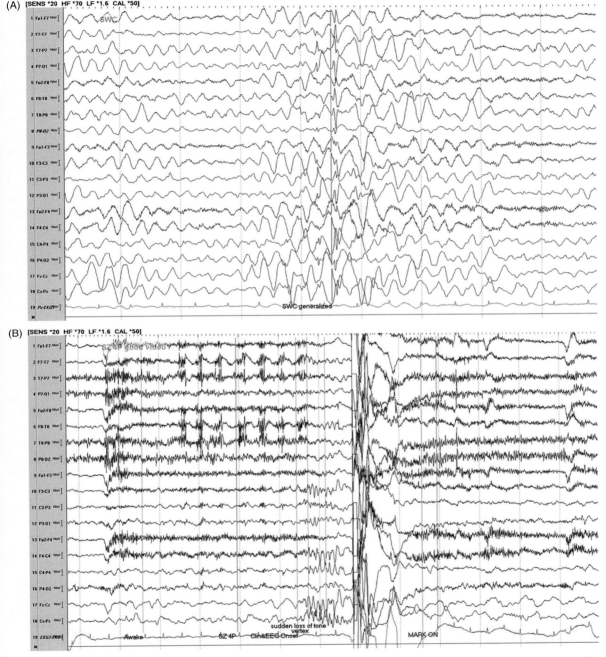

Figure 13.10 (A) Inter-ictal EEG of a three-year-old female with new onset of drop attacks. She has normal neurodevelopment, normal neurological exam and normal waking and sleeping background rhythms in the EEG. Her brother and uncles had febrile seizures. (B) Ictal EEG during an atonic seizure with polyspikes maximum fronto-central followed by a drop artifact.

control, learning deterioration, memory difficulties, poor executive function, poor coordination and poor socialization skills. Oral motor dysfunction can also occur. These problems are very challenging and require not only behavioural therapy and medications but full support from school personnel.

As CSWS is an age-related encephalopathy, clinical improvement and then resolution is seen after reaching adolescence. Nevertheless, the neuropsychiatric syndrome associated with CSWS can leave devastating consequences.

LKS represents a severe epileptic encephalopathy in which, in addition to the seizures, neurocognitive deterioration and severe behavioural problems, there is an acquired aphasia due to verbal auditory agnosia. The typical pattern is characterized by an initial inability to understand spoken language that is followed by loss of ability to use spoken language. As in CSWS, partial seizures or GTC seizures are easily controlled and typically resolve during the teenage years, along with the EEG abnormalities, but language and behavioural problems can persist in children with LKS [111].

CSWS and LKS are considered the severe end of the spectrum of epileptic encephalopathies in which there is potentiation of the epileptogenic activity in the transition from wakefulness to sleep. During recordings in patients with CSWS and LKS, the typical EEG pattern is electrographic status epilepticus of sleep (ESES) (Figure 13.11). ESES is characterized by near continuous slow spike and wave discharges that appear when the patient falls asleep. Spikes are seen mainly during non-REM sleep and can be bilateral or unilateral. These spikes at times are maximum in the centro-temporal and mid-temporal regions. Spikes can be present during wakefulness, but during non-REM sleep there is activation of the spikes, which can be generalized or focal. There is disagreement within the medical community about the best definition of ESES and the best method to quantify the spikes [112]. A broad range of spike and wave index (SWI) of 25–85% during slow wave sleep has been discussed [113]. Nevertheless, a study by Van Hirtum-Das et al. found that an SWI greater than 50% was associated with global developmental deficit [114].

The aetiology of CSWS and LKS is usually non-lesional, but some children with known brain structural lesions develop ESES [114]. Early developmental lesions that involve the thalamus alone or the thalamus and the cerebral hemispheres have been found on brain MRI of nearly 50% of patients with ESES and include malformation of cortical development and the sequelae of ischaemia, haemorrhage or infectious disease.

A family history of epilepsy is present in one-sixth of patients [112,115]. A number of case reports support genetic factors as potential contributors to the CSWS phenotype [116]. The recent discovery of a mutation in the N-methyl-D-aspartate receptor subunit gene GRIN2A in chromosome 16p13.1 adds support to the notion of a continuum or variation of phenotypes in patients with epilepsy, cognitive, and speech and language disorders, the epilepsy–aphasia spectrum [117]. In addition to CSWS and LKS, this gene abnormality has been found in patients with atypical benign focal epilepsy and autosomal dominant rolandic epilepsy with speech dyspraxia, but is rare in patients with benign epilepsy with centro-temporal spikes (BECTS) [117]. The absence of GRIN2A in adults with idiopathic generalized epilepsy and temporal lobe epilepsy confirms that this genetic mutation is most likely associated with a childhood-onset epilepsy phenotype [118]. Other genetic defects recently described as predisposing to disease in CSWS are RBFOX1 or RBFOX3 and copy number variants that include deletions and duplications in chromosomes 1–3, 5–11, 13–16, 20, 22 and the X chromosome [117].

Hormonal treatment is considered the first line of treatment for CSWS and LKS by Vigevano et al. [119]. In patients with CSWS of unknown aetiology, structural or metabolic causes, treatment with steroids is favoured early in the diagnosis by some [120]. The rationale for this approach is early intervention for prevention of the subsequent cognitive and behaviour abnormalities. Other groups propose treatment with anti-seizure medications with known efficacy (valproate, ethosuximide, levetiracetam, sulthiame, lamotrigine and high-dose benzodiazepines) before the use of hormonal treatment and have used steroids after other failed choices [121–123]. Wilson et al. reported the experience of one centre with the use of amantadine 200 mg/day in the treatment of ESES and found near complete resolution of ESES in 30% of the cases and a reduction in SWI in almost 25% [124]. Some studies focus on the use of prednisone, hydrocortisone and methylprednisolone for the management of ESES. A few studies have focused in the use of ACTH in the treatment of ESES [121,125,126]. Immunomodulation with intravenous immunoglobulin can also be used, but the level of evidence remains limited to case reports and the response rate has been variable [127,128]. In cases with focal brain lesions, lesionectomy and hemispherectomy can result in successful termination of ESES [115]. Multiple subpial transection has been recommended

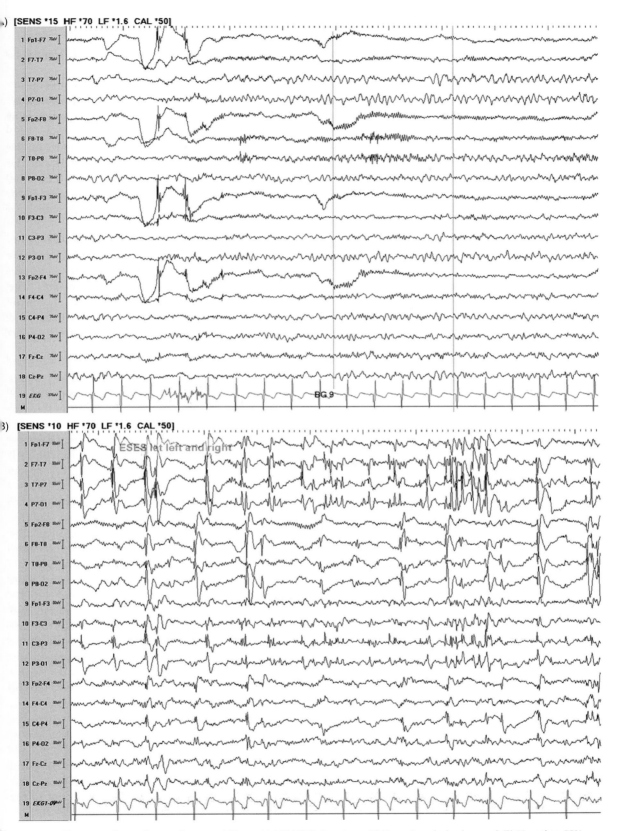

Figure 13.11 These samples are from a nine-year-old boy with LKS/ESES phenotype. (A) Normal awake background. (B) More than 85% activation of the spikes during sleep with a bilateral independent centro-temporal distribution.

in patients with non-lesional ESES or lesions in the dominant hemisphere [129].

Future randomized studies will clarify whether NMDA antagonists, currently used in the treatment of Alzheimer's dementia, will offer the clinical benefits to patients with GRIN2A mutation that are hypothesized, based on its mechanism of action [130].

Treatment of ESES beyond seizure control and eliminating the frequent spikes during sleep is critical for the improvement of cognitive function and other neurobehavioural conditions, such as ADHD. The importance of eliminating spikes in ESES has been supported by findings in animal studies. Several animal studies suggest that the induction of spikes by different methods result in memory, spatial orientation and cognitive changes [131–134]. These studies offer a possible explanation for the need to preserve cognitive function in children with ESES. A recent study documented reduction in inattention symptoms when ACTH was administered to rats with early onset interictal spiking [135].

Juvenile Absence Epilepsy

Juvenile absence epilepsy (JAE) begins in late childhood and early adolescence, typically at age 9–13 years. As its name implies, the predominant seizure type is absence seizures that are less frequent, but longer than those in children with childhood absence epilepsy. Presentation with an early morning generalized convulsion is not uncommon for this syndrome. Around one-fifth of these patients also have myoclonic seizures. Both genders are affected equally.

EEG shows 3 Hz spike and wave complexes activated by hyperventilation in a background normal for age when awake and asleep.

Seizures may respond well to treatment with ethosuximide or valproate. Some patients will need treatment for life. There are reports of non-convulsive status epilepticus in adults with this epilepsy type [77,136].

Juvenile Myoclonic Epilepsy

Juvenile myoclonic epilepsy (JME) was initially described by Janz [137]. JME is a common epilepsy, frequent in teenagers. JME accounts for 5–10% of all epilepsies. The age of onset is during puberty and there is a female predominance. There is controversy

among neurologists as to whether JME should be considered a refractory epilepsy.

A typical presentation is with GTC seizures occurring in the setting of sleep deprivation, stressful situations or exposure to bright lights. Upon careful observation, the convulsions in JME often begin with a quick succession of myoclonic jerks of the upper limbs that lead to faster clonic jerks of the body, at times with clear asymmetry of the limbs, before finally evolving into a tonic–clonic convulsion, so typical GTC seizures in patients with JME have multiple phases.

While GTC seizures occur in almost all patients with JME, the main seizure type that defines this syndrome is myoclonus, which is more common after awakening in the morning or from naps. The jerks typically involve the upper extremities, but myoclonus of the lower extremities can also occur and result in falls. Myoclonus is typically symmetric but focal features have been described.

In addition to myoclonus and GTC seizures, absence seizures are present in one-third of patients with JME. Some children with childhood absence epilepsy who do not go into remission can develop JME during their teenage years [138].

In addition to sleep deprivation, stress and strobe lights, other seizure precipitants in patients with JME are alcohol intake, highly caffeinated energy drinks and menses.

Neurological exam and cognitive performance are normal [139].

EEG is the only test necessary to confirm the diagnosis. Waking and sleeping rhythms are normal for age and frequently interrupted by generalized irregular polyspikes and fast spike and wave complexes, usually at a frequency around 4–6 Hz (Figure 13.12). Focal features can be present and do not exclude the diagnosis in the appropriate clinical setting. Activation manoeuvers with photic stimulation at 15 Hz or higher elicits a photoparoxysmal response in many cases. Photo-convulsive episodes with myoclonus or a GTC seizure can be also seen in the EEG laboratory. Ictal patterns during myoclonus include polyspikes or polyspikes and fast wave patterns. During the convulsions, initial polyspikes can quickly evolve to high-voltage spikes or fast spike and wave complexes, and then the EEG becomes obscured by muscle artifacts, but some interruptions corresponding to the clonic phases can be seen.

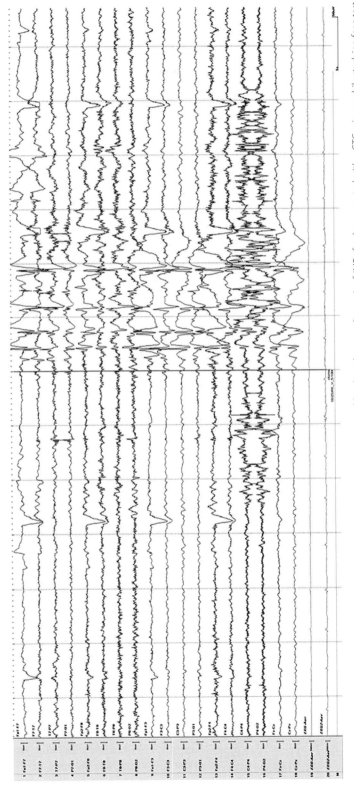

Figure 13.12 This figure shows the EEG during early morning myoclonus in an 18-year-old male with a new diagnosis of JME after he presented with a GTC seizure while studying for a test. Video-EEG confirmed the presence of early morning myoclonus interfering with his preparation of breakfast.

There is no need to perform neuroimaging in JME. Depression is a common comorbidity and almost half the patients need treatment with antidepressants [140].

Regarding treatment, there is no current class A, B or C evidence for the treatment of JME. There is class D evidence for the effectiveness of valproate and topiramate in the treatment of JME [141]. There is FDA indication for levetiracetam and clonazepam for the treatment of JME. Despite the lack of best evidence and well-designed studies, zonisamide, primidone, phenobarbital and lacosamide can also be effective drugs for this epilepsy. There has been a report of lamotrigine worsening myoclonus in patients with JME. Carbamazepine, oxcarbazepine, gabapentin, tiagabine, vigabatrin and phenytoin can aggravate all seizure types in these patients and should be avoided. Valproate should be avoided in women of reproductive age due to its teratogenic effect.

Even though JME is considered a life-long epilepsy, myoclonic seizures seem to subside in the fourth decade [142,143]. A detailed long-term outcome study from Nova Scotia followed 23 patients with JME for 25 years. They reported seizure freedom in 78% of the cases, with 48% reporting discontinuation of the treatment. All seizure types were in remission in 17% of the patients. Only myoclonus persisted in 13% and a few of these patients were able to stop treatment with ASMs. Convulsive status epilepticus occurred in 36% of the patients and 3 of 23 had intractable epilepsy. One patient died from drowning. No SUDEP was reported in this cohort [140]. In addition to depression, social isolation, social impulsivity and unemployment resulted in a less than satisfactory life for around 30% of the patients, even though 87% graduated from high school education.

Jeavons Syndrome

Jeavons syndrome (JS) is known as a medically refractory generalized epilepsy that is not recognized by the ILAE as an independent epileptic syndrome. This epilepsy is often mistaken for JME or juvenile absence epilepsy and is probably lumped together with these generalized idiopathic epilepsies in research studies. In fact, at the Cleveland Clinic, 35% of the patients with a diagnosis of JME and photoparoxysmal response in the EEG had clinical features of JS (personal communication; Abstract 2.081, American Epilepsy Society Meeting, 2016).

In the 1989 ILAE Classification of Epilepsies and Syndromes, this epilepsy was classified under epilepsies precipitated by other modes of activation or reflex epilepsies [144].

More recently, a new seizure type, eyelid myoclonia with or without absences, has been accepted as a seizure type present in many idiopathic or symptomatic epileptic syndromes [145].

Providing a correct diagnosis of JS is very important so that the prognosis of the epilepsy can be properly discussed. In this group of patients, seizures are often difficult to control, even with polytherapy. Counselling on avoidance of precipitant factors and lifestyle modification is important to provide the best seizure control.

JS was initially describes by Jeavons in 1977 [146] and is defined by frequent occurrence of eyelid myoclonia with or without brief absences, often in combination with a history of visually induced seizures and eye-closure-induced seizures. JS has onset in childhood, typically with a peak at six to eight years of age (range 2–14 years). Seizures induced by bright light environments and photic stimulation in the EEG laboratory are common. This epilepsy is predominant in girls and prevalence is around 2.7% among adult epileptic disorders and 12.9% among idiopathic generalized epilepsies (IGE) with typical absences. Prevalence in children is unknown [139].

EEG shows generalized epileptiform activity triggered by eye closure with occipital predominance (Figure 13.13A), generalized photoparoxysmal response to photic stimulation, generalized polyspikes and SWC with variable frequency from 3–6 Hz (Figure 13.13B). Hyperventilation also can trigger generalized spike and wave discharges.

Eye-closure sensitivity is a common feature of this epilepsy phenotype and must be distinguished from eye-closed sensitivity. In eye-closure sensitivity, the inter-ictal epileptiform discharges occur as soon as the eyes are closed at a slower speed than a simple eye blink (see Figure 13.13). The associated epileptiform discharges are generalized and the phenomenon extinguishes after 1–3 seconds or when associated with clinical seizures when the seizure is over. Eye-closed sensitivity is also known as the fixation-off phenomenon. It is characterized by continuous epileptiform discharges, mainly in the posterior head regions that appear 1–3 seconds following eye closure and disappear once the eyes are open or when fixation returns.

(A)

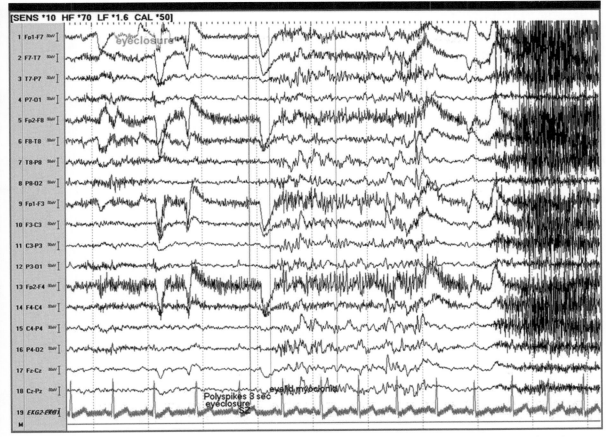

Figure 13.13 (A) Eye closure with eyelid myoclonus in a female adolescent with Jeavons syndrome. (B) EEG with 3 Hz spike and wave complex during an absence seizure. Both seizures are triggered by eye closure.

Yang et al. studied the difference between eye-*closure* sensitivity and eye-*closed* sensitivity. They found that eye-closure sensitivity is more common in epileptic syndromes and has a stronger association with photosensitivity than eye-closed sensitivity, but both can be present in the same epileptic syndrome; nevertheless the pathophysiological mechanisms could be different [147]. Eye-closed sensitivity is seen in idiopathic or symptomatic focal occipital epilepsies.

The aetiology is probably related to a genetic contribution, as suggested by reports of identical twins affected [148,149]. A malfunction of the alpha rhythm generator in the occipital cortex has been suggested as a possible pathophysiology [150].

Treatment of JS has been poorly studied. A study of levetiracetam monotherapy reported 80% seizure control in patients with JS [151]. However, caution must be used when prescribing levetiracetam to

teenage females with possible undiagnosed and untreated depression or a strong family history of depression, as levetiracetam can worsen depressive symptoms and even lead to suicidal ideation, suicide attempts or successful suicide [152,153]. Valproate is another useful drug that should be avoided in females of reproductive age. A combination of valproate with a benzodiazepine or ethosuximide can control the seizures. Phenobarbital is another excellent anti-myoclonic medication that is often forgotten. Lamotrigine can be used with some success, but in some patients worsens the myoclonus. As in other generalized idiopathic epilepsies, the use of carbamazepine, oxcarbazepine, gabapentin, phenytoin, tiagabine and vigabatrin must be avoided due to the high risk of worsening seizures [154]. Our approach to the treatment is based on the predominant seizure type.

(B)

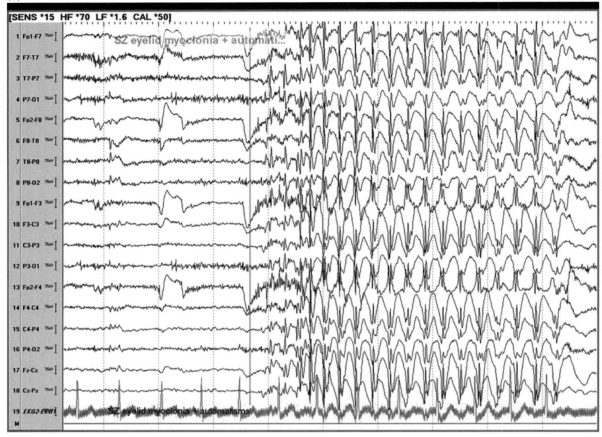

Figure 13.13 (cont)

Blue lenses have been recommended for the treatment of JS, but lifestyle modification, including avoidance of bright light situations and treatment adherence are important for successful control of the seizures [155].

A Word about Epilepsy Surgery in Patients with Epileptic Encephalopathy

Despite specific criteria for the referral of children with medically refractory seizure for epilepsy surgery evaluation [156], epilepsy surgery remains an under-utilized treatment for children with epilepsy in the United States [157,158]. Epilepsy surgery as a treatment option for children with epileptic encephalopathies has been established for a long time [159–164] and today is considered a safe and quality-of-life changing treatment.

Epilepsy surgery should be considered in infants with onset focal seizures and unilateral brain abnormalities and in infants with persistent seizures despite treatment with two appropriate anti-seizure medications [30]. Nevertheless, it is important to consider that infantile spasm is the predominant epilepsy phenotype for this age group, so the possibility of a surgical resolution must be considered even when there is no evidence of focal seizures or focal findings on the EEG [162,163]. In other words, the presence of generalized EEG findings is not an exclusion criteria for epilepsy surgery in children with early brain lesions [86].

The same principle applies for children with the Lennox–Gastaut phenotype and lesional electro-graphic status epilepticus of sleep [86,87,115,165].

Today, it is well known that resective epilepsy surgery in children with LGS offers an opportunity of 60–80% seizure freedom, as reported in series with short- and long-term follow-up [86,87,166–168]. The benefits of epilepsy surgery in this epileptic encephalopathy goes beyond seizure freedom, as the majority of patients are able to walk independently, attend school and for some even gain employment [165].

A pooled analysis that evaluated the treatment outcome in 575 cases with ESES reported cognitive, EEG and other improvements that were nearly equivalent for patients treated with epilepsy surgery compared to those who received steroids. Surgery or steroids resulted in better treatment effects than benzodiazepines and conventional ASMs [169].

A Word about Transition of Care in Patients with Epileptic Encephalopathy

Around 50% of epilepsies with onset in childhood will persist into adulthood [170]. Therefore, a knowledge of medically refractory epilepsies with onset in childhood becomes very important for adult epileptologists and neurologists who will be providing adult care once these patients reach adulthood and are transferred to adult hospitals and facilities.

Data from studies on young adults with medical needs shows that around 60% do not receive transition care, in particular those with major medical care needs and functional limitations. At particular risk are youths who are male, non-Caucasian and lack health insurance [171]. In recent years, there has been a greater effort from the epilepsy community to educate patients, their families and health professionals on the need for proper transition of care.

Limitations in transition of care are caused by all involved in the process from the family to the paediatric neurologist/epileptologist and the adult neurologist/epileptologist, including adult care facilities and hospitals. A study by the Child Neurology Society showed that even though the majority of those surveyed had trained to transfer their patients to adult care (87%), only 13% had used a transition clinic. Methods of transfer of care are not standardized and most providers use a letter of referral (67%), a phone call (39%) or leave the transfer in the hands of the paediatrician (23%) [172].

A study by Falcone et al. (Project CARE: Parent and Youth Attitudes about Transition and Care Coordination, HRSA grant, personal communication), also documented that most families, even knowing that their child will be reaching adult age, have not thought about transition of care and do not have a plan in place.

Currently there are different models for transition of care that include: disease-based models, care coordination models and adolescent medicine programs based on medical needs [173,174]. The selection of one model over another depends largely on the characteristics of the setting in which the patient has been receiving care and where the patient is being transferred to, as some children's hospitals and paediatric care facilities are not affiliated with or close to adult facilities. Nevertheless, the appropriate steps and discussion regarding transition of care should start early, in particular for patients with chronic conditions such as epilepsy.

Key Points

- Medically refractory epilepsies affect 20–30% of patients evaluated at an epilepsy centre. Over 50% of childhood-onset epilepsies persist into adulthood.
- A variable degree of developmental delay and cognitive impairment, from mild to severe, is a common denominator of childhood-onset medically refractory epilepsies, especially those with the earliest onset.
- Brain MRI and genetic testing are the main diagnostic tests to clarify the aetiology of early-onset epileptic syndromes that are refractory to medical treatment.
- Ohtahara syndrome, or early infantile epileptic encephalopathy (EIEE) with suppression burst, and early myoclonic epileptic encephalopathy (EMEE) are rare forms of early infantile encephalopathy that typically present with refractory epilepsy in the first week of life, with tonic or segmental myoclonic seizures that occur in isolation or in clusters. EEG shows a suppression-burst pattern.
- Infantile spasms (IS) are an age-specific seizure type of early infancy and the type most commonly associated with epileptic encephalopathy in this age group. Clinical presentation varies from classic flexor or extensor spasms to subtle spasms, requiring a high index of clinical suspicion for early diagnosis. Similarly, the EEG may show findings consistent with classic hypsarrhythmia, but multiple variations of the hypsarrhythmia can be present instead, so familiarity with this range of

presentation is important to ensure early diagnosis. Treatment in children with epileptic spasms should be started as soon as possible with ACTH (Class B evidence), prednisone, or vigabatrin (Class C evidence).

- Malignant migrating partial seizures of infancy (MPSI) is a rare and newly recognized epileptic encephalopathy syndrome with onset between six and seven months of age. Seizures are typically a mixture of epileptic spasms, tonic seizures, myoclonic seizures and partial seizures with ictal onsets independently in the right and left hemispheres. Genetic work-up is important to clarify the aetiology, as initially the brain MRIs of children with MPSI are normal. Seizures are typically difficult to control with anti-seizure medications.

- Dravet syndrome is one of the sodium channelopathies that causes infant-onset epileptic encephalopathies with high-temperature susceptibility. Febrile convulsions and status epilepticus are common forms of presentation. Myoclonus can be present, but it is not the only seizure type, and it may be absent in some patients. Seizures in Dravet syndrome are refractory to medical treatment. The long-term prognosis of Dravet syndrome includes high mortality (16–20.8%). Patients with Dravet syndrome have increased susceptibility to SUDEP.

- Epilepsy with myoclonic absences is a genetic generalized epilepsy syndrome recognized by the ILAE. The age at onset is variable from the first year of life until the pre-teenage years, but most commonly it is seen in early-school-age children. Clinically, there is a combination of absence seizures with superimposed myoclonic seizures. This epilepsy can be refractory to monotherapy with some anti-myoclonic seizure drugs. Children may require combination treatment with ethosuximide, valproate, topiramate or levetiracetam.

- Progressive myoclonic epilepsy (PME) represents a group of genetic diseases in which there is a clinical combination of myoclonus, generalized tonic–clonic seizures, cognitive decline and ataxia. EEG shows inter-ictal generalized spikes and polyspikes with a variable frequency from 2.5–6 Hz. Photoparoxysmal response and photoconvulsion are common.

- Lennox–Gastaut syndrome (LGS) is a severe epileptic encephalopathy in children with onset during the first two to four years of life. Seizure types include tonic seizures, atonic seizures, atypical absences, myoclonic seizures, generalized tonic–clonic seizures and partial seizures. Most patients are refractory to traditional anti-seizure medications, and polytherapy is often needed. FDA approval for adjunctive treatment of LGS exists for topiramate, felbamate, lamotrigine, rufinamide, clonazepam and clobazam. Valproate in combination with lamotrigine can be effective. Zonisamide and levetiracetam may have some efficacy. Diets, neurostimulation and surgery become necessary treatments in patients with LGS who respond poorly to medical treatment. In patients with early focal or hemispheric brain lesions on MRI, the possibility of epilepsy surgery must be considered, despite the presence of generalized inter-ictal and ictal patterns on EEG.

- Myoclonic astatic epilepsy (MAE) or Doose syndrome presents with myoclonic, atonic or a combination of seizures between the ages of two and five years. A family history of epilepsy is present in some cases. Some patients evolve into a LGS phenotype with tonic seizures, generalized tonic–clonic seizures, and poor response to anti-seizure medications, but 50–70% of the patients eventually become seizure-free.

- Epilepsy with continuous spike wave of sleep (CSWS) and Landau–Kleffner syndrome (LKS) are rare epileptic encephalopathies that affect school-aged children and adolescents. Seizures typically are easier to control with conventional drugs, but more troublesome than the seizures are the behavioural and cognitive problems associated with the syndrome. The aetiology of CSWS and LKS is usually non-lesional and often seen with self-limited childhood epilepsy with centro-temporal spikes, but some children with known brain structural lesions develop ESES and genetic causes are being found more frequently. Hormonal treatment is considered the first line of treatment for CSWS and LKS by some experts in the field. Other groups propose treatment with anti-seizure medications with known efficacy (valproate, ethosuximide, levetiracetam, sulthiame, lamotrigine and high-dose benzodiazepines). Surgery may be effective for lesional cases.

- Juvenile absence epilepsy begins in late childhood and early adolescence, typically between the ages of 9 and 13 years, with absence seizures being the predominant but not exclusive seizure type. EEG shows 3 Hz spike and wave complexes activated by hyperventilation. Seizures may respond well to treatment with ethosuximide or valproate, but polytherapy may be necessary.

- Juvenile myoclonic epilepsy (JME) is a common epilepsy, frequently with onset in the teenage years. Myoclonic seizures upon awakening are the predominant seizure type, but typically the first recognition of the epilepsy follows a generalized tonic–clonic seizure occurring in the setting of sleep deprivation, stressful situations or exposure to bright lights. EEG shows generalized irregular polyspikes and fast spike and wave complexes, usually at a frequency around 4–6 Hz, but focal EEG features can be present as well.

- There is controversy among neurologists as to whether JME should be considered a refractory epilepsy or not. Valproate and topiramate have Class D evidence for the treatment of JME. There is FDA indication for levetiracetam and clonazepam. Despite the lack of Class A, B or C evidence and well-designed studies, zonisamide, primidone, phenobarbital and lacosamide can also be effective drugs for this epilepsy. Carbamazepine, oxcarbazepine, gabapentin, tiagabine, vigabatrin and phenytoin can aggravate all seizure types in these patients.

- Jeavons syndrome (JS) is known as medically refractory generalized epilepsy that is not recognized by the ILAE as an independent epileptic syndrome. This epilepsy is often mistaken for JME or juvenile absence epilepsy, and it is probably lumped together with these generalized idiopathic epilepsies in research studies. More recently, a new seizure type, eyelid myoclonia with or without absences, has been accepted as a seizure type present in many idiopathic or symptomatic epileptic syndromes. The main clinical feature is eyelid myoclonia with or without brief absences, often in combination with a history of visually induced seizures and eye-closure-induced seizures. Seizures induced by bright light environments and photic stimulation in the EEG laboratory are common.

- EEG in JS shows generalized epileptiform activity with occipital predominance triggered by eye closure, generalized or posterior photoparoxysmal response, generalized polyspikes and SWC with a variable frequency from 3–6 Hz. Hyperventilation also can trigger generalized spike and wave discharges. Levetiracetam, valproate, ethosuximide and benzodiazepines can be used for treatment. Sometimes polytherapy is needed, but seizures can be controlled in many patients.

References

1. Berg AT, Vickrey BG, Testa FM, et al. How long does it take for epilepsy to become intractable?: a prospective investigation. *Ann Neurol* 2006;**60**(1):73–79

2. Ohtahara S, Yamatogi Y. Ohtahara syndrome: with special reference to its developmental aspects for differentiating from early myoclonic encephalopathy. *Epilepsy Res* 2006;**70**(Suppl 1):S58–S67

3. Pavone P, Spalice A, Polizzi A, Parisi P, Ruggieri M. Ohtahara syndrome with emphasis on recent genetic discovery. *Brain Dev* 2012;**34**(6):459–468

4. Nieh SE, Sherr EH. Epileptic encephalopathies: new genes and new pathways. *Neurotherapeutics* 2014;**11**(4):796–806

5. Van Karnebeek CD, Tiebout SA, Niermeijer J, et al. Pyridoxine-dependent epilepsy: an expanding clinical spectrum. *Pediatr Neurol* 2016;**59**:6–12

6. Chien YH, Lin MI, Weng WC, Du JC, Lee WT. Dextromethorphan in the treatment of early myoclonic encephalopathy evolving into migrating partial seizures in infancy. *J Formos Med Assoc* 2012;**111**(5):290–294

7. Djukic A, Lado FA, Shinnar S, Moshe SL. Are early myoclonic encephalopathy (EME) and the Ohtahara syndrome (EIEE) independent of each other? *Epilepsy Res* 2006;**70**(Suppl 1):S68–S76

8. Allen NM, Mannion M, Conroy J, et al. The variable phenotypes of KCNQ-related epilepsy. *Epilepsia* 2014;**55**(9):e99–105

9. Maljevic S, Lerche H. Potassium channel genes and benign familial neonatal epilepsy. *Prog Brain Res* 2014;**213**:17–53

10. Orhan G, Bock M, Schepers D, et al. Dominant-negative effects of KCNQ2 mutations are associated with epileptic encephalopathy. *Ann Neurol* 2014;**75**(3):382–394

11. Millichap JJ, Park KL, Tsuchida T, et al. KCNQ2 encephalopathy: features, mutational hot spots, and ezogabine treatment of 11 patients. *Neurol Genet* 2016;**2**(5):e96

12. Numis AL, Angriman M, Sullivan JE, et al. KCNQ2 encephalopathy: delineation of the electroclinical

phenotype and treatment response. *Neurology* 2014;**82**(4):368–370

13. Pisano T, Numis AL, Heavin SB, et al. Early and effective treatment of KCNQ2 encephalopathy. *Epilepsia* 2015;**56**(5):685–691

14. Pan Z, Kao T, Horvath Z, et al. A common ankyrin-G-based mechanism retains KCNQ and NaV channels at electrically active domains of the axon. *J Neurosci* 2006;**26**(10):2599–2613

15. Cowan LD, Hudson LS. The epidemiology and natural history of infantile spasms. *J Child Neurol* 1991;**6**(4):355–364

16. Riikonen R, Donner M. Incidence and aetiology of infantile spasms from 1960 to 1976: a population study in Finland. *Dev Med Child Neurol* 1979;**21**(3):333–343

17. Sidenvall R, Eeg-Olofsson O. Epidemiology of infantile spasms in Sweden. *Epilepsia* 1995;**36**(6):572–574

18. Gaily E, Lommi M, Lapatto R, Lehesjoki AE. Incidence and outcome of epilepsy syndromes with onset in the first year of life: a retrospective population-based study. *Epilepsia* 2016;**57**(10):1594–1601

19. Cone TE, Jr. On a peculiar form of infantile convulsions (hypsarrhythmia) as described in his own infant son by Dr W.J. West in 1841. *Pediatrics* 1970;**46**(4):603

20. Gibbs EL, Fleming MM, Gibbs FA. Diagnosis and prognosis of hypsarhythmia and infantile spasms. *Pediatrics* 1954;**13**(1):66–73

21. Cerullo A, Marini C, Carcangiu R, Baruzzi A, Tinuper P. Clinical and video-polygraphic features of epileptic spasms in adults with cortical migration disorder. *Epileptic Disord* 1999;**1**(1):27–33

22. Watanabe K, Negoro T, Okumura A. Symptomatology of infantile spasms. *Brain Dev* 2001;**23**(7):453–466

23. Lortie A, Plouin P, Chiron C, Delalande O, Dulac O. Characteristics of epilepsy in focal cortical dysplasia in infancy. *Epilepsy Res* 2002;**51**(1–2):133–145

24. Donat JF, Wright FS. Simultaneous infantile spasms and partial seizures. *J Child Neurol* 1991;**6**(3):246–250

25. Donat JF, Wright FS. Unusual variants of infantile spasms. *J Child Neurol* 1991;**6**(4):313–318

26. Hrachovy RA, Frost JD, Jr, Kellaway P. Hypsarrhythmia: variations on the theme. *Epilepsia* 1984;**25**(3):317–325

27. Caraballo RH, Ruggieri V, Gonzalez G, et al. Infantile spams without hypsarrhythmia: a study of 16 cases. *Seizure* 2011;**20**(3):197–202

28. Hussain SA, Kwong G, Millichap JJ, et al. Hypsarrhythmia assessment exhibits poor interrater reliability: a threat to clinical trial validity. *Epilepsia* 2015;**56**(1):77–81

29. Fusco L, Vigevano F. Ictal clinical electroencephalographic findings of spasms in West syndrome. *Epilepsia* 1993;**34**(4):671–678

30. Wilmshurst JM, Gaillard WD, Vinayan KP, et al. Summary of recommendations for the management of infantile seizures: Task Force Report for the ILAE Commission of Pediatrics. *Epilepsia* 2015;**56**(8):1185–1197

31. Wirrell EC, Shellhaas RA, Joshi C, et al. How should children with West syndrome be efficiently and accurately investigated?: results from the National Infantile Spasms Consortium. *Epilepsia* 2015;**56**(4):617–625

32. Mercimek-Mahmutoglu S, Patel J, Cordeiro D, et al. Diagnostic yield of genetic testing in epileptic encephalopathy in childhood. *Epilepsia* 2015;**56**(5):707–716

33. Helbig KL, Farwell Hagman KD, Shinde DN, et al. Diagnostic exome sequencing provides a molecular diagnosis for a significant proportion of patients with epilepsy. *Genet Med* 2016;**18**(9):898–905

34. Mackay MT, Weiss SK, Adams-Webber T, et al. Practice parameter: medical treatment of infantile spasms: report of the American Academy of Neurology and the Child Neurology Society. *Neurology* 2004;**62**(10):1668–1681

35. Knupp KG, Coryell J, Nickels KC, et al. Response to treatment in a prospective national infantile spasms cohort. *Ann Neurol* 2016;**79**(3):475–484

36. Riikonen RS. Favourable prognostic factors with infantile spasms. *Eur J Paediatr Neurol* 2010;**14**(1):13–18

37. Camfield P, Camfield C. Long-term prognosis for symptomatic (secondarily) generalized epilepsies: a population-based study. *Epilepsia* 2007;**48**(6):1128–1132

38. Riikonen R. Long-term outcome of West syndrome: a study of adults with a history of infantile spasms. *Epilepsia* 1996;**37**(4):367–372

39. Riikonen R. Long-term outcome of patients with West syndrome. *Brain Dev* 2001;**23**(7):683–687

40. Coppola G, Plouin P, Chiron C, Robain O, Dulac O. Migrating partial seizures in infancy: a malignant disorder with developmental arrest. *Epilepsia* 1995;**36**(10):1017–1024

41. McTague A, Appleton R, Avula S, et al. Migrating partial seizures of infancy: expansion of the electroclinical, radiological and pathological disease spectrum. *Brain* 2013;**136**(Pt 5):1578–1591

42. Coppola G. Malignant migrating partial seizures in infancy: an epilepsy syndrome of unknown etiology. *Epilepsia* 2009;**50**(Suppl 5):49–51

43. Freilich ER, Jones JM, Gaillard WD, et al. Novel SCN1A mutation in a proband with malignant migrating partial seizures of infancy. *Arch Neurol* 2011;**68**(5):665–671

44. Poduri A, Chopra SS, Neilan EG, et al. Homozygous PLCB1 deletion associated with malignant migrating partial seizures in infancy. *Epilepsia* 2012;**53**(8): e146–e150

45. Milh M, Falace A, Villeneuve N, et al. Novel compound heterozygous mutations in TBC1D24 cause familial malignant migrating partial seizures of infancy. *Hum Mutat* 2013;**34**(6):869–872

46. Poduri A, Heinzen EL, Chitsazzadeh V, et al. SLC25A22 is a novel gene for migrating partial seizures in infancy. *Ann Neurol* 2013;**74**(6):873–882

47. Dhamija R, Wirrell E, Falcao G, Kirmani S, Wong-Kisiel LC. Novel de novo SCN2A mutation in a child with migrating focal seizures of infancy. *Pediatr Neurol* 2013;**49**(6):486–488

48. Barcia G, Fleming MR, Deligniere A, et al. De novo gain-of-function KCNT1 channel mutations cause malignant migrating partial seizures of infancy. *Nat Genet* 2012;**44**(11):1255–1259

49. Ohba C, Kato M, Takahashi S, et al. Early onset epileptic encephalopathy caused by de novo SCN8A mutations. *Epilepsia* 2014;**55**(7):994–1000

50. Coppola G, Veggiotti P, Del Giudice EM, et al. Mutational scanning of potassium, sodium and chloride ion channels in malignant migrating partial seizures in infancy. *Brain Dev* 2006;**28**(2):76–79

51. Lim BC, Hwang H, Kim H, et al. Epilepsy phenotype associated with a chromosome 2q24.3 deletion involving SCN1A: migrating partial seizures of infancy or atypical Dravet syndrome? *Epilepsy Res* 2015;**109**:34–39

52. Iyer RS, Thanikasalam, Krishnan M. Migrating partial seizures in infancy and 47XYY syndrome: cause or coincidence? *Epilepsy Behav Case Rep* 2014;**2**:43–45

53. De Filippo MR, Rizzo F, Marchese G, et al. Lack of pathogenic mutations in six patients with MMPSI. *Epilepsy Res* 2014;**108**(2):340–344

54. Merdariu D, Delanoe C, Mahfoufi N, Bellavoine V, Auvin S. Malignant migrating partial seizures of infancy controlled by stiripentol and clonazepam. *Brain Dev* 2013;**35**(2):177–180

55. Djuric M, Kravljanac R, Kovacevic G, Martic J. The efficacy of bromides, stiripentol and levetiracetam in two patients with malignant migrating partial seizures in infancy. *Epileptic Disord* 2011;**13**(1):22–26

56. Vendrame M, Poduri A, Loddenkemper T, et al. Treatment of malignant migrating partial epilepsy of infancy with rufinamide: report of five cases. *Epileptic Disord* 2011;**13**(1):18–21

57. Caraballo R, Noli D, Cachia P. Epilepsy of infancy with migrating focal seizures: three patients treated with the ketogenic diet. *Epileptic Disord* 2015;**17**(2):194–197

58. Caraballo RH, Valenzuela GR, Armeno M, et al. The ketogenic diet in two paediatric patients with refractory myoclonic status epilepticus. *Epileptic Disord* 2015;**17**(4):491–495

59. Cilio MR, Bianchi R, Balestri M, et al. Intravenous levetiracetam terminates refractory status epilepticus in two patients with migrating partial seizures in infancy. *Epilepsy Res* 2009;**86**(1):66–71

60. Irahara K, Saito Y, Sugai K, et al. Effects of acetazolamide on epileptic apnea in migrating partial seizures in infancy. *Epilepsy Res* 2011;**96**(1–2):185–189

61. Unver O, Incecik F, Dundar H, et al. Potassium bromide for treatment of malignant migrating partial seizures in infancy. *Pediatr Neurol* 2013;**49**(5):355–357

62. Saade D, Joshi C. Pure cannabidiol in the treatment of malignant migrating partial seizures in infancy: a case report. *Pediatr Neurol* 2015;**52**(5):544–547

63. Bearden D, Strong A, Ehnot J, et al. Targeted treatment of migrating partial seizures of infancy with quinidine. *Ann Neurol* 2014;**76**(3):457–461

64. Mikati MA, Jiang YH, Carboni M, et al. Quinidine in the treatment of KCNT1-positive epilepsies. *Ann Neurol* 2015;**78**(6):995–999

65. Bearden D, DiGiovine M, Dlugos D, Goldberg E. Reply. *Ann Neurol* 2016;**79**(3):503–504

66. Engel J, Jr. A proposed diagnostic scheme for people with epileptic seizures and with epilepsy: report of the ILAE Task Force on Classification and Terminology. *Epilepsia* 2001;**42**(6):796–803

67. Fujiwara T, Sugawara T, Mazaki-Miyazaki E, et al. Mutations of sodium channel alpha subunit type 1 (SCN1A) in intractable childhood epilepsies with frequent generalized tonic–clonic seizures. *Brain* 2003;**126**(Pt 3):531–546

68. Berkovic SF, Harkin L, McMahon JM, et al. De-novo mutations of the sodium channel gene SCN1A in alleged vaccine encephalopathy: a retrospective study. *Lancet Neurol* 2006;**5**(6):488–492

69. Jansen FE, Sadleir LG, Harkin LA, et al. Severe myoclonic epilepsy of infancy (Dravet syndrome): recognition and diagnosis in adults. *Neurology* 2006;**67**(12):2224–2226

70. Wolff M, Casse-Perrot C, Dravet C. Severe myoclonic epilepsy of infants (Dravet syndrome): natural history and neuropsychological findings. *Epilepsia* 2006;**47**(Suppl 2):45–48

71. Scheffer IE, Turner SJ, Dibbens LM, et al. Epilepsy and mental retardation limited to females: an

under-recognized disorder. *Brain* 2008;**131** (Pt 4):918–927

72. Devinsky O, Nabbout R, Miller I, et al. Long-term cannabidiol treatment in patients with Dravet syndrome: an open-label extension trial. *Epilepsia* 2019;**60**(2):294–302

73. Bialer M, Johannessen SI, Koepp MJ, et al. Progress report on new antiepileptic drugs: a summary of the Fourteenth Eilat Conference on New Antiepileptic Drugs and Devices (EILAT XIV). I. Drugs in preclinical and early clinical development. *Epilepsia* 2018;**59**(10):1811–1841

74. Genton P, Velizarova R, Dravet C. Dravet syndrome: the long-term outcome. *Epilepsia* 2011;**52**(Suppl 2):44–49

75. Akiyama M, Kobayashi K, Yoshinaga H, Ohtsuka Y. A long-term follow-up study of Dravet syndrome up to adulthood. *Epilepsia* 2010;**51**(6):1043–1052

76. Camfield PR. Definition and natural history of Lennox-Gastaut syndrome. *Epilepsia* 2011;**52**(Suppl 5):3–9

77. Proposal for revised classification of epilepsies and epileptic syndromes: Commission on Classification and Terminology of the International League Against Epilepsy. *Epilepsia* 1989;**30**(4):389–399

78. Scheffer IE, Berkovic S, Capovilla G, et al. ILAE classification of the epilepsies: position paper of the ILAE Commission for Classification and Terminology. *Epilepsia* 2017;**58**(4):512–521

79. Cherian A, Jabeen SA, Kandadai RM, et al. Epilepsy with myoclonic absences in siblings. *Brain Dev* 2014;**36**(10):892–898

80. Bureau M, Tassinari CA. Epilepsy with myoclonic absences. *Brain Dev* 2005;**27**(3):178–184

81. Kalviainen R. Progressive myoclonus epilepsies. *Semin Neurol* 2015;**35**(3):293–299

82. Vaca GF, Lenz T, Knight EM, Tuxhorn I. Gaucher disease: successful treatment of myoclonic status epilepticus with levetiracetam. *Epileptic Disord* 2012;**14**(2):155–158

83. Gastaut H, Tassinari CA. Triggering mechanisms in epilepsy: the electroclinical point of view. *Epilepsia* 1966;**7**(2):85–138

84. Arzimanoglou A, Resnick T. All children who experience epileptic falls do not necessarily have Lennox-Gastaut syndrome … but many do. *Epileptic Disord* 2011;**13**(Suppl 1):S3–S13

85. Arzimanoglou A, Resnick T. Diagnosing and treating epileptic drop attacks, atypical absences and episodes of nonconvulsive status epilepticus. *Epileptic Disord* 2011;**13**(Suppl 1):S1-S2

86. Wyllie E, Lachhwani DK, Gupta A, et al. Successful surgery for epilepsy due to early brain lesions despite generalized EEG findings. *Neurology* 2007;**69**(4):389–397

87. Gupta A, Chirla A, Wyllie E, et al. Pediatric epilepsy surgery in focal lesions and generalized electroencephalogram abnormalities. *Pediatr Neurol* 2007;**37**(1):8–15

88. Carvill GL, Heavin SB, Yendle SC, et al. Targeted resequencing in epileptic encephalopathies identifies de novo mutations in CHD2 and SYNGAP1. *Nat Genet* 2013;**45**(7):825–830

89. Allen AS, Berkovic SF, Cossette P, et al. De novo mutations in epileptic encephalopathies. *Nature* 2013;**501**(7466):217–221

90. Dravet C, Natale O, Magaudda A, et al. [Status epilepticus in the Lennox-Gastaut syndrome]. *Rev Electroencephalogr Neurophysiol Clin* 1986;**15**(4):361–368

91. Sinclair DB. Prednisone therapy in pediatric epilepsy. *Pediatr Neurol* 2003;**28**(3):194–198

92. Yamatogi Y, Ohtsuka Y, Ishida T, et al. Treatment of the Lennox syndrome with ACTH: a clinical and electroencephalographic study. *Brain Dev* 1979;**1**(4):267–276

93. Bello-Espinosa LE, Rajapakse T, Rho JM, Buchhalter J. Efficacy of intravenous immunoglobulin in a cohort of children with drug-resistant epilepsy. *Pediatr Neurol* 2015;**52**(5):509–516

94. Billiau AD, Witters P, Ceulemans B, et al. Intravenous immunoglobulins in refractory childhood-onset epilepsy: effects on seizure frequency, EEG activity, and cerebrospinal fluid cytokine profile. *Epilepsia* 2007;**48**(9):1739–1749

95. Kossoff EH, Krauss GL, McGrogan JR, Freeman JM. Efficacy of the Atkins diet as therapy for intractable epilepsy. *Neurology* 2003;**61**(12):1789–1791

96. Kossoff EH, McGrogan JR, Bluml RM, et al. A modified Atkins diet is effective for the treatment of intractable pediatric epilepsy. *Epilepsia* 2006;**47**(2):421–424

97. Sirven J, Whedon B, Caplan D, et al. The ketogenic diet for intractable epilepsy in adults: preliminary results. *Epilepsia* 1999;**40**(12):1721–1726

98. Lancman G, Virk M, Shao H, et al. Vagus nerve stimulation vs. corpus callosotomy in the treatment of Lennox-Gastaut syndrome: a meta-analysis. *Seizure* 2013;**22**(1):3–8

99. Iwasaki M, Uematsu M, Nakayama T, et al. Parental satisfaction and seizure outcome after corpus callosotomy in patients with infantile or early childhood onset epilepsy. *Seizure* 2013;**22**(4):303–305

100. Maehara T, Shimizu H. Surgical outcome of corpus callosotomy in patients with drop attacks. *Epilepsia* 2001;**42**(1):67–71

101. Park MS, Nakagawa E, Schoenberg MR, Benbadis SR, Vale FL. Outcome of corpus callosotomy in adults. *Epilepsy Behav* 2013;**28**(2):181–184

102. Roger J, Remy C, Bureau M, et al. [Lennox-Gastaut syndrome in the adult]. *Rev Neurol (Paris)* 1987;**143** (5):401–405

103. Boyer JP, Deschatrette A, Delwarde M. [Convulsive autism?: apropos of 9 cases of primary autism associated with the Lennox-Gastaut syndrome]. *Pediatrie* 1981;**36**(5):353–368

104. Camfield C, Camfield P. Twenty years after childhood-onset symptomatic generalized epilepsy the social outcome is usually dependency or death: a population-based study. *Dev Med Child Neurol* 2008;**50**(11):859–863

105. Doose H, Gerken H, Leonhardt R, Volzke E, Volz C. Centrencephalic myoclonic-astatic petit mal. Clinical and genetic investigation. *Neuropadiatrie* 1970;**2** (1):59–78

106. Guerrini R, Aicardi J. Epileptic encephalopathies with myoclonic seizures in infants and children (severe myoclonic epilepsy and myoclonic-astatic epilepsy). *J Clin Neurophysiol* 2003;**20**(6):449–461

107. Harkin LA, McMahon JM, Iona X, et al. The spectrum of SCN1A-related infantile epileptic encephalopathies. *Brain* 2007;**130**(Pt 3):843–852

108. Kilaru S, Bergqvist AG. Current treatment of myoclonic astatic epilepsy: clinical experience at the Children's Hospital of Philadelphia. *Epilepsia* 2007;**48** (9):1703–1707

109. Oguni H, Tanaka T, Hayashi K, et al. Treatment and long-term prognosis of myoclonic-astatic epilepsy of early childhood. *Neuropediatrics* 2002;**33**(3):122–132

110. Camfield P, Camfield C. Epileptic syndromes in childhood: clinical features, outcomes, and treatment. *Epilepsia* 2002;**43**(Suppl 3):27–32

111. Caraballo RH, Cejas N, Chamorro N, et al. Landau-Kleffner syndrome: a study of 29 patients. *Seizure* 2014;**23**(2):98–104

112. Sánchez Fernández I, Loddenkemper T, Peters JM, Kothare SV. Electrical status epilepticus in sleep: clinical presentation and pathophysiology. *Pediatr Neurol* 2012;**47**(6):390–410

113. Fernandez IS, Chapman KE, Peters JM, et al. The tower of Babel: survey on concepts and terminology in electrical status epilepticus in sleep and continuous spikes and waves during sleep in North America. *Epilepsia* 2013;**54**(4):741–750

114. Van Hirtum-Das M, Licht EA, Koh S, et al. Children with ESES: variability in the syndrome. *Epilepsy Res* 2006;**70**(Suppl 1):S248–S258

115. Loddenkemper T, Cosmo G, Kotagal P, et al. Epilepsy surgery in children with electrical status epilepticus in sleep. *Neurosurgery* 2009;**64**(2):328–337

116. Sánchez Fernández I, Chapman KE, Peters JM, et al. Continuous spikes and waves during sleep: electroclinical presentation and suggestions for management. *Epilepsy Res Treat* 2013;**2013**:583531

117. Turner SJ, Morgan AT, Perez ER, Scheffer IE. New genes for focal epilepsies with speech and language disorders. *Curr Neurol Neurosci Rep* 2015;**15**(6):35

118. Lal D, Steinbrucker S, Schubert J, et al. Investigation of GRIN2A in common epilepsy phenotypes. *Epilepsy Res* 2015;**115**:95–99

119. Vigevano F, Arzimanoglou A, Plouin P, Specchio N. Therapeutic approach to epileptic encephalopathies. *Epilepsia* 2013;**54**(Suppl 8):45–50

120. Veggiotti P, Pera MC, Teutonico F, et al. Therapy of encephalopathy with status epilepticus during sleep (ESES/CSWS syndrome): an update. *Epileptic Disord* 2012;**14**(1):1–11

121. Inutsuka M, Kobayashi K, Oka M, Hattori J, Ohtsuka Y. Treatment of epilepsy with electrical status epilepticus during slow sleep and its related disorders. *Brain Dev* 2006;**28**(5):281–286

122. Mikati MA, Shamseddine AN. Management of Landau-Kleffner syndrome. *Paediatr Drugs* 2005;**7** (6):377–389

123. Okuyaz C, Aydin K, Gucuyener K, Serdaroglu A. Treatment of electrical status epilepticus during slow-wave sleep with high-dose corticosteroid. *Pediatr Neurol* 2005;**32**(1):64–67

124. Wilson RB, Eliyan Y, Sankar R, Hussain SA. Amantadine: a new treatment for refractory electrical status epilepticus in sleep. *Epilepsy Behav* 2018;**84**:74–78

125. Gross-Selbeck G. Treatment of "benign" partial epilepsies of childhood, including atypical forms. *Neuropediatrics* 1995;**26**(1):45–50

126. Raybarman C. Landau-Kleffner syndrome: a case report. *Neurol India* 2002;**50**(2):212–213

127. Fainberg N, Harper A, Tchapyjnikov D, Mikati MA. Response to immunotherapy in a patient with Landau-Kleffner syndrome and GRIN2A mutation. *Epileptic Disord* 2016;**18**(1):97–100

128. Mikati MA, Saab R. Successful use of intravenous immunoglobulin as initial monotherapy in Landau-Kleffner syndrome. *Epilepsia* 2000;**41** (7):880–886

129. Irwin K, Birch V, Lees J, et al. Multiple subpial transection in Landau-Kleffner syndrome. *Dev Med Child Neurol* 2001;**43**(4):248–252

130. Pierson TM, Yuan H, Marsh ED, et al. GRIN2A mutation and early-onset epileptic encephalopathy: personalized therapy with memantine. *Ann Clin Transl Neurol* 2014;**1**(3):190–198

131. Ben-Ari Y, Holmes GL. Effects of seizures on developmental processes in the immature brain. *Lancet Neurol* 2006;**5**(12):1055–1063

132. Holmes GL, Lenck-Santini PP. Role of interictal epileptiform abnormalities in cognitive impairment. *Epilepsy Behav* 2006;**8**(3):504–515

133. Holmes GL. Clinical evidence that epilepsy is a progressive disorder with special emphasis on epilepsy syndromes that do progress. *Adv Neurol* 2006;**97**:323–331

134. Shatskikh TN, Raghavendra M, Zhao Q, Cui Z, Holmes GL. Electrical induction of spikes in the hippocampus impairs recognition capacity and spatial memory in rats. *Epilepsy Behav* 2006;**9**(4):549–556

135. Hernan AE, Alexander A, Lenck-Santini PP, Scott RC, Holmes GL. Attention deficit associated with early life interictal spikes in a rat model is improved with ACTH. *PLoS One* 2014;**9**(2):e89812

136. Nordli DR, Jr. Idiopathic generalized epilepsies recognized by the International League Against Epilepsy. *Epilepsia* 2005;**46**(Suppl 9):48–56

137. Janz D. Epilepsy with impulsive petit mal (juvenile myoclonic epilepsy). *Acta Neurol Scand* 1985;**72**(5):449–459

138. Wirrell EC, Camfield CS, Camfield PR, Gordon KE, Dooley JM. Long-term prognosis of typical childhood absence epilepsy: remission or progression to juvenile myoclonic epilepsy. *Neurology* 1996;**47**(4):912–918

139. Panayiotopoulos CP. Idiopathic generalized epilepsies: a review and modern approach. *Epilepsia* 2005;**46**(Suppl 9):1–6

140. Camfield CS, Camfield PR. Juvenile myoclonic epilepsy 25 years after seizure onset: a population-based study. *Neurology* 2009;**73**(13):1041–1045

141. Glauser T, Ben-Menachem E, Bourgeois B, et al. Updated ILAE evidence review of antiepileptic drug efficacy and effectiveness as initial monotherapy for epileptic seizures and syndromes. *Epilepsia* 2013;**54**(3):551–563

142. Camfield C, Camfield P. Management guidelines for children with idiopathic generalized epilepsy. *Epilepsia* 2005;**46**(Suppl 9):112–116

143. Baykan B, Altindag EA, Bebek N, et al. Myoclonic seizures subside in the fourth decade in juvenile myoclonic epilepsy. *Neurology* 2008;**70**(22 Pt 2):2123–2129

144. Striano S, Capovilla G, Sofia V, et al. Eyelid myoclonia with absences (Jeavons syndrome): a well-defined idiopathic generalized epilepsy syndrome or a spectrum of photosensitive conditions? *Epilepsia* 2009;**50**(Suppl 5):15–19

145. Engel J, Jr. Report of the ILAE classification core group. *Epilepsia* 2006;**47**(9):1558–1568

146. Jeavons PM. Nosological problems of myoclonic epilepsies in childhood and adolescence. *Dev Med Child Neurol* 1977;**19**(1):3–8

147. Yang ZX, Cai X, Liu XY, Qin J. Relationship among eye condition sensitivities, photosensitivity and epileptic syndromes. *Chin Med J (Engl)* 2008;**121**(17):1633–1637

148. Striano S, Striano P, Nocerino C, et al. Eyelid myoclonia with absences: an overlooked epileptic syndrome? *Neurophysiol Clin* 2002;**32**(5):287–296

149. Adachi N, Kanemoto K, Muramatsu R, et al. Intellectual prognosis of status epilepticus in adult epilepsy patients: analysis with Wechsler Adult Intelligence Scale-revised. *Epilepsia* 2005;**46**(9):1502–1509

150. Viravan S, Go C, Ochi A, et al. Jeavons syndrome existing as occipital cortex initiating generalized epilepsy. *Epilepsia* 2011;**52**(7):1273–1279

151. Striano P, Sofia V, Capovilla G, et al. A pilot trial of levetiracetam in eyelid myoclonia with absences (Jeavons syndrome). *Epilepsia* 2008;**49**(3):425–430

152. Jung DE, Yu R, Yoon JR, et al. Neuropsychological effects of levetiracetam and carbamazepine in children with focal epilepsy. *Neurology* 2015;**84**(23):2312–2319

153. Molokwu OA, Ezeala-Adikaibe BA, Onwuekwe IO. Levetiracetam-induced rage and suicidality: two case reports and review of literature. *Epilepsy Behav Case Rep* 2015;**4**:79–81

154. Menon R, Baheti NN, Cherian A, Iyer RS. Oxcarbazepine induced worsening of seizures in Jeavons syndrome: lessons learnt from an interesting presentation. *Neurol India* 2011;**59**(1):70–72

155. Capovilla G, Gambardella A, Rubboli G, et al. Suppressive efficacy by a commercially available blue lens on PPR in 610 photosensitive epilepsy patients. *Epilepsia* 2006;**47**(3):529–533

156. Cross JH, Jayakar P, Nordli D, et al. Proposed criteria for referral and evaluation of children for epilepsy surgery: recommendations of the Subcommission for Pediatric Epilepsy Surgery. *Epilepsia* 2006;**47**(6):952–959

157. Pestana Knight EM, Schiltz NK, Bakaki PM, et al. In response: epilepsy surgery trends in the U.S. – differences between kids and adults. *Epilepsia* 2015;**56**(8):1321–1322

158. Pestana Knight EM, Schiltz NK, Bakaki PM, et al. Increasing utilization of pediatric epilepsy surgery in the United States between 1997 and 2009. *Epilepsia* 2015;**56**(3):375–381

159. Dunkley C, Kung J, Scott RC, et al. Epilepsy surgery in children under 3 years. *Epilepsy Res* 2011;**93**(2–3):96–106

160. Gowda S, Salazar F, Bingaman WE, et al. Surgery for catastrophic epilepsy in infants 6 months of age and younger. *J Neurosurg Pediatr* 2010;**5**(6):603–607

161. Wyllie E, Comair YG, Kotagal P, Raja S, Ruggieri P. Epilepsy surgery in infants. *Epilepsia* 1996;**37**(7):625–637

162. Wyllie E, Comair Y, Ruggieri P, Raja S, Prayson R. Epilepsy surgery in the setting of periventricular leukomalacia and focal cortical dysplasia. *Neurology* 1996;**46**(3):839–841

163. Wyllie E. Surgery for catastrophic localization-related epilepsy in infants. *Epilepsia* 1996;**37**(Suppl 1):S22–S25

164. Chugani HT, Shields WD, Shewmon DA, et al. Infantile spasms: I. PET identifies focal cortical dysgenesis in cryptogenic cases for surgical treatment. *Ann Neurol* 1990;**27**(4):406–413

165. Moosa AN, Jehi L, Marashly A, et al. Long-term functional outcomes and their predictors after hemispherectomy in 115 children. *Epilepsia* 2013;**54**(10):1771–1779

166. Lee YJ, Kang HC, Lee JS, et al. Resective pediatric epilepsy surgery in Lennox–Gastaut syndrome. *Pediatrics* 2010;**125**(1):e58–e66

167. Lee YJ, Lee JS, Kang HC, et al. Outcomes of epilepsy surgery in childhood-onset epileptic encephalopathy. *Brain Dev* 2014;**36**(6):496–504

168. Moosa AN, Gupta A, Jehi L, et al. Longitudinal seizure outcome and prognostic predictors after hemispherectomy in 170 children. *Neurology* 2013;**80**(3):253–260

169. Van den Munckhof B, van D, V, Sagi L, et al. Treatment of electrical status epilepticus in sleep: a pooled analysis of 575 cases. *Epilepsia* 2015;**56**(11):1738–1746

170. Sillanpaa M, Jalava M, Kaleva O, Shinnar S. Long-term prognosis of seizures with onset in childhood. *N Engl J Med* 1998;**338**(24):1715–1722

171. Looman WS, Lindeke LL. Children and youth with special health care needs: partnering with families for effective advocacy. *J Pediatr Health Care* 2008;**22**(2):134–136

172. Camfield PR, Gibson PA, Douglass LM. Strategies for transitioning to adult care for youth with Lennox–Gastaut syndrome and related disorders. *Epilepsia* 2011;**52**(Suppl 5):21–27

173. Blum RW. Introduction: improving transition for adolescents with special health care needs from pediatric to adult-centered health care. *Pediatrics* 2002;**110**(6 Pt 2):1301–1303

174. Kelly AM, Kratz B, Bielski M, Rinehart PM. Implementing transitions for youth with complex chronic conditions using the medical home model. *Pediatrics* 2002;**110**(6 Pt 2):1322–1327

Medication-Resistant Epilepsy in Adults

Martin Holtkamp and Felix Benninger

Mesial Temporal Lobe Epilepsy

The temporal lobe epilepsies (TLE) are widely heterogeneous with regard to aetiology, age at onset, prognosis and response to treatment. An important distinction on topographic grounds is made between mesial (MTLE) and lateral temporal lobe epilepsy (LTLE).

Introduction

MTLE is the most common form of focal epilepsy in adults. It is usually sporadic without a family history, but can present with clear familial occurrence. The unique connectivity in the mesial temporal lobe (MTL) is responsible for the high epileptogenic potential, and the entorhinal cortex and amygdalo-hippocampal complex have particular importance. The temporal lobe is the most epileptogenic region of the human brain, and about 80% of temporal lobe seizures originate in the hippocampus. Its epileptogenic potential has been studied extensively and includes channelopathies, as well as cell-type-specific malfunction (e.g. interneuronopathies) all converging towards a hippocampal circuitry dysfunction characterized by neuronal hyperexcitability.

Seizure Semiology

The majority (up to 90%) of seizures with impaired awareness arising from the MTL manifest with various simple or complex illusions or auras [1]. These can also occur in isolation, and the most common auras generated in the MTL are characterized by autonomic symptoms like abdominal discomfort or nausea rising towards the throat (epigastric aura). Further ictal psychic symptoms, especially fear but also other emotions and distorted memories (déjà-vu, déjà-vecu, déjà-entendu, jamais vu, jamais entendu), flashbacks or rapid recollections of memories from the past are common [2,3]. Dysphasic symptoms can occur, but might be difficult to distinguish from negative motor symptoms (speech arrest). Besides those subjective ictal

phenomena typical for seizures arising in the MTL (also termed limbic seizures), automatisms are classic early motor symptoms. Often believed to involve neighbouring limbic structures, these consist of swallowing, lip smacking and chewing (oroalimentary automatisms) or more complex repetitive movements like gestures, picking of clothes or stereotypical verbalizations (calling a name, 'mmh, mmh', 'oh no'). Dystonic posturing and versive movements are often observed, but are not specific for MTL seizures and can be seen in frontal lobe seizures as well. Early head or body turning can be directed towards the side of seizure origin. These clinical signs are not considered to be of high lateralizing value, yet their occurrence just before secondary generalization is correlated well with ictal onset in the contralateral hemisphere. Loss of awareness during seizures and especially post-ictal confusion are typical for seizures with onset in limbic structures propagating to other parts of the temporal lobe, but propagation to produce a tonic–clonic seizure is infrequent with ASM treatment [4].

Inter-Ictal and Ictal EEG Patterns

In MTLE, spikes or sharp waves are seen in up to 90% of inter-ictal EEGs. These are usually located in the anterior temporal regions, and basal electrodes or additional cheek or sphenoidal electrodes can improve detection. Spike frequency has been suggested as a useful biomarker for the extent of epileptogenicity, as its increase is correlated with unfavourable surgical outcome [5]. Up to one-third of patients show bilateral temporal inter-ictal epileptiform discharges. Intermittent slowing in the theta or delta range (lateralized rhythmic delta activity) is seen in a minority of patients, but is highly associated with TLE. In up to 60% of patients, the EEG can be normal at the beginning of the seizure. The typical ictal EEG pattern consists of regular rhythmic focal anterior temporal theta activity and has a high lateralizing value. The rhythmic theta activity usually

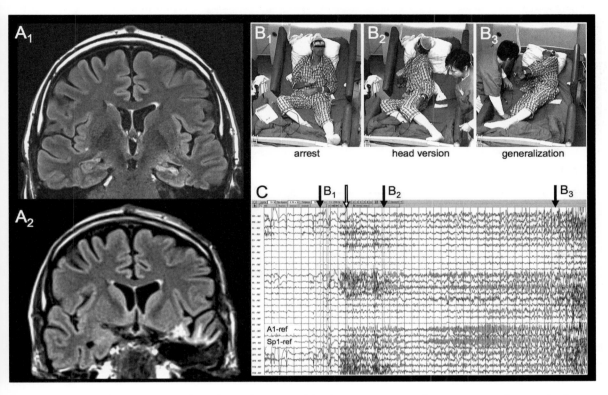

Figure 14.1 Case 1: Mesial temporal lobe epilepsy. This 57-year-old male patient experienced at age 28 years a first episode of unresponsiveness and staring, undirected activities of his hands and chewing movements. These episodes occurred repeatedly with increasing frequency; they were further followed by arbitrary actions in which different objects fell from his hands, leading to spilled coffee or broken dishes. Occasionally, he would fall causing injuries. Rarely, these episodes were trailed by generalized tonic–clonic convulsions and a post-ictal period of aphasia with right hand weakness. His inter-ictal scalp EEG showed a normal background rhythm of 8 Hz with left temporal slowing and epilepsy-typical potentials in left anterior temporal recordings. A 3 T MRI of his brain exposed an atrophic left hippocampus and an enhanced signal on the FLAIR sequence (A₁) compatible with left hippocampal sclerosis. He was treated with carbamazepine, reducing seizure frequency, but he never gained seizure freedom. After unsuccessful therapeutic trials with two more anti-seizure medications, he was admitted to pre-surgical epilepsy monitoring. Two typical episodes were captured presenting with arrest of the patient and orofacial automatisms (B₁), forced head version to the right (B₂) followed by seizure generalization (B₃). The correlating surface EEG seizure pattern started 3 seconds after the first behavioural changes with high-amplitude rhythmic theta activity in left anterior temporal electrodes (C; white arrow indicates seizure onset at electrodes SP1 and A1). The patient underwent left anterior temporal lobectomy with amygdalohippocampectomy as demonstrated in the post-operative MRI (A₂). Histopathology revealed hippocampal sclerosis Wyler IV. A slight left facial nerve paresis was observed post-surgery, but the patient has become free of seizures on a combination therapy of levetiracetam and lacosamide for now more than one year (Engel Ia).

evolves, but can be waxing–waning [4] and, unlike seizures from other brain regions, fast spikes or other high-frequency rhythmic discharges are relatively uncommon. Ictal EEG changes at the onset of clinical signs or symptoms were reported by Williamson et al. in only 6% of 67 patients [6]. In MTLE, the seizure-onset zone is difficult to determine using surface EEG in some cases. This might be due to early spread to extratemporal structures or to the contralateral MTL, thus providing discordant information on EEG changes and seizure semiology.

Intra-cranial EEG recordings using subdural strip electrodes or depth electrodes are necessary to localize the seizure-onset zone in such cases. Especially in patients undergoing epilepsy surgery, correct localization of the seizure-onset zone is crucial for favourable post-surgical outcome.

Pathomorphological entities

By far the most common cause of seizures originating in the MTL is hippocampal sclerosis (HS). Other causes include hamartomas or glial tumours, vascular

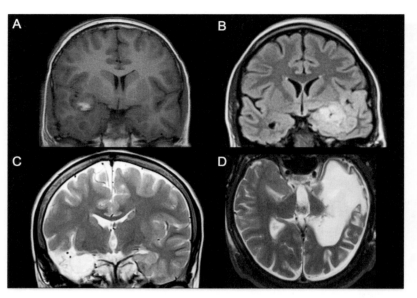

Figure 14.2 Examples of pathologies underlying mesial temporal lobe epilepsy. (A) Right-sided histologically verified ganglioglioma in a 20-year-old male patient with epilepsy since the age of 13 years. (B) Histologically verified DNET in the left temporal lobe with mesial preponderance in a 19-year-old female patient with epilepsy since the age of 12 years. (C) Right-sided mesio-temporal and temporo-basal post-encephalitic lesion in an 18-year-old female patient with PCR-proven herpes simplex type I encephalitis at the age of 11 months and epilepsy since then. (D) Extended left temporal post-traumatic lesion involving mesio-temporal structures in a 41-year-old male patient with traumatic brain injury at the age of 18 years and epilepsy since the age of 23 years.

and congenital malformations, and gliotic lesions due to trauma or infections, but all those have been less common than HS.

Hippocampal Sclerosis

In MTLE, atrophy combined with astrogliosis of the amygdala, hippocampus, parahippocampal gyrus and entorhinal cortex is the most common pathology found in pre-operative MRI studies, as well as in histopathology after epilepsy surgery. This pathologic entity HS is found in about 65% of all patients with MTLE. Prolonged febrile seizures have been associated with the development of HS as they may induce hippocampal oedema. Up to two-thirds of patients with MTLE report a febrile seizure history [1]. The FEBSTAT study included 226 children with febrile status epilepticus and identified an association with acute hippocampal changes on MRI imaging (T2 hyperintensity). When compared to controls with simple febrile seizures, reduced hippocampal growth and imaging features of HS were present after one year [7].

High-resolution MRI imaging is sufficient to visualize most HS in vivo, based on features of reduced hippocampal volume, increased signal intensity on T2-weighted or FLAIR imaging, and disturbed internal architecture. MRI evidence of HS is not necessarily related to seizure severity. Similar changes have been described in individuals who never experienced seizures. FDG-PET in HS demonstrates inter-ictal hypometabolism that appears more widespread than the pathology seen on structural MRI. Without MRI, it is practically impossible to make the correct intra vitam diagnosis of HS with exclusion of other aetiologies underlying MTLE.

Dual pathology indicates the presence of HS and an additional pathology and occurs in 5–20% of patients with HS. It can include cortical developmental tumours (dysembryoplastic neuroepithelial tumour or DNET), malformations of cortical development (MCD) and acquired brain lesions. In cases of dual pathology, bilateral hippocampal atrophy is more common.

Other Aetiologies

Semiologically, MTL seizures caused by HS are indistinguishable from those caused by other aetiologies. Regarding specific aetiologies, tumours are a common identifiable cause of new-onset epilepsy, and the site and spatial distance of the tumour to the cortex determine seizure incidence. Low-grade and slow-growing tumours are the most epileptogenic, and Le Blanc and Rasmussen showed that oligodendrogliomas had the highest epileptogenic potential (92%) followed by astrocytomas (70%) and glioblastomas (35%) [8]. The reason for the high epileptogenicity of rather benign tumours is still debated.

Gangliogliomas have a predilection for the frontal and temporal lobes and are found to be over-represented in patients with chronic epilepsy. DNETs followed represent approximately 8% of all lesional cases of TLE. They occur mainly in the temporal lobe, but can be found in the frontal lobe as well. Surgical outcomes can be excellent, and, in some series, have a higher seizure freedom rate than that of other MTLE aetiologies. Focal cortical dysplasia (FCD) is a common cause of medically intractable epilepsy in children and young adults. In various studies on TLE, the prevalence of FCD ranges from 9–45% and can either present alone or additionally to other pathologies, such as HS or developmental tumours. Vascular malformations, including arteriovenous malformations (AVM) or cavernous angiomas, present a seizure risk of approximately 1.5% per person-year. For AVMs, seizures are the second most common presenting sign – after new-onset neurological deficits due to haemorrhage – and occur in about 40 to 70% of cavernous angioma instances. Infectious causes for MTL seizures have been described. The association between the human herpes virus 6 (HHV6) and the development of HS is still debated. During viral encephalitis, acute-symptomatic temporal lobe seizures can be observed, and, depending on the lesion extent, chronic TLE may develop. This is especially seen after herpes simplex virus 1 (HSV1) encephalitis, typically involving the temporal lobe and has been described in HHV6 encephalitis in the immune-compromised host. Neurocysticercosis (NCC) is worldwide the most common infectious neurological disorder, and in recent years an association between NCC and the development of MTLE has been suggested.

Response to Treatment

More than 60% of patients with focal epilepsy will become seizure-free with the use of ASMs. Once the first drug fails, the chances of becoming seizure-free are drastically reduced, and only about 10% achieve seizure freedom with additional ASMs. In a hospital-based observational study, patients with MTLE achieved seizure freedom in only 20%, and HS and dual pathology were associated with the lowest rate of seizure freedom [9]. Thus, all patients proving to be resistant to medical treatment should undergo thorough evaluation for epilepsy surgery. In two randomized prospective trials comparing medical to surgical treatment for medication-resistant MTLE, seizure freedom was achieved in 58% and 73% in the surgical groups, compared to 8% and 0% in the medical treatment groups [10,11]. In light of this overwhelming superiority of epilepsy surgery compared to medical

treatment in intractable epilepsy, the low referral rate of patients for epilepsy surgery evaluation leaves enormous space for improvement [12].

Neocortical Epilepsies

Introduction

Epilepsies confined to neocortical structures by nature are highly heterogeneous with regard to seizure semiology, and detailed history-taking on auras and other seizure types, as well as analysis of video-EEG may contribute to identifying the localization of the seizure-onset zone. Aetiologies cover a broad spectrum, from congenital abnormalities to acquired lesions; furthermore, a relevant number of patients suffer from neocortical epilepsy of unknown cause. Autosomal dominant frontal or temporal lobe epilepsies commonly demonstrate a favourable response to pharmacological treatment and therefore are not covered in this chapter. In intractable neocortical epilepsies, application of potential surgical treatment approaches is determined by the localization and extent of the seizure-onset zone regarding overlap with functionally relevant brain structures and technical feasibility.

Seizure Semiology

Lateral Temporal Lobe Seizures

In partial epilepsies, temporal lobe seizures make up approximately 60% of all seizures and they predominantly arise in mesial structures. It is estimated that only 10% of temporal lobe seizures are confined to the neocortex. The International League against Epilepsy (ILAE) recognizes a distinction between mesial and lateral forms of TLE. Focal seizures from lateral structures are characterized by auditory hallucinations or illusions, visual misperceptions, or language disorders, when affecting the language-dominant hemisphere. Psychic alterations comprising déjà and jamais vu, fear and depersonalization may also occur. These may progress to complex partial seizures if propagation to mesiotemporal or extratemporal structures occur [13]. Ictal clinical signs supporting MTLE in contrast to lateral onset include manual and oral automatisms, body shifting and dystonic posturing. However, differentiation between lateral and mesial TLE based on seizure semiology alone may be difficult and of limited reliability, as some ictal signs and symptoms can occur in both conditions.

Frontal Lobe Seizures

In patients with intractable partial epilepsy, approximately 20–25% of all seizures arise from frontal lobe structures. Due to the diverse functional anatomy of the frontal lobe, seizure semiology accordingly is heterogeneous. The ILAE orders frontal lobe seizures following distinction into seven anatomical regions: primary motor cortex, dorsolateral region, operculum, anterior frontopolar region, orbitofrontal region, cingulate gyrus and supplementary motor area [13]. Applying a rougher allocation, the latter two regions are referred to as the medial frontal lobe and the former four regions are summarized as the lateral frontal lobe, while the orbitofrontal region is not combined with another region. However, there is some overlap between these three groups.

Primary motor cortex: Focal motor seizures are characterized by unilateral clonic twitching – rather than tonic contractions – of contralateral muscle groups with fully preserved consciousness. Propagation of epileptic activity may follow the motor homunculus and manifest clinically as the well-known Jacksonian march.

Dorsolateral region: This brain area comprises the premotor and the prefrontal cortex, and, according to some authors, the primary motor cortex, which has already been discussed above. Seizures from the premotor area are typically characterized by contralateral deviation of the eyes and head version. If seizure activity spreads further, version extends to the trunk, commonly resulting in secondary generalization of the seizure.

Seizures arising in prefrontal areas are more prominent. They ordinarily commence with a somatosensory aura followed by hypermotor activity, including bizarre gestures, shouting, bicycle peddling and thrashing of the extremities [14]. These seizures are usually of short duration and they commonly manifest in sleep. In both premotor and prefrontal seizures, consciousness in not impaired.

Operculum: Typical ictal signs are mastication, salivation, swallowing and speech arrest. Patients may experience epigastric aura, fear or autonomic phenomena. Partial clonic facial seizures may be seen ipsilaterally.

Anterior frontopolar region: Ictal seizure patterns include forced thinking or initial loss of contact, and adversive movements of head and eyes possibly evolving into contraversive movements.

Orbitofrontal region: This structure generates complex partial seizures with initial motor and gestural automatisms. Auras are very common and consist of olfactory sensations. Autonomic seizures may also be seen; these comprise cardiovascular, respiratory, gastrointestinal, cutaneous or urogenital signs.

Cingulate gyrus: Typical are complex partial seizures with impaired consciousness and complex stereotypic movements, such as thrashing, kicking, grasping and running, with or without vocalization at onset. Autonomic signs are common, as are changes in mood and affect. A semiological study from the Epilepsy-Center Bonn compared frontal lobe seizures with either lateral frontal, orbitofrontal or medial frontal onset. Medial frontal seizures were, among other ictal signs, significantly associated with facial expression of anxiety and fear, restlessness, and body turning along the horizontal axis, all of which reliably distinguished seizure onset in medial from lateral frontal and orbitofrontal structures [15].

Supplementary motor area: Typical semiological seizure patterns are postural, focal tonic, with vocalization, speech arrest and autonomic signs. Seizures are frequent and often occur during sleep [13]. They are characterized by sudden, brief and asymmetric tonic posturing commonly of bilateral extremities. Ictal manifestations include the 'fencing posture' with extended contralateral upper extremity, flexed ipsilateral arm abducted at the shoulder and the head rotated contralateral to the seizure-onset zone, as well as the 'figure of four' with extension of the contralateral upper extremity across the chest and ipsilateral arm flexion at the elbow [16]. Consciousness is preserved during seizures.

Parieto-Occipital Lobe Seizures

Seizures in parieto-occipital structures are predominantly sensory with many different characteristics. In part, this variability in auras is due to the abundance of association cortex allowing for rapid spread of ictal activity within and beyond these structures.

In the landmark report from the Montréal Epilepsy Group, summarizing 82 patients with parietal lobe epilepsy who underwent surgery, 94%

exhibited auras. The most common were somatosensory (64% of patients); a quarter of those patients also described pain. Further auras comprised disturbances of body image, visual illusions, vertiginous sensations, and aphasia or dysphasia. Commonly, ictal semiology indicated seizure spread to frontal or mesio-temporal structures [17]. In the vast majority of patients, somatosensory auras are contralateral to the seizure focus, but manifestation may also be ipsilateral or bilateral.

In occipital lobe epilepsy, clinical seizure manifestation usually includes visual symptoms. In more than half of the cases, elementary visual hallucinations with blurred vision, blindness, flashing or field defects may occur. Sensations in elementary visual seizures appear in the visual field contralateral to the seizure focus in the specific visual cortex, but ictal activity can spread to the entire visual field [13]. Impaired consciousness or motor signs even at seizure onset may indicate rapid spread of activity to temporal or frontal structures.

Inter-Ictal and Ictal EEG Patterns

In TLE, inter-ictal epileptiform activity detected by scalp EEG is seen in 80–90% of patients. When the epileptogenic abnormality is mesial, the inter-ictal activity is commonly observed over the anterior temporal lobe because of projection laterally. Scalp EEG seizure patterns are often characterized by rhythmic theta activity and this is not specific when differentiating lateral from mesial temporal onset. Extratemporally generated seizures may exhibit a misleading lateral temporal seizure pattern.

Inter-ictal EEG in frontal lobe epilepsy (FLE) often is non-diagnostic; in up to 40% of patients, no discharges in surface EEG can be demonstrated. Identification of the epileptogenic zone by inter-ictal surface EEG is significantly less precise in medial frontal compared to dorsolateral structures. This is due to the distance between mesial frontal cortex and electrodes, and due to the tangential orientation of dipoles to the scalp hindering successful surface recording [18].

Frontal lobe seizures are more difficult to characterize by surface EEG than temporal lobe seizures, which is why intra-cranial EEG is more often undertaken in the evaluation of epilepsy from frontal structures. Reasons for these difficulties include the difficulty visualizing ictal scalp EEG patterns when seizures originate from medial and orbitofrontal regions, often abrupt manifestation of motor activity with massive movement artifacts, and common occurrence of rapid bilateral synchrony. All this impedes regionalization, lateralization and sometimes detection of seizure onset in FLE.

In dorsolateral FLE, ictal scalp EEG demonstrates correct localization of the epileptogenic zone in two-thirds of patients. The most frequent EEG seizure onset patterns are repetitive epileptiform activity, rhythmic delta activity and EEG suppression, while rhythmic theta activity, the most frequent pattern in TLE, is seen in less than 10% of frontal lobe seizures [19].

In medial FLE, the broad spectrum of ictal EEG findings includes rhythmic delta to beta activity, repetitive epileptiform discharges and diffuse attenuation. In the vast majority of seizures, the ictal EEG pattern occurs in a generalized fashion, which is seen here significantly more often than in any other brain region [19].

In the surgical evaluation of FLE, intra-cranial EEG recording is frequently required in order to define the epileptogenic zone and to delineate functional cortex. Subdural grids and strips and/or depth electrodes are applied according to the hypothesis for seizure focus localization. In intra-cranial EEG, rapid seizure spread is an independent predictor for poor surgical outcome [20].

In parieto-occipital epilepsies, surface inter-ictal and ictal EEG findings may be inconclusive in a considerable number of patients. In the Montréal study on surgery for parietal lobe epilepsy, surface EEG was available in 66 patients; the region demonstrating inter-ictal epileptiform activity most frequently was fronto-centro-parietal (22 patients), 3 patients had bilateral discharges and 5 patients had none [17]. Ictal discharges were predominantly lateralized; localized parietal seizure onset was recorded in 4 out of 66 patients, only.

The Montréal epilepsy group reported 42 patients with occipital lobe epilepsy who underwent pre-surgical assessment between 1930 and 1991. In 39 of these, scalp EEG recordings were available, and inter-ictal epileptiform activity was restricted to the occipital lobe in only 7 patients (18%). The most common location of inter-ictal epileptiform discharges was the posterior temporal-occipital region (46%) [21]. Scalp ictal EEG recordings revealed few

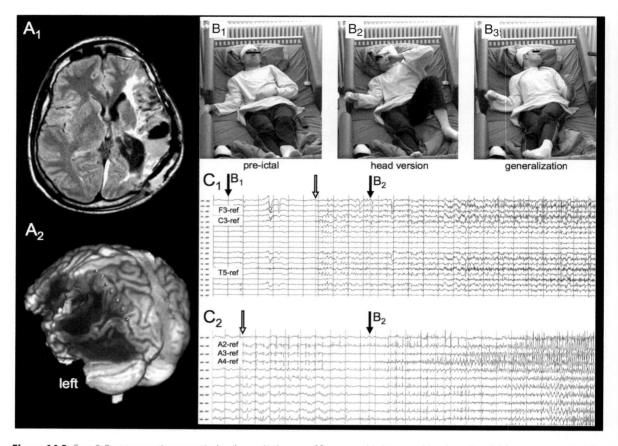

Figure 14.3 Case 2: Post-traumatic neocortical epilepsy. At the age of five years, this 34-year-old male patient fell from an open third-floor window and suffered severe left hemispheric traumatic brain injury. In addition to a moderate right-sided spastic hemiparesis and homonymous hemianopsia, he started to suffer from monthly epileptic seizures initiated by a non-specific aura, turning of the head to the right and rhythmic right arm movements without loss of consciousness, lasting approximately two minutes. About once a year, these fits develop into generalized tonic–clonic seizures. Previously, he failed to respond to anti-convulsant treatment with phenobarbital, carbamazepine, oxcarbazepine, valproic acid, levetiracetam and lacosamide in adequate doses. MRI imaging of his brain showed an extended left hemispheric lesion with enlarged lateral ventricles and hippocampal volume loss (A$_1$ and A$_2$). Inter-ictal EEG demonstrated a diffuse left-sided slowing, with fronto-central-temporal spikes and polyspikes. During video-EEG recordings with surface electrodes, one seizure was captured. Four seconds before any clinical changes (B$_1$), an EEG seizure correlate with rhythmic epileptiform discharges was seen left fronto-centro-temporally (C$_1$; white arrow indicates seizure onset at electrodes C3, F3, T5) followed by a forced head and body version to the right (B$_2$) and clonic right arm movements, which further on generalized (B$_3$). Due to the extent of the lesion and the undefined localization of seizure onset by surface EEG, subdural strip electrodes were implanted on left frontal, temporal and parietal brain structures. Two behavioural seizures were recorded; ictal EEG demonstrated seizure onset with high-amplitude spiking (C$_2$; white arrow indicates seizure onset at electrodes A2 to A4; latency to first clinical signs 8 seconds and thus 4 seconds earlier compared to scalp recording) and secondary spread of activity to adjacent electrodes within the next 5–10 seconds. A tailored cortical resection of brain structures underneath electrodes A2 to A6 and just below the sulcus parallel to the upper posterior margin of the lesion was performed. During follow-up of, so far, six months, the patient has remained free of epileptic seizures on stable ASM medication. Interestingly, he had experienced post-operatively two new-onset psychogenic non-epileptic seizures with bilateral undulating motor signs of upper and lower extremities, accompanied by closed eyes.

patients demonstrating onset within one occipital lobe, and most patients having ictal onsets involving adjacent parietal and temporal structures [21]. Intra-cranial EEG frequently shows widespread areas of seizure onset with rapid spread into temporal and frontal structures.

Correlation of intra-cranial EEG ictal onset patterns to the underlying pathology recently demonstrated that periodic spikes were specific for mesial temporal sclerosis, and delta brush (rhythmic delta waves at 1–2 Hz with superimposed brief bursts at 20–30 Hz) occurred more often in focal cortical dysplasia [22].

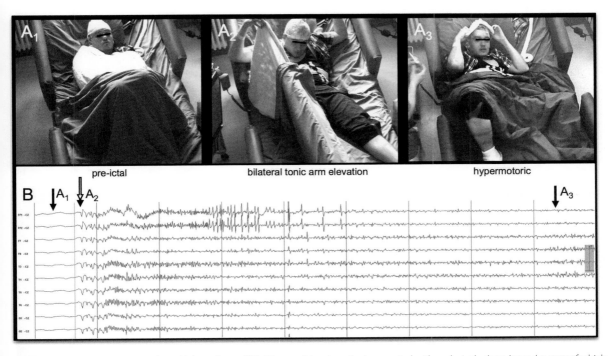

Figure 14.4 Case 3: Cryptogenic frontal lobe epilepsy. This 27-year-old male patient presented with exclusively sleep-bound events of which he does not have any recollection. Family members described a sudden awakening, both arms violently raised, then rhythmic arm movements with opened eyes and rarely followed by unrest, after which the patient continues sleeping. These events started at age two years, but today frequency could not be determined as he lives alone. An MRI of his brain was not showing any pathology, and awake inter-ictal EEG was read as normal. Medical treatment with high doses of topiramate, stiripentol, phenobarbital, oxcarbazepine, phenytoin, felbamate, levetiracetam and lacosamide failed to control the events or caused significant side effects. During admission and long-term video-EEG monitoring over seven days, up to 40 stereotypical events with sudden eye opening and bilateral tonic raising of his arms (A$_2$) occasionally followed by hypermotor movements (A$_3$) were captured. The first clinical signs suggest seizure onset in the supplemental motor area, then propagation into prefrontal structures, no clear hints for lateralization. First ictal EEG changes (B, white arrow) occur simultaneously with clinical onset; they are characterized by rhythmic discharges with bifrontal preponderance at 10–12 Hz for <0.5 seconds, then generalized low-amplitude fast activity, and after another 2 seconds bifrontal epileptiform discharges. The patient was recommended implantation of depth electrodes in bilateral mesial and dorsolateral frontal lobe structures; his decision is pending.

Pathomorphological Entities

Malformation of Cortical Development and Vascular Malformations

In intractable partial epilepsy, malformations of cortical development (MCD) are found as the underlying cause in approximately 8% of patients [9]. The most frequent MCDs are heterotopia and FCDs. Heterotopia are commonly located in subcortical structures or periventricularly. When periventricular, the intrinsic epileptogenicity may be in either the periventricular heterotopion, the overlying neocortex or both. FCDs are highly variable with regard to the localization and extent of the lesion. FCD type I may be invisible on MRI, may be focal or affect a larger region or multiple lobes, and has a diversity of epilepsy

severity and age of onset. FCD Type II is typically focal, but may be part of a larger malformation of cortical development, and also has a diversity of epilepsy severity. Neurologic dysfunction for both FCD I and II often relates to the anatomic extent of the abnormality.

Vascular malformations such as AVM or cavernoma may be found in 1–2% of patients with medication-resistant focal epilepsy. They are primarily located in the white matter, but may have close proximity to cortical structures, allowing them to generate epileptic seizures. Vascular malformations may occur in all brain lobes.

Neoplasms

In half of patients with primary brain tumours, epileptic seizures are the first clinical manifestation. Benign tumours are more likely associated with epilepsy than

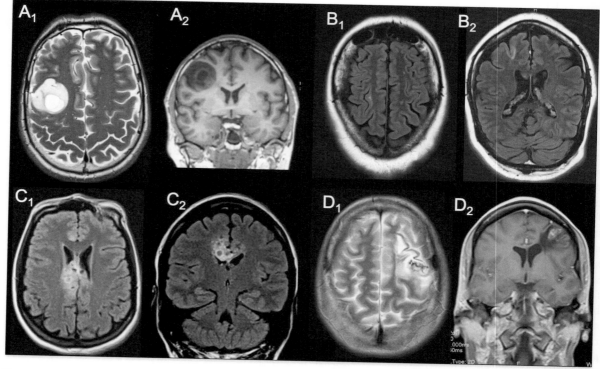

Figure 14.5 Examples of pathologies underlying neocortical epilepsies. (A) Right fronto-temporal astrocytoma II in a 49-year-old male patient with epilepsy since the age of 44 years. (B) Right frontal focal cortical dysplasia in a 41-year-old male patient with epilepsy since the age of six years. Some months before the scheduled resection, the patient had died of probable SUDEP (sudden unexplained death in epilepsy). (C) Space-occupying, polycystic bilateral mesial frontal lesion (with left-sided preponderance) in a 37-year-old female patient with partial epilepsy since the age of six years. Histology demonstrated DNET of complex variant with focally increased proliferation rate. (D) Arterio-venous malformation with surrounding post-haemorrhagic defect zone in left lateral frontal structures in a 29-year-old female patient with partial epilepsy since the age of 21 years.

malignant variants. Almost all patients with DNET and with gangliogliomas have epilepsy. In contrast, glioblastoma multiforme, primary central nervous system lymphoma and metastasis are associated with epilepsy in less than 50% of cases. While new-onset focal epilepsy may be caused by brain tumours in 7% of cases, intractable epilepsy can be attributed to neoplasia in only 1%.

Traumatic Brain Injury

Severe traumatic brain injury (TBI) is associated with a 20% risk of developing epilepsy within 30 years. TBI is the cause of either new-onset or intractable focal epilepsy in 5% of patients. Location of the post-traumatic lesion is determined by how the initial trauma affected the brain.

Cerebrovascular Lesions

In new-onset epilepsy, stroke is the most likely aetiology in 10% of cases. In patients 65 years and older,

epilepsy is caused by remote cerebrovascular accidents in 23%. Intractable focal epilepsy can be attributed to former stroke in 3–4% of cases. The vast majority of ischaemic strokes affect the anterior circulation, most likely resulting in frontal or temporal lobe epilepsy. Interestingly, thalamic strokes in adults do not seem to be associated with increased epileptogenicity.

Post-Encephalitic Lesions

Infectious or autoimmune-mediated encephalitis is followed by epilepsy in 25–30% of patients. HSV1 encephalitis has a predilection for the temporal lobe, which in particular has a low threshold for the generation of epileptic seizures. It is difficult to estimate in how many cases refractory partial epilepsy is caused by post-encephalitic lesions, as available data report MRI findings such as non-specific 'scars' or 'lesions' rather than underlying aetiologies.

Response to Treatment

In neocortical epilepsy, seizure freedom rates are determined by the brain structure affected and, even more, by the underlying pathology. Seizures arising from the temporal lobe seem to be less likely controlled (20%) than extratemporal seizures (35%) [9]. More than 50% of patients with post-stroke epilepsy are seizure-free, but this is true for only 30% of patients with post-traumatic epilepsy and for 24% of patients with MCDs [9]. All patients with medication-resistant focal epilepsies should undergo comprehensive pre-surgical assessment; however, only a minority of those patients is eligible for surgery. Sustained post-surgery seizure freedom is reported in 50–70% of patients; main predictors are a well-defined lesion as underlying cause and seizure onset in temporal structures. If patients with medication-resistant epilepsy do not qualify for or fail resective surgery, neurostimulation may be considered. Among all stimulation treatments currently licensed in Europe or the USA, i.e. vagus nerve stimulation, deep brain stimulation of the anterior thalamus and responsive stimulation of the epileptogenic focus, seizure freedom rates are 10% or less and may only be temporary; short-term responder rates (>50% reduction in seizure frequency) are 30–40% and thus comparable to a new anti-seizure medication.

Gelastic Epilepsy with Hypothalamic Hamartoma

Introduction

Hypothalamic hamartomas (HH) are a rare congenital malformation located in the ventral hypothalamus. HH are often associated with epileptic seizures, a clinico-pathological syndrome with a prevalence of 0.5 to 1 in 100 000 individuals. The semiological hallmark is seizures with mirthless laughter for which the term 'gelastic seizures' has been used. Intrinsic epileptogenicity of the HH is capable of generating gelastic seizures, as has been proven by depth electrode recordings [23].

The clinical spectrum is heterogeneous, ranging from severe forms with childhood onset and occurrence of multiple seizure types, epileptic encephalo-pathy with deteriorating behaviour and cognitive functions, and precocious puberty to milder forms with adult onset lacking progressive functional impairment.

Though our understanding of mechanisms underlying HH associated with epilepsy has improved within the last decades, we are still confronted with questions of why the response to therapeutic resection or destruction of the hamartoma is poor.

Seizure Semiology

Gelastic seizures – as defined by Gascon and Lombroso in 1971 – are 'stereotypic recurrence of ictal laughter, unrelated to context, associated with other signs compatible with seizure and with ictal/inter-ictal EEG abnormalities' [24]. Those other ictal signs comprise loss of muscle tone, running, crying ('dacrystic seizure'), and ballisto-choreic movements. Laughter or sometimes just a smile is mechanical and lacks a sense of mirth. Gelastic seizures are usually of short duration (<10 seconds), frequency may be up to several times daily and seizure clusters are not uncommon. In young children with HH and epilepsy, gelastic seizures or gelastic components of seizures are predominant, while they are less frequent in adult patients. Gelastic seizures are almost pathognomonic for HH, as they are rarely seen in frontal or temporal lobe epilepsy.

Other seizure types are commonly seen in HH-related epilepsy, including unilateral tonic, clonic and tonic–clonic, as well as atonic and complex partial seizures. These seizures may have an initial gelastic component and then evolve to other semiologies. Secondarily generalized tonic–clonic seizures do not occur in children, but are frequent in adolescents and adults with childhood onset. This finding may argue for secondary epileptogenesis in initially normal brain structures beyond HH.

EEG Patterns

Inter-ictal and ictal scalp EEG findings seem to be of limited value in hypothalamic hamartoma-associated epilepsy. Depth electrode recordings from within the hamartoma have been reported in two patients. In one patient, focal spikes were recorded and stimulation resulted in habitual seizures with a funny feeling in the head followed by laughing for 15 seconds [25]. In the other patient, multiple gelastic seizures were recorded from the hamartoma demonstrating low-amplitude fast activity at seizure onset followed by rapid spike-wave discharges with decreasing frequency [23].

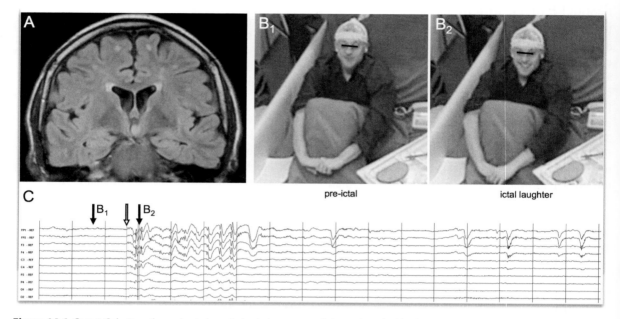

Figure 14.6 Case 4: Gelastic epilepsy due to hypothalamic hamartoma. Seizures described by this 27-year-old male patient consist of sudden unrest followed by laughter lasting 2–3 seconds after which the patient returns to his previous activities. Additionally, he has rare seizures with an unspecific aura, bilateral tonic arm elevations and generalization since four years of age. Previous medication with phenytoin, carbamazepine and oxcarbazepine did reduce frequency but did not achieve seizure freedom. A vagus nerve stimulator did not improve his seizure situation. During video-EEG monitoring, several seizures were captured, including a sudden upright sitting in the bed (B$_1$) followed by laughter (B$_2$) without impaired awareness. During those events, the surface EEG at onset (1 second prior to behavioural changes) showed non-lateralized fronto-central low-amplitude fast activity, which is directly followed by a bilateral frontal polyspikes and spike-wave complexes for the period of laughter (C). A 3 T MRI of his brain revealed a hyperintense lesion on FLAIR in the hypothalamus consistent with a hypothalamic hamartoma (A). The patient was treated by iodine-125 seed implant at age 19 years; he improved temporarily, but now he still suffers ongoing seizures.

Imaging and Neuropathology

With structural MRI, HH are hyperintense on T2-weighted images, and in the majority of patients, hypointense on T1-weighted images. Commonly, HH are nestled between the fornix, the mammillary body and the mamillo-thalamic tract. HH volume is approximately 1–3 cm^3; volume does not depend on the duration of epilepsy, demonstrating a lack of growth over time. Morphological changes beyond the HH, which are detectable by MRI, are rather rare. Functional neuroimaging using PET and SPECT has demonstrated ictal hyperperfusion in HH further arguing that seizures are directly generated in that structure.

Neuropathologically, HH at first hand is a developmental, non-neoplastic disorganized network of astrocytes and neurons that is conceptually comparable to cortical dysplasia and lesions in tuberous sclerosis complex. Small gamma-aminobutyric acid

(GABA)-expressing neurons which discharge spontaneously and drive the synchrony of large pyramidal-like neurons constitute the pathophysiological basis of intrinsic HH epileptogenicity [26,27].

Response to Treatment

Commonly, epilepsy in HH is medication resistant. Therefore, the general treatment concept is based on resection, disconnection or destruction of the HH. As open resective surgery is associated with significant endocrine, neurological and vascular morbidity, endoscopic resections are preferred, resulting in seizure freedom in every third patient. Alternative minimally invasive surgical approaches are gamma-knife ablation [28], stereotactic thermo-ablation, and stereotactic implantation of iodine-125 radioactive seeds. Seizure freedom rates of the different therapeutic methods employed are 30–40% after follow-up of one to two years. HH ablation by stereotactic laser application is a newer treatment approach: the largest series so far reported 71 children and adolescents; 93% were free of gelastic seizures one year after the procedure, 23 patients required more than one laser intervention; safety was favourable, 1 patient had significant memory problems, another had worsening of diabetes insipidus [29].

Key Points

- Mesial temporal lobe epilepsy is the most frequent type of medication-resistant partial epilepsy; resective surgery may result in seizure freedom in 60–70% of patients.
- Neocortical epilepsies are heterogeneous with regard to seizure semiology and ictal EEG patterns. Feasibility and success of surgery is determined by size and localization of the seizure-onset zone.
- Gelastic epilepsy with hypothalamic hamartoma is a rare clinico-pathological syndrome with an ictal hallmark of laughter. The response to destruction or resection of the lesion can be poor.

References

1. French JA, Williamson PD, Thadani VM, et al. Characteristics of medial temporal lobe epilepsy: I. Results of history and physical examination. *Ann Neurol* 1993;**34**:774–780

2. Sperling MR. Autonomic Seizures. In: CP Panayiotopoulos *(ed.), Atlas of Epilepsies.* London: Springer; 2010:467–470.

3. Stern JM. Focal Seizures with Olfactory Hallucinations. In: CP Panayiotopoulos *(ed.), Atlas of Epilepsies.* London: Springer; 2010;453–455.

4. ILAE Commission on Neurosurgery of Epilepsy, Wieser HG. ILAE Commission Report: Mesial temporal lobe epilepsy with hippocampal sclerosis. *Epilepsia* 2004;**45**(6):695-714

5. Krendl R, Lurger S, Baumgartner C. Absolute spike frequency predicts surgical outcome in TLE with unilateral hippocampal atrophy. *Neurology* 2008;**71**:413–418

6. Williamson PD, French JA, Thadani VM, et al. Characteristics of medial temporal lobe epilepsy: II. Interictal and ictal scalp electroencephalography, neuropsychological testing, neuroimaging, surgical results, and pathology. *Ann Neurol* 1993;**34**:781–787

7. Lewis DV, Shinnar S, Hesdorffer DC, et al. Hippocampal sclerosis after febrile status epilepticus: the FEBSTAT study. *Ann Neurol* 2014;**75**:178–185

8. Le Blanc FE, Rasmussen T. Cerebral seizures and brain tumors. In: P Vinken, GW Bruyn (eds.), *Handbook of Clinical Neurology.* Amsterdam: Elsevier, 1974;295–301

9. Semah F, Picot MC, Adam C, et al. Is the underlying cause of epilepsy a major prognostic factor for recurrence? *Neurology* 1998;**51**:1256–1262

10. Engel J, McDermott MP, Wiebe S, et al. Early surgical therapy for drug-resistant temporal lobe epilepsy: a randomized trial. *J Am Med Assoc* 2012;**307**:922–930

11. Effectiveness and Efficiency of Surgery for Temporal Lobe Epilepsy Study Group, Wiebe S, Blume WT, Girvin JP, Eliasziw M. A randomized, controlled trial of surgery for temporal-lobe epilepsy. *N Engl J Med* 2001;**345**:311–318

12. Jobst BC, Cascino GD. Resective epilepsy surgery for drug-resistant focal epilepsy: a review. *J Am Med Assoc* 2015;**313**:285–293

13. [No authors listed] Proposal for revised classification of epilepsies and epileptic syndromes. Commission on Classification and Terminology of the International League Against Epilepsy. *Epilepsia* 1989;**30**:389–399

14. Manford M, Fish DR, Shorvon SD. An analysis of clinical seizure patterns and their localizing value in frontal and temporal lobe epilepsies. *Brain* 1996;**119**:17–40

15. Leung H, Schindler K, Clusmann H, et al. Mesial frontal epilepsy and ictal body turning along the horizontal body axis. *Arch Neurol* 2008;**65**:71–77

16. Unnwongse K, Wehner T, Foldvary-Schaefer N. Mesial frontal lobe epilepsy. *J Clin Neurophysiol* 2012;**29**:371–378

17. Salanova V, Andermann F, Rasmussen T, et al. Parietal lobe epilepsy: clinical manifestations and outcome in 82 patients treated surgically between 1929 and 1988. *Brain* 1995;**118**:607–627

18. Beleza P, Pinho J. Frontal lobe epilepsy. *J Clinl Neuroscience* 2011;**18**:593–600

19. Foldvary N, Klem G, Hammel J, et al. The localizing value of ictal EEG in focal epilepsy. *Neurology* 2001;**57**:2022–2028

20. Holtkamp M, Sharan A, Sperling MR. Intracranial EEG in predicting surgical outcome in frontal lobe epilepsy. *Epilepsia* 2012;**53**:1739–1745

21. Salanova V, Andermann F, Olivier A, et al. Occipital lobe epilepsy: electroclinical manifestations, electrocorticography, cortical stimulation and outcome in 42 patients treated between 1930 and 1991. Surgery of occipital lobe epilepsy. *Brain* 1992;**115**:1655–1680

22. Perucca P, Dubeau F, Gotman J. Intracranial electroencephalographic seizure-onset patterns: effect of underlying pathology. *Brain* 2014;**137**:183–196

23. Munari C, Kahane P, Francione S, et al. Role of the hypothalamic hamartoma in the genesis of gelastic fits (a video-stereo-EEG study). *Electroencephalogr Clin Neurophysiol* 1995;**95**:154–160

24. Gascon GG, Lombroso CT. Epileptic (gelastic) laughter. *Epilepsia* 1971;**12**:63–76

25. Kuzniecky R, Guthrie B, Mountz J, et al. Intrinsic epileptogenesis of hypothalamic hamartomas in gelastic epilepsy. *Ann Neurol* 1997;**42**:60–67

26. Fenoglio KA, Wu J, Simeone TA, et al. Hypothalamic hamartoma: basic mechanisms of intrinsic epileptogenesis. *Semin Pediatr Neurol* 2007;**14**:51–59

27. Kim DY, Fenoglio KA, Simeone TA, et al. GABAA receptor-mediated activation of L-type calcium channels induces neuronal excitation in surgically resected human hypothalamic hamartomas. *Epilepsia* 2008;**49**:861–871

28. Drees C, Chapman K, Prenger E, et al. Seizure outcome and complications following hypothalamic hamartoma treatment in adults: endoscopic, open, and Gamma Knife procedures. *J Neurosurg* 2012;**117**:255–261

29. Curry DJ, Raskin J, Ali I, Wilfong AA. MR-guided laser ablation for the treatment of hypothalamic hamartomas. *Epilepsy Res* 2018;**142**:131–134

Chapter 15

Approach to the Treatment of Medication-Resistant Epilepsy

John M. Stern

Introduction

This chapter provides an overview of a conceptual approach to providing care for the patient with medication-resistant epilepsy (MRE), with consideration of the care sequence and components. This discussion of the gestalt is not intended to provide one established algorithm, as one treatment pathway cannot serve the needs of the diverse MRE patient population. Nevertheless, the considerations described below comprise a generally accepted care process aimed to improve the MRE clinical outcome. Detailed discussions of the care elements are provided in other chapters.

Diagnostic Accuracy

The patient with MRE does not present with MRE. Moreover, MRE is not one condition and, unfortunately, there is no biomarker for it at this time. Essentially, the MRE diagnosis follows failure of standard pharmacotherapy to provide seizure freedom. As such, the patient with MRE first presents as any patient with epilepsy presents, and the usual approach to epilepsy diagnosis and care is the initial approach. This includes the inherent shortcomings to the epilepsy diagnostic process, including the dependence on the seizure history because of the lack of a diagnostic test that can supplant this dependence. Therefore, the MRE diagnosis is sometimes not accurate because the patient's epilepsy diagnosis is not accurate.

To expound on the diagnostic limitations, diagnosing epilepsy can be based entirely upon only the history of seizures and without any abnormal diagnostic test [1]. This path to the epilepsy diagnosis ultimately depends on the description by the patient or witnesses of two or more episodes that have convincing features of epileptic seizures. However, patients often have difficulty describing the episodes, and witnesses, even medically trained witnesses, often are inaccurate in their descriptions of epileptic

seizures [2,3]. Considering these limitations in the seizure history, the episodes that lead to the initial presentation are prone to misrepresentation and thereby misdiagnosis.

Diagnostic tests supportive of the epilepsy diagnosis can improve the diagnostic accuracy, but the two most commonly used tests, EEG and MRI, each have considerable limitations. An EEG demonstrating epileptiform abnormalities is useful in supporting the epilepsy diagnosis of a patient presenting with episodes suspected to be seizures. However, EEG is subjective and dependent on the interpreting physician's visual recognition of epileptiform abnormalities, normal variants and recording artifacts. Because this recognition depends on education and experience, inter-rater variability can be high in EEG interpretation [4,5]. That is, one interpreter may see an abnormality supportive of the epilepsy diagnosis, while another sees a normal variant. The problem is compounded when non-epileptic episodes that are behaviourally similar to epileptic seizures are interpreted as indicating epilepsy because of normal EEG findings that are seemingly similar to epileptiform abnormality.

MRI also is problematic as a diagnostic test in epilepsy, essentially because the MRI depicts brain structure and epilepsy is a disease of brain function. The functional abnormality of epilepsy may be related to a structural abnormality, which often is visible on MRI, but the presence of an MRI abnormality, even one that can be a cause for epilepsy, does not necessarily indicate an epilepsy diagnosis. For example, the MRI finding of encephalomalacia is not rare in populations at risk for epilepsy, but it may still be an incidental finding and interpreted as supportive of an epilepsy diagnosis simply because it is an abnormality. Overall, the epilepsy diagnosis is inherently vulnerable to misdiagnosis, even with advanced diagnostic testing, and especially when the diagnosis is provided by a non-expert clinician.

Based on this risk for misdiagnosis, an important, initial question to consider after diagnosing MRE is whether epilepsy is actually the diagnosis. The essential question is whether the failure of anti-seizure medications (ASMs) is due to treatment being targeted toward the wrong diagnosis? Numerous other conditions present with paroxysmal behavioural abnormalities similar to epileptic seizures, and these are worthy of consideration when diagnosing MRE. Reconsidering the diagnosis can begin with retaking the original history and personally reviewing the diagnostic tests. That is a fresh look may be more helpful to the patient than trying another ASM. Reconsidering the diagnosis may require additional diagnostic testing, and video-EEG recordings of the patient's habitual seizures is the most reliable test when a seizure recording is feasible. The time and expense of video-EEG seizure recording is easily preferred to ongoing treatment with ineffective medications that can have adverse effects and the continuation of the actual disorder because it is not being treated.

The diagnostic term non-epileptic seizure is now the most commonly used for conditions where apparent MRE is found not to be epilepsy. However, the term non-epileptic seizure indicates a misdiagnosis and not a specific condition. Moreover, this term would not be applied for the same condition if that condition was diagnosed correctly at the outset. Epilepsy misdiagnosis is commonly discovered at epilepsy referral centres, as is demonstrated by the revision of the diagnosis to non-epileptic seizures for about 30% of patients admitted to adult video-EEG monitoring units with the diagnosis of MRE [6,7]. This 30% prevalence is commonly cited, but the percentage varies across epilepsy centres, presumably because of the referral patterns and criteria for inpatient diagnostic testing. Centres focused on differential diagnosis that are not highly active in epilepsy surgery may have higher percentages, and surgical centres with narrower admission criteria may have lower percentages.

Among the patients with non-epileptic seizures, conversion disorder is the most frequent and this form of non-epileptic seizure is now most commonly called psychogenic non-epileptic seizures. Other terms that have been or are used include psychogenic non-epileptic attack, psychogenic non-epileptic episode, and dissociative seizure. In an adult video-EEG monitoring unit, psychogenic non-epileptic seizures is the diagnosis for more than 90% of the patients with non-epileptic seizures (UCLA adult epilepsy experience). Psychogenic non-epileptic seizures may present with a variety of behaviours that is as broad as epileptic seizures, spanning behavioural arrest with minimal movement, to loss of awareness with minor movements, to generalized convulsions. Differentiation from epileptic seizures depends on expert knowledge of seizure behaviours and EEG interpretation.

Other non-epileptic seizures include several entities that are each seen occasionally. These include: parasomnias with an abrupt arousal during sleep with convulsive movements, physiological abnormalities with loss of consciousness because of hypotension, hypoglycaemia or other metabolic disturbances, migraine or other pain syndromes with loss of engagement along with stereotyped movements, pharmaceutical misuse, and parent or care-partner misidentification of activity in patients who are unable to communicate. In each situation, establishing the correct diagnosis eliminates the diagnosis of MRE and leads to more appropriate treatment, as needed, with a second chance at a good clinical outcome.

Lifestyle Impact on Seizure Control

In parallel to reconsideration of the epilepsy diagnosis, the impact of behaviours and choices on seizure control also should be reviewed because they can produce a situation that appears as MRE but is not truly MRE. MRE is predicated on the failure of medications to provide benefit, but this requires adherence to the medication plan. Adherence is difficult for all patients and especially so for patients requiring chronic therapy with multiple doses daily. Essentially, inquiring about adherence is an important aspect of care when treatment fails. Rather than asking whether treatment is taken as directed, which may make some patients defensive, questions may be phrased to expect the difficulty while inquiring about specific difficulties with the regimen. Poor adherence can be due to numerous causes including: forgetfulness, cost, expense, access to refills, misunderstanding of the dosing regimen, concern about safety of the treatment, complexity of polytherapy, inconvenience of the dose time, lack of understanding of the need for every dose, denial of need for treatment and avoidance of adverse effects [8]. Of course, other reasons can occur, but the point is that identifying and then addressing the reason for poor adherence can be an effective means to improve seizure control.

MRE also may be due to seizures that are related to avoidable triggers or circumstances. A simple and important consideration is whether a medication taken by the patient is associated with a risk of seizure exacerbation. Another situation is the patient who is seizure-free except after physiologically stressing circumstances, such as excessive sleep deprivation or extreme alcohol consumption. Such patients may not truly have MRE because a change to lifestyle may produce seizure freedom. The key question for consideration of circumstances is whether an indefinite avoidance of the circumstance is possible. This question arises from the reality that excessive sleep deprivation can be avoided by better planning, but minor sleep deprivation may not be avoidable. As such, circumstances that cannot be realistically avoided may not be correctly targeted as a means to achieve better seizure control. Stress is another common example of this. Many patients identify stress as a cause for worsening seizures. Whereas improved stress management may be achieved, especially for extreme stress and with professional counselling, stress cannot be completely avoided. In circumstances of unavoidable triggers, MRE may be the correct diagnosis and pursuit of better treatment is likely to be more effective than Herculean efforts at lifestyle modification.

Anti-Seizure Medication Selection and Utilization

When the patient truly has epilepsy and is engaged in treatment as well as can be expected, the next question is whether the ASMs have failed because of inadequate doses or appropriateness for the patient. An ASM is considered to have failed only after it has been tried at a typically efficacious dose, and this can be hampered by adverse effects. A patient who has tried many ASMs and could not reach typically efficacious doses due to intolerable adverse effects may not be considered as having MRE, but this patient may still require the advancing of care that is provided for MRE. Failure of many ASMs due to adverse effects at low doses does not necessarily indicate that other ASMs will similarly fail, but the consideration of non-pharmacological treatments would be reasonable in this situation, just as it would for MRE.

A well-tolerated ASM may fail at an appropriate dose because it is not efficacious for the patient's seizure type. The ASMs are arguably better described as anti-seizure instead of anti-epileptic because their benefit is seizure control, as measured by their respective clinical trials. These trials use the seizure type as a main selection criterion, so matching the patient's seizure type to the evidence of the ASM for that seizure type is an important consideration in MRE. A straightforward example is the patient with juvenile myoclonic epilepsy who has freedom from generalized tonic–clonic seizures but has medication-resistant myoclonus because the ASM has efficacy for tonic–clonic seizures but not myoclonus. Another example is the patient who has seizures manifested as lapses of awareness that are believed to be focal seizures with impaired awareness (formerly called complex partial seizures) and is on a medication with efficacy for focal seizures when the actual seizure is absence, a generalized seizure type. Essentially, MRE can be incorrectly diagnosed because some ASMs have a narrow spectrum of efficacy across seizure types.

Lastly, appropriate ASMs can fail at typically efficacious doses, which is the essence of MRE. In this situation, additional ASM treatments should be considered along with non-pharmacologic treatments. For the selection of the next ASM, there is a philosophy of considering ASMs with other mechanisms of action. Although many ASMs have multiple mechanisms of action and presumably many ASMs may have mechanisms of action that are not yet identified, each ASM has at least one mechanism that is likely contributing to its efficacy. A simplified, lumper's listing of these mechanisms can be according to whether the action involves the sodium channel, calcium channel, intra-cellular calcium release, GABA receptor, glutamate receptor or SV2a protein. According to this philosophy, if several sodium channel modulating ASMs have failed, trying an ASM that is not a sodium channel modulator is a reasonable consideration. Sometimes this principle is termed 'rational polypharmacy' and prescribes using ASMs with differing mechanisms when combining ASMs. 'Rational' implies a fundamental justification, but the general approach has not yet been supported through clinical research. Some ASM combinations have limited evidence of benefit from their combination, but the overarching principle is a belief and not evidence-based. Nevertheless, it is commonly used in practice and particularly reasonable for patients with narrow ASM mechanism treatment histories. More importantly, the question should be whether a range of ASM mechanisms of action have been used. If not, common sense supports doing so.

Specific Epilepsy Diagnoses

Multiple ASM options are available for all forms of epilepsy, but several epilepsies have treatments that are more specific and should be considered, even early in the course of MRE treatment. The most important of these are the autoimmune epilepsies. These conditions include several forms that each are identified by their respective autoantibody. Some produce a limbic encephalitis and some present as epilepsy without obvious concomitant abnormality, as discussed in Chapter 12. Nevertheless, immuno-suppression treatment is recommended because of the potential benefits to seizure control and, depending on the condition, concomitant abnormalities. An auto-immune epilepsy is generally recommended for consideration when the patient has frequent focal seizures at the onset of epilepsy, with early development of MRE and has associated neurologic or psychiatric findings, such as with memory, mood and clarity of thought [9,10]. Early diagnosis of auto-immune epilepsy is important because of potential treatment with immuno-suppression, which is a major change to treatment.

Over the decades since the characterization of the epilepsy syndromes, childhood absence epilepsy and juvenile myoclonic epilepsy, each has been associated with one ASM that has been believed to be particularly effective and worth trying when other ASMs fail. For childhood absence epilepsy, ethosuximide was considered to be best for many years before a randomized comparison trial confirmed superiority to valproate (tolerability) and lamotrigine (efficacy), which are two of the other commonly used ASMs for absence seizures [11]. For juvenile myoclonic epilepsy, valproate has been considered to be best, but an analogous comparison trial has not been conducted. Valproate use has decreased over recent years, especially among women with childbearing potential, because of its greater metabolic toxicity when compared with other ASMs and its greater rate of teratogenicity and association with reduction in IQ and increased autism prevalence with in utero exposure [12–14]. Nevertheless, conventional practice includes consideration of a treatment attempt with valproate for medication-resistant juvenile myoclonic epilepsy.

Dravet syndrome is an uncommon genetic epilepsy with onset in early childhood. It often presents with febrile convulsions and then MRE associated with convulsive seizures and intellectual disability or behavioural disorders. Establishing the diagnosis of Dravet syndrome is clinically impactful to ASM selection because ASMs that are in the sodium channel class have been identified as less effective and to be avoided because of potential to be detrimental to the clinical course [15]. Glucose transporter 1 deficiency (GLUT1) is another uncommon genetic epilepsy with childhood onset. It is associated with absence seizures that are sometimes early onset and can be associated with motor and intellectual impairments [16]. For this epilepsy, ketogenic diet therapy is recommended and is expected to be superior to ASMs.

Tuberous sclerosis complex (TSC) is a more common genetic cause for epilepsy. Its seizures are usually due to cerebral malformations (tubers), but TSC includes other brain malformations and neoplasia, along with malformations of the skin, heart, lungs and kidneys. The underlying genetic causes of TSC are genetic abnormalities that impact the protein kinase mTORC1, and several of the tuberous sclerosis malformations and neoplasia can be treated with everolimus, which inhibits mTORC1. Important for the treatment of MRE due to TSC, everolimus has been found to be beneficial for seizure control in a prospective clinical trial, so everolimus can be considered to be an ASM specific to TSC [17,18].

Treatments Beyond Anti-Seizure Medications

Ultimately, the treatment of MRE leads to the question of when to consider non-pharmacologic treatments. MRE is defined by the failure of two or more ASMs, but attempts at pharmacologic treatment usually continue beyond two ASMs [19,20]. Clearly, other treatment approaches should not wait until all pharmacologic options have been exhausted because expanding the range of treatment possibilities is reasonable as soon as ASMs are no longer preferred. Moreover, all pharmacologic treatment options cannot possibly be tried, given more than 20 ASM options, the possibility of ASM combinations and the requisite time for determining a treatment response. A calculation of the time needed for ASM treatments, based on 20 ASMs and six months for each ASM treatment found that 10 years would be needed for all 20 monotherapy treatments, 95 years for all combinations of duotherapy and 570 years for all combinations of three ASMs [21].

ASM is the preferred initial treatment for epilepsy because of efficacy for the newly diagnosed, safety and reversibility. That is, medications can be discontinued, but surgical treatments cannot be undone. Once the likelihood of ASM success is reduced, other options are appropriate. The canonical paper by Kwan and Brody is the most often cited source for the likelihood of seizure freedom as a function of the number of failed ASMs [22]. The relevant results are that about 36% of patients with newly diagnosed epilepsy have MRE, 44% obtain seizure freedom from the first ASM, 9% from the second ASM (after the first failed) and 4% from additional ASMs. These results are not unique to this one publication. Similar results were identified 20 years earlier in the Veterans Cooperative Study of treatment of new-onset epilepsy and the response rate has not substantially changed in the 20 years since the publication, as identified in a follow-up study at the same centre [23,24].

Fundamentally, treatments that have a possibility of seizure freedom with at least the same likelihood as an ASM are worth considering and discussing with patients when two or more appropriate ASMs have failed to produce seizure freedom at typically efficacious doses. These treatments are discussed in the subsequent chapters and include resective surgery, ablative surgery, stimulation and diet. Deciding which of the treatments to consider is the next question when providing care. Shifting to another treatment approach usually requires additional diagnostic testing, especially the recording of seizures with video-EEG, and the results of this testing will influence the decision-making. Most importantly, the evaluation determines whether a patient is a candidate for surgical treatment. Overall, clinical decision-making at this timepoint centres on the treatment options for the specific patient, the expected benefit for the patient from a treatment, the patient's risk tolerance or other personal factors will allow for the treatment, whether the patient has particular vulnerabilities to the adverse effects of the treatment and whether the patient's lifestyle or circumstances would allow for the treatment. In the end, the answer to each of these questions should be considered in the context of the treatment's likelihood of producing seizure freedom or at least a substantial improvement. Sometimes, the high likelihood for a great gain leads patients to rethink what is acceptable, so the benefits of each treatment needs to be explained to each patient as clearly as the risks.

Seizure Burden Goals

The universally accepted goal when treating epilepsy is expeditious seizure freedom without adverse effects. This goal is indispensable at the time of epilepsy onset, but the treatment of MRE often leads to an expansion of the goals. As large case series have shown, sustained seizure freedom is unlikely when multiple treatments have been ineffective, so treatment should include consideration of the clinically meaningful goals that are more likely to be achievable. As an example, a patient whose treatment change reduces the seizure burden from weekly bilateral tonic–clonic seizures to monthly focal seizures still has MRE, but that patient's overall burden of epilepsy, including risk of morbidity and mortality, is meaningfully reduced. As another example, a patient whose treatment change does not change the seizures but minimizes an ASM adverse effect burden that impacts school or employment performance because of fatigue, memory impairment and concentration difficulty still has MRE, but that patient's epilepsy burden, by way of the treatment burden, has been reduced.

Several elements of the seizure burden are worth routinely discussing with patients who have MRE. Seizure frequency obviously impacts seizure burden and it is a good starting point, but the discussion should include consideration of different seizure manifestations, including the seizure severity, seizure duration, and post-ictal recovery duration for each of the manifestations. For some patients, the different manifestations follow the established seizure classification. For example, if a patient has atypical absence seizures, myoclonic (non-drop) seizures and tonic (drop) seizures, knowing the frequency for each seizure type can lead to prioritizing treatment toward improvement of the seizure that is most disabling, based on each seizure type's frequency and impact. Other patients may differentiate the seizures according to a personal measure of the severity, regardless of whether the seizure classification system would place all of the seizures as the same type. For example, a patient may have some focal seizures that follow one type of aura and produce a two-second gap in awareness and other focal seizures that follow a different aura and produce a two-minute gap in awareness. Clearly, monitoring the frequency of each would allow for more meaningful understanding of the impact of treatment changes. Fortunately, human nature leads most patients to make the severity distinction, so the clinician needs only to listen to the descriptions while putting aside the classification system. Shortening the post-ictal recovery duration is one more opportunity for decreasing the seizure burden. For some patients, the seizure is not as disabling as the protracted post-ictal recovery, and a better treatment can be one that shortens the post-ictal recovery. This dissection of the seizure burden into frequency, severity, duration and recovery adds detail to the ongoing care that provides opportunities for improving outcome even if seizure freedom is not achieved.

Additional Treatment Goals

MRE often includes comorbidities, and attention to the entirety of the epilepsy, including the comorbidities, should be implicit to treating MRE. The consideration of the entirety of the epilepsy is based on the conceptualization of epilepsy as a cerebral disorder that produces seizures and also the comorbidities, the most common of which are mood disorders and cognitive impairments. Recognizing a patient's specific behavioural or cognitive impairments benefits the localization process of focal epilepsy, which is important when evaluating for epilepsy surgery, but, also importantly, it can allow for these non-seizure aspects of MRE to be addressed. Among the comorbidities, depression and memory impairment are the most common, in part because of the high prevalence with mesial temporal lobe epilepsy, which is localized to the limbic system. Addressing each of these comorbidities can substantially improve overall outcomes and clearly benefits quality of life, as measured with validated instruments. Successfully treating mood disorders can have a greater impact on quality-of-life measures than a reduction in seizure frequency that does not produce seizure freedom. For MRE, epilepsy quality-of-life measures track with mood measures more than seizure frequency [25]. This, alone, should be convincing for the need to integrate emotional health treatment into MRE treatment. Addressing the cognitive impairments begins with neuropsychological testing to best identify the specific difficulty, and this can lead to counselling for maximizing cognitive strengths to offset the impairments. The testing also can provide the specifics for accommodations, as needed. As such, comprehensive epilepsy centres should include the expertise of psychologists, neuropsychologists and psychiatrists.

MRE treatment must include counselling to minimize the risk of seizure-related injury. A central goal of ASM or other seizure treatment is the reduction in risk of seizure-related injury, but this risk also may be reduced by safety discussion with the patient. The discussion is most effective when it reviews situations that are specific to the patient, because the resulting understanding of the risk reality will allow the patient to make better decisions. The discussion has to include the acceptance that elimination of all risk is not possible, but a risk reduction is realistically achievable and highly impactful, especially with attention to the relative risks of different activities. One way to differentiate activities according to risk is by judging whether an injury would be permanent (death included) if a seizure occurred during that activity. Such high-risk activities include driving and some recreational activities. However, other recreational activities may produce a minor, self-limited injury if a seizure occurs, and the patient has to judge whether the activity is worth the risk. This approach can help avoid over-restriction, which can create more burden from epilepsy than is absolutely needed.

Additional Care Elements

As with any chronic illness that has considerable potential to produce disability, best care for MRE extends beyond the clinician's office to daily life. Ideally, daily life with MRE should not be unnecessarily focused on MRE. That is, life should be broad and impacted only as much as absolutely needed. For the aspects of MRE that extend into daily life, resources outside the office can be important. This can include social support structures, such as engagement of family or others who are close to the patient. These should be encouraged as a means to reduce isolation, balance any stigma that is experienced and also assist with navigating the safety restrictions. The support can be explored and encouraged during routine MRE care. Beyond those who are close to the patient, the larger epilepsy community also can provide benefit. This includes epilepsy-patient-oriented organizations, which can provide a sense of community, narratives from other patients about their experiences, an opportunity to share one's own experiences to an understanding group and updates on research and care. The International Bureau for Epilepsy is the umbrella organization for many such organizations around the world, including the United States Epilepsy Foundation. The websites for these organizations provide an important common ground in numerous countries, and the Epilepsy Foundation's website epilepsy.com is an expansive and reliable educational resource for those who read English.

Community engagement for the patient with MRE can extend beyond the patient community to the research community. Patients who show interest in contributing to advancing epilepsy care should be encouraged to pursue this, and participating in research can be personally meaningful to the patient. Contributing to research can be through any one of a variety of mechanisms, including financial support by donations or fundraising, sharing one's anonymized medical history and diagnostic test results, volunteering for diagnostic test research and volunteering to participate in a clinical trial. As such, a range of opportunities exists, and some may ultimately provide direct clinical benefit to the patient, even if this cannot be known when deciding to participate.

Conclusion

MRE is a diverse and challenging condition, and an algorithmic approach to maximize the clinical outcome is, unfortunately, not yet available. However, the general approach to care for MRE is clear. This begins with reconsidering the epilepsy diagnosis, the seizure type diagnosis, and the appropriateness and dosing of the medication interventions. When MRE is clearly present, care should include consideration of the larger range of treatment options, which includes surgeries, devices and diets. Much is available for MRE. Beyond treatments targeting seizure control, care for MRE should include attention to the other aspects of epilepsy, including emotional and cognitive needs, and the essential goal of continuing to live a full life.

Key Points

- If considering the diagnosis of MRE, reconsider the diagnosis of epilepsy and the type or cause of the epilepsy. The treatment may be incorrect or suboptimal for the patient.
- Maximize the response to medication by addressing the impacts of lifestyle and behaviours on seizure control.
- Treatment selection for MRE should include discussion of the non-pharmacologic approaches, including epilepsy surgery for potential candidates.
- Care goals should include minimizing each of the multiple factors that relate to the burden of MRE. These include seizure features, treatment adverse effects, and emotional, cognitive and social challenges.

References

1. Fisher RS, Acevedo C, Arzimanoglou A, et al. ILAE official report: a practical clinical definition of epilepsy. *Epilepsia* 2014;**55**:475–482

2. Rugg-Gunn FJ, Harrison NA, Duncan JS. Evaluation of the accuracy of seizure descriptions by the relatives of patients with epilepsy. *Epilepsy Res* 2001;**43**:193–199

3. Mannan JB, Wieshmann UC. How accurate are witness descriptions of epilepsy seizures? *Seizure* 2003;**12**:444–447

4. Benbadis SR, Tatum WO. Overinterpretation of EEGs and misdiagnosis of epilepsy. *J Clin Neurophysiol* 2003;**20**:42–44

5. Hussain SA, Kwong G, Millichap JJ, et al. Hypsarrhythmia assessment exhibits poor interrater reliability: a threat to clinical trial validity. *Epilepsia* 2015;**56**:77–81

6. Mohan KK, Markand ON, Salanova V. Diagnostic utility of video EEG monitoring in paroxysmal events. *Act Neurol Scand* 1996;**94**:320–325

7. Benbadis SR, O'Neill E, Tatum WO, Heriaud L. Outcome of prolonged video-EEG monitoring at a typical referral epilepsy center. *Epilepsia* 2004;**45**:1150–1153

8. World Health Organization, 2003. Adherence to long-term therapies: Evidence for action. https://apps.who.int/iris/bitstream/handle/10665/42682/9241545992.pdf (accessed March 2020)

9. Quek AML, Britton JW, McKeon A, et al. Autoimmune epilepsy: clinical characteristics and response to immunotherapy. *Arch Neurol* 2012;**69**:582–593

10. Graus F, Titulaer MJ, Balu R, et al. A clinical approach to diagnosis of autoimmune encephalitis. *Lancet Neurol* 2016;**15**:391–404

11. Glauser TA, Cnaan A, Shinnar S, et al. Ethosuximide, valproic acid, and lamotrigine in childhood absence epilepsy. *N Engl J Med* 2010;**362**:790–799

12. Vinten J, Adab N, Kini U, et al. Neuropsychological effects of exposure to anticonvulsant medication in utero. *Neurology* 2005;**64**:949–954

13. Christensen J, Grønborg TK, Sørensen MJ, et al. Prenatal valproate exposure and risk of autism spectrum disorders and childhood autism. *J Am Med Assoc* 2013;**309**:1696–1703

14. Gerard EE, Meador KJ. An update on maternal use of antiepileptic medications in pregnancy and neurodevelopment outcomes. *J Pediatr Genet* 2015;**4**:94–110

15. De Lange IM, Gunning B, Sonsma ACM, et al. Influence of contraindicated medication use on

cognitive outcome in Dravet syndrome and age at first afebrile seizure as a clinical predictor in SCNA1A-related seizure phenotypes. *Epilepsia* 2018;**59**:1154–1165

16. Suls A, Mullen SA, Weber YG, et al. Early-onset absence epilepsy caused by mutations in the glucose transporter GLUT1. *Ann Neurol* 2009;**66**:415–419

17. French JA, Lawson JA, Yapici Z, et al. Adjunctive everolimus therapy for treatment-resistant focal-onset seizures associated with tuberous sclerosis (EXIST-3): a phase 3, randomised, double-blind, placebo-controlled study. *Lancet* 2016;**388**:2153–2163

18. Krueger DA, Wilfong AA, Mays M, et al. Long-term treatment of epilepsy with everolimus in tuberous sclerosis. *Neurology* 2016;**87**:2408–2415

19. De Flon P, Kumlien E, Reuterwall C, Mattsson P. Empirical evidence of underutilization of referrals for epilepsy surgery evaluation. *Eur J Neurol* 2010;**17**:619–625

20. Haneef Z, Stern J, Dewar S, Engel J, Jr. Referral pattern for epilepsy surgery after evidence-based recommendations: a retrospective study. *Neurology* 2010;**75**:699–704

21. Montenegro MA, Novals A, Hirsch LJ. How long would it take to try all the antiepileptic drugs available? *Epilepsy Res* 2019;**154**:77–78

22. Kwan P, Brodie MJ. Early identification of refractory epilepsy. *N Engl J Med* 2000;**342**:314–319

23. Mattson RH, Cramer JA, Collins JF, et al. Comparison of carbamazepine, phenobarbital, phenytoin, and primidone in partial and secondarily generalized tonic–clonic seizures. *N Eng J Med* 1985;**313**:145–151

24. Chen Z, Brodie MJ, Liew D, et al. Treatment outcomes in patients with newly diagnosed epilepsy treated with established and new antiepileptic drugs: a 30-year longitudinal cohort study. *JAMA Neurol* 2018;**75**:279–286

25. Tracy JI, Dechant V, Sperling MR, et al. The association of mood with quality of life ratings in epilepsy. *Neurology* 2007;**68**:1101–1107

Chapter 16

Pharmacotherapy for Medication-Resistant Epilepsy

Graham A. Powell and Anthony G. Marson

ASM Treatment for Epilepsy

First-Line Treatment with ASMs

Anti-seizure medications (ASMs) remain the mainstay of the treatment of epilepsy and the majority of patients with epilepsy (60–70%) will achieve a sustained remission from seizures. The number of ASMs has increased dramatically in recent years and there are now over 20 ASMs licensed and available [1]. Given that epilepsy is a chronic condition, often requiring years of treatment, a choice among these drugs requires evidence about longer-term clinical and cost-effectiveness, which will come largely from randomized controlled trials (RCTs), in which treatments are compared head to head. Much of this evidence comes from publically funded trials rather than those sponsored by the pharmaceutical industry, whose trials are designed to meet regulatory requirements rather than to inform clinical decision-making. In the EU this currently results in non-inferiority trials assessing six-month remission rate [2,3], whilst in the USA this resulted in short-term trials using a historical control design [4]. More recently, the US FDA has allowed extrapolation of adjunctive therapy RCT data. Approval requires pharmacokinetic studies and recommendations for dosing to achieve levels similar to those obtained in adjunctive therapy. This approach has resulted in approvals for monotherapy for perampanel, eslicarbazepine and brivaracetam, without the need for a separate efficacy trial.

Traditionally, carbamazepine and sodium valproate have been the recommended first-line ASMs for focal and generalized epilepsy, respectively. However, longer-term RCTs such as the Standard and New Antiepileptic Drugs Trial (SANAD) provide evidence to support lamotrigine as a first-line treatment for focal epilepsy, whilst also demonstrating that gabapentin and topiramate are poor first-line treatments. Similarly topiramate and lamotrigine were shown to be inferior to valproate as a first-line treatment for generalized or unclassified epilepsy [5,6]. Whilst other ASMs (levetiracetam, zonisamide) have a monotherapy indication, current evidence is insufficient to recommend them as first-line treatments.

A number of treatment guidelines have been published by national bodies such as the National Institute for Health and Care Excellence (NICE)[7] and medical associations such as the International League Against Epilepsy (ILAE) [8]. Guidelines aim to consider the available evidence and make appropriate recommendations, but the strength of recommendations is necessarily limited by the quality of evidence available. Due to the limited evidence available, rather than recommend a single drug, NICE, in their most recent update of their epilepsy guidelines, recommend a number of ASMs that should be considered 'first-line' in the treatment of a range of seizure types [7]. Clinician and patient can then discuss the pros and cons of the various options. Perhaps the most important choice is for women of child-bearing age with genetic generalized epilepsy, where sodium valproate should be used with caution due to the risks of teratogenicity and greater risks of neurodevelopmental sequelae [9], where likely less effective, but safer options such as levetiracetam and lamotrigine may be chosen [10]. Although there are some important limitations in the evidence that informs ASM monotherapy choices, the evidence base that informs treatment decisions later in the patient's trajectory is even more limited.

From First Treatment Failure to Medication-Resistant Epilepsy?

Deriving an operational definition of medication-resistant epilepsy that is useful for both clinical practice and research has proved challenging. This should not be surprising, as it requires dichotomizing a continuum, whilst also taking time into account and the evolution of and certainty about refractoriness.

The first-line ASM will fail in a significant proportion of patients due to lack of efficacy, intolerability or a combination of both, regardless of ASM [11]. Given the heterogeneous nature of epilepsy, it is not surprising that a number of clinical factors have been found to be associated with treatment failure, for example a multi-variable analysis of data from the SANAD trial generated a prognostic model for time to treatment failure that included the following factors: seizure type, EEG result and ASM treatment prior to randomization. Notably, choice of ASM is not a significant predictor of treatment failure, indicating that the differences in efficacy between ASMs is small, and that clinical factors are much more important determinants of treatment failure [12].

Further analyses of the SANAD cohort have also allowed assessment of outcome following a first treatment failure and clinical factors that affect outcome [13]. Following a first treatment failure, the probability of a 12-month remission remains fairly high; overall 70% of patients will achieve a 12-month remission, 80% with a first treatment failure due to adverse events and 65% with treatment failure due to inadequate seizure control. A range of clinical factors were included in a prognostic model, including age at treatment failure, gender, seizure type, total number of tonic–clonic seizures before starting treatment, time on randomized treatment and MRI result. For example, a 40-year-old male with 10 focal-onset generalized seizures and a normal MRI has a 63% (95% CI: 55–71) chance of a 12-month remission if the first treatment failed due to adverse events, and 44% (95% CI: 37–52) if the first treatment failed due to inadequate seizure control. Thus, whilst outcome following a first treatment failure can be estimated for patients with a range of characteristics, specific patient groups that will develop medication-resistant epilepsy cannot be reliably identified.

Inevitably, the more treatments that fail due to lack of seizure control, the less likely that subsequent treatment trials will be successful [14,15]. The ILAE has defined medication resistance as 'failure of adequate trials of two tolerated, appropriately chosen and used anti-epileptic drug schedules whether as monotherapy or in combination to achieve sustained seizure freedom' [16]. The rationale behind this definition is that following adequate therapeutic trials of two ASMs, the chance of achieving seizure freedom is modest. Following failure of first ASM due to lack of efficacy, 11% of patients subsequently become seizure-free; 41% subsequently become seizure-free when failure of first ASM was due to intolerable adverse events [14]. However, some patients do achieve seizure control following further ASM changes [13,17].

Monotherapy or Polytherapy Following a First or Subsequent Treatment Failure?

There is general agreement that initial treatment should be with ASM monotherapy for most patients, and that for those with treatment-refractory epilepsy, seizure control is most likely to be achieved with polytherapy. There is, however, limited evidence regarding when in the patient trajectory to switch from mono- to polytherapy. Whilst these are everyday pragmatic clinical questions, few RCTs have been undertaken in an attempt to inform treatment policies. One RCT has recruited patients following a first treatment failure (n = 157) [18], who were randomized to alternative monotherapy or to polytherapy. The trial was underpowered and found no significant advantage for either policy, but was unable to exclude the possibility of important differences (HR: 1.06 95% CI: 0.68–1.66). The evidence discussed in the previous section highlights the high subsequent remission rates for those failing their first ASM due to adverse events, and for such patients, alternative monotherapy may be appropriate. For patients with a first ASM failure due to inadequate seizure control, the probability of subsequent remission is lower, and if they failed an appropriate first-line ASM for their seizure type and syndrome, early polytherapy may be in their best interest. Guidelines such as those published by NICE recommend alternative monotherapy after failure of a first ASM [7].

There are no RCT data to inform treatment policy following failure of a second monotherapy. Epidemiological studies show that following each successive treatment failure, the probability of seizure control with subsequent ASM regimens diminishes. For example, in one study, 67% achieved seizure freedom with initial monotherapy. Of those whose seizures were not controlled in the first ASM, 11% achieved seizure freedom with the second ASM [14]. It is data from such studies that underpin the ILAE's definition of medication-resistant epilepsy [16]. It is important to highlight however, that whilst such studies can estimate prognosis for cohorts of patients, they cannot, given their observational design, provide reliable evidence about the likely efficacy of any particular treatment policy, ASM or treatment regimen.

When making such treatment decisions, it is clearly paramount to discuss the various options and possible outcomes with the patient to enable them to state a preference. The drive for seizure control with polytherapy may come with a risk of adverse events that is unacceptable to the patient.

Overview of RCT Methods to Assess Anti-Seizure Medications for Treatment-Refractory Epilepsy and the Shortcomings of Regulatory Trials

Most ASM RCTs are undertaken to meet the requirements of regulatory authorities such as the United States Food and Drug Administration (FDA) or the European Medicines Agency (EMA). Trials will usually be undertaken first in adults with drug-refractory focal epilepsy who have failed multiple previous ASMs and who are having at least four seizures per month. The comparison is typically with placebo in order to demonstrate statistically significant superiority for efficacy. Once a drug is licensed for use as an add-on treatment for refractory focal epilepsy, trials may be taken in other populations, including children, patients with drug-refractory generalized seizures, specific epilepsy syndromes and as monotherapy.

Very few head-to-head trials have been undertaken that compare differing add-on regimens. Similarly, no longer-term pragmatic studies have been undertaken that assess the clinical or cost effectiveness of differing ASMs when used as add-on treatments. As a result, the majority of the RCT evidence regarding the efficacy of ASMs when used as add-on treatments in patients with medication-resistant epilepsy comes from regulatory placebo-controlled add-on trials. Given that these trials are designed to inform regulatory decisions, it is important to highlight their shortcomings from the perspective of informing everyday treatment choices in the clinic.

Epilepsy is a chronic condition, and treatment decisions will be best informed by trials that measure longer-term outcomes that are valid and meaningful to patients. Regulatory add-on trials typically have an eight-week baseline followed by a treatment period of 16 weeks' duration, which is too short to provide evidence about longer-term effectiveness that patients and health services require. Also, the outcome reported is a measure of change in seizure frequency, the FDA preferring median reduction in seizure frequency and the EMA preferring the proportion of patients with a 50% or greater reduction in seizure frequency. Neither outcome is particularly meaningful to patients. Placebo-controlled studies are often followed by open-label extension studies which may provide longer-term, but uncontrolled, data about new ASMs. Whilst such designs may provide additional safety data, they are uninterpretable from the point of view of efficacy due to selection bias, heterogeneity and their uncontrolled design [19].

Clinicians and patients need to make a choice among available alternatives, but placebo-controlled trials do not provide head-to-head data to inform such decisions. Indirect comparisons can be made, which can be done in the context of a network meta-analysis [20]. Whilst this approach uses data from RCTs (placebo controlled) it is important to emphasize that any comparison is indirect and not randomized. Network meta-analyses make several assumptions, in particular that the population of patients recruited to trials is similar and consistent across trials. This assumption is most likely violated in refractory epilepsy as the typical patient recruited to trials in the late 1980s and early 1990s is systematically different to a current typical patient. Current patients are likely more refractory given the range of treatments now available to try before considering joining a trial, and trials are conducted over many more centres worldwide than was previously the case. Good evidence for the change in case mix comes from the work exploring the escalating placebo response rate in these trials [21].

The highly selected nature of cohorts recruited into regulatory add-on trials results in very limited external validity. In particular, the patients recruited do not represent the majority of patients with refractory epilepsy who may, for example, have a lower seizure rate or comorbidities that prevent participation in a trial. Clinicians will need to make a judgment as to whether data can be extrapolated to specific patients they see in routine practice. Whilst it may be reasonable to extrapolate to patients with similar seizure types or syndromes, data on refractory focal seizures cannot be extrapolated to refractory generalized-onset seizures.

There are no RCT data that provide reliable evidence about specific ASM combinations that are most effective. One popular approach has been called 'rational polytherapy'. The aim here is to combine drugs that have differing mechanisms of action, aiming to maximize efficacy and minimize adverse events. Whilst this approach may be logical, there is only scarce data from RCTs to support it [22,23], the interpretation of which is confounded by selection biases. Identifying the most effective ASM combinations will remain a huge challenge, as at present there are over 400 dual-therapy regimens, which cannot feasibly be assessed within the context of RCTs.

Finally, it is important to highlight that important safety data will come from designs other than RCTs, and that coordinated post-marketing surveillance is required to minimize risk to patients. This is particularly important for rare but life-threatening events such as felbamate-associated liver failure, long-term events such as vigabatrin retinopathy [24] and retigabine (ezogabine) pigmentation and retinopathy [25], and several ASM teratogenic effects [26].

Efficacy and Tolerability of Add-On ASMs

Despite the limitations of the evidence base highlighted above, placebo-controlled add-on trials remain the best source of evidence about the efficacy and tolerability of ASMs when used as add-on therapy. Much of the available evidence has been summarized in systematic reviews undertaken by members of the Cochrane Epilepsy group. A summary of the results assessing licensed add-on treatments for refractory focal epilepsy is presented in Table 16.1. All have greater efficacy when compared to placebo and have differing adverse effect profiles.

Given the inadequate evidence base, it is inevitable that individual treatment choices will be based on a range of factors, including clinician experience, views about rational polytherapy, patient comorbidities and patient preference. One concern is that the evidence vacuum leaves clinical practice more open to the influence of marketing from pharmaceutical companies.

The Future

'Novel' ASMs

Although the majority of patients enter a sustained remission from seizures on ASM treatment, there is little evidence that the proportion of patients with treatment-refractory epilepsy has diminished over time, despite the development of newer ASMs [27]. There is therefore no doubt about ongoing patient and societal burden, underpinning a desire to develop new treatments.

There are several novel compounds that have either recently been considered for licensing, are approaching licensing or are in development with potential to contribute to the treatment of medication-resistant epilepsy, summarized briefly:

Cenobamate is a novel therapeutic agent with broad anti-convulsant activity and unclear mechanism of action. At the time of this publication, it was recently approved by the US FDA for partial-onset seizures.

2-Deoxy-D-glucose acts as an intra-cellular inhibitor of glycolysis and is thought to have a similar mechanism of action as the ketogenic diet.

Elpetrigine is an analogue of lamotrigine and is a potent sodium and voltage-gated calcium channel blocker. Its efficacy and tolerability profile are broadly similar to lamotrigine.

Fluorofelbamate is an analogue of felbamate developed with the aim of reducing the bone marrow and hepatic toxicities associated with felbamate.

Ganaxolone is a novel neuroactive steroid acting by modulating the extrasynaptic GABA-A receptor complex. Phase I and II trials in patients with focal-onset epilepsy have demonstrated some efficacy with reasonable tolerability. An interesting ganaxalone trial targets young women with PCDH19 gene mutations who harbour associated deficits in the gene for the aldo-keto reductase that plays a role in the conversion of progesterone to allopregnanolone, a neurosteroid that is an agonist at the extrasynaptic GABA receptor [28]. Ganaxalone is a methylated form that can be used orally, unlike allopregnanolone.

Padsevonil is a compound with affinity for the SV2A synaptic vesicle protein and the GABA-A receptor. It is being investigated for efficacy against focal-onset seizures.

Safinamide is a sodium channel blocker and an inhibitor of the excessive release of glutamate. A further mechanism of action is the reversible inhibition of MAO-B and as such this compound may also have clinical use in Parkinson's disease.

T2000 (1,3-dimethoxymethyl-5,5-diphenyl-barbituric acid) is a pro-drug, its active metabolite possessing a mechanism of action similar to phenytoin and phenobarbitone. Efficacy and the associated adverse event profile are similar, including the effects on cytochrome P450 liver enzymes.

Tonabersat is a novel anti-seizure medication with a mechanism of action thought to involve selective

Table 16.1 Summary of meta-analysis results from cochrane systematic reviews assessing add-on ASM treatment of refractory focal epilepsy

ASM	50% responders (RR 95% CI)	Withdrawal (RR 95% CI)	Significant adverse events (RR 99% CI)
Eslicarbazepine	All doses: 1.86 (1.46–2.36)	1.07 (0.73–1.57)	Dizziness 3.09 (1.76–5.43) Nausea 3.06 (1.07–8.74) Diplopia 3.73 (1.19–11.64)
Gabapentin	All doses: 1.89 (1.40–2.55)	1.05 (0.74–1.49)	Dizziness 2.43 (1.44–4.12) Somnolence 1.93 (1.22–3.06)
Lacosamide	All doses: 1.70 (1.38–2.10) 200 mg: 1.41 (1.07–1.85) 400 mg: 1.80 (1.43–2.25) 600 mg: 1.98 (1.43–2.73)	1.88 (1.40–2.52)	Uncoordination 6.12 (1.35–27.77) Diplopia 5.29 (1.97–14.23) Dizziness 3.53 (2.20–5.68) Nausea 2.37 (1.23–4.58) Vomiting 3.49 (1.43–8.54)
Lamotrigine	All doses: 1.80 (1.45–2.23) 300 mg: 1.23 (0.57–2.67) 500mg: 2.13 (1.08–4.20)	1.11 (0.90–1.36)	Ataxia 3.34 (2.01–5.55) Dizziness 2.00 (1.51–2.64) Diplopia 3.79 (2.15–6.68) Nausea 1.81 (1.22–2.68)
Levetiracetam	Children 60 mg/kg/day: 1.91 (1.38–2.63) Adults 1000 mg: 2.49 (1.78–3.50) Adults 2000 mg: 4.91 (2.75–8.77) Adults 3000 mg: 2.59 (2.01–3.33)	Adults: 0.98 (0.73–1.32) Children: 0.80 (0.43–1.46)	Somnolence 1.51 (1.06–2.17) Infection 1.76 (1.03–3.02)
Oxcarbazepine	All doses: OR 2.96 (2.20–4.00) 600 mg: OR 2.41 (1.42–4.11) 1200 mg: OR 4.18 (2.61–6.68) 2400 mg: OR 5.62 (3.57–8.83)	OR 2.17 (1.59–2.97)	Ataxia OR 2.93 (1.72–4.99) Dizziness OR 3.05 (1.99–4.67) Fatigue OR 1.80 (1.02–3.19) Nausea OR 2.88 (1.77–4.69) Somnolence OR 2.55 (1.84–3.55) Diplopia OR 4.32 (2.65–7.04)
Pregabalin	All doses: 2.61 (1.70–4.01) 50 mg: 1.06 (0.52–2.12) 150 mg: 2.22 (1.36–3.63) 300 mg: 2.86 (0.65–4.94) 600 mg: 2.86 (2.32–3.54) Titrated 150–600 mg: 2.86 (1.42–5.76)	1.39 (1.13 to 1.72)	Ataxia 3.90 (2.05–7.42) Dizziness 3.06 (2.16–4.34) Somnolence 2.08 (1.45–2.99) Weight gain 4.92 (2.41–10.03)
Tiagabine	All doses: 3.16 (1.97–5.07)	1.81 (1.25–2.62)	Dizziness 1.69 (1.31–2.51) Fatigue 1.38 (0.89–2.14) Nervousness 10.65 (0.78–146.08) Tremor 4.56 (1.00–20.94)
Topiramate	All doses: 2.97 (2.38–3.72)	2.44 (1.64–3.62)	Ataxia 2.29 (1.10 to 4.77) Concentration difficulties 7.81 (2.08–29.29) Dizziness 1.54 (1.07–2.22) Fatigue 2.19 (1.42–3.40) Paraesthesia 3.91 (1.51–10.12) Somnolence 2.29 (1.49–3.51) 'Thinking abnormally' 5.70 (2.26–14.38) Weight loss 3.47 (1.55–7.79)
Vigabatrin	All doses: 2.58 (1.87 to 3.57)	2.49 (1.05–5.88)	Dizziness 1.64 (1.01–2.65) Fatigue 1.85 (1.31–2.60) Depression 2.81 (1.12–7.07)
Zonisamide	All Doses: 1.92 (1.52–2.42) 300 to 500 mg: 2.00 (1.58–2.54)	1.47 (1.07–2.01)	Ataxia 3.77 (1.28–11.11) Somnolence 1.83 (1.08–3.11) Agitation 2.35 (1.05–5.27) Anorexia 2.71 (1.29–5.69)

modulation of gap junctions. There is limited evidence to suggest indication in generalized and complex partial epilepsies.

Valrocemide, a valproic acid/glycinamide conjugation, has an unclear mechanism of action. In development until 2004, valrocemide offered some promise in the treatment of focal epilepsy.

Alternative Approaches to the Treatment of Medication-Resistant Epilepsy

The recent generation of new ASMs has largely been developed via the NIH anti-seizure medication screening programme [29], in which thousands of chemicals have been assessed in animal models. In Figure 16.1 we attempt to show the likely additional benefit of new ASMs as they come onto the market. Successive drugs developed using current paradigms are less likely to have impact than their predecessors in an overcrowded market. We clearly need a paradigm shift in our understanding of the basic biology of epilepsy and of drug development in order to develop new treatments likely to have a significant impact on patient outcome. Ideally such drugs will be disease-modifying rather than merely anti-seizure. In the final section of this chapter we will briefly discuss two routes to developing new treatments that are currently being investigated.

There is increasing evidence from both experimental animal epilepsy models and subsequently resected human brain tissue, that several inflammatory pathways are implicated in the pathogenesis of epilepsy, including epileptogenesis and the long-term consequences of epilepsy. This is perhaps as expected; it has long been recognized that febrile seizures can herald the later development of focal epilepsy and systemic infection and fever can precipitate seizures in patients with known epilepsy. However, the identification of the hallmarks of chronic inflammation in resected brain tissue, together with the identification of abnormal inflammatory pathways has provided insight into the underlying pathogenesis of some focal epilepsies [30]. Mediators include interleukin-1β, high-mobility group box protein 1 (HMGB1), and

Toll-like receptor (TLR) signalling. Identification of such abnormal inflammatory pathways raises the possibility of novel, anti-inflammatory approaches to the treatment of certain epilepsies. The evidence is currently limited; however, inhibitors of interleukin converting enzyme (ICE)/caspase-1, the protease that catalyses the conversion of the inactive precursor pro-IL-1β to active IL-1β, demonstrate the greatest potential in animal models.

The development of such treatments for human epilepsy poses a number of significant challenges and questions to be resolved. For example, where in the patient trajectory should such treatments be evaluated? Immediately after a brain injury or insult? Following a first seizure? Similarly, the best trial designs and outcomes measures are yet to be agreed upon.

We also need to investigate how inflammatory markers might be used as stratifying tools, both in terms of prognosis and treatment choice. Ideally, inflammatory biomarkers would help identify those with active inflammation who might best benefit from treatment. This will be particularly important if such treatments are associated with significant risks or side effects.

Advances in genomics, and our understanding of the genetic architecture of the epilepsies is starting to have an impact for a small number of patients, mainly those with severe epilepsies with onset in childhood [31]. For example, Dravet's syndrome is associated with a mutation in the type 1 voltage-gated sodium channel-encoding SCN1A gene, expressed in GABAergic interneurons. Avoidance of sodium- channel-blocking ASMs can avoid an exacerbation of seizures and improve outcome. For those with a progressive myoclonic epilepsy, genotyping for the Lafora-associated genes (EMP2A and EMP2B) and the Unverricht–Lundborg PME-associated cystatin B gene early in the course can lead to an earlier diagnosis and treatment with gentamicin, which facilitates normal transcription, eliminating pathological Lafora inclusion bodies from neurons. Also, an abnormal glucose transport protein type 1 (GLUT1) can impair glucose transport across the blood–brain barrier, resulting in seizures and developmental delay in infancy. Testing for mutations in GLUT1/SLC2A1 can aid diagnosis, followed by use of the ketogenic diet. And finally, patients positive for KCNT1 mutations may benefit from treatment with quinidine [32]. The latter is a good example of how genetic findings can

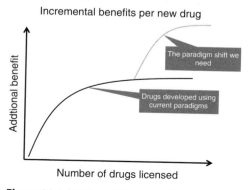

Incremental benefits per new drug

The paradigm shift we need

Drugs developed using current paradigms

Additional benefit

Number of drugs licensed

Figure 16.1 Paradigm shift required for new drug development.

be taken into in vitro models in order to identify potential treatments, and in this case quinidine, a known anti-arrhythmic drug, was repurposed, based on in vitro physiology. However, it is sobering to note that an RCT of quinidine in patients with KCNT1 mutations presenting with autosomal dominant nocturnal frontal lobe epilepsy failed dramatically [33].

Whilst the above findings may herald the dawn of precision medicine in epilepsy, considerable caution is required, given that the common epilepsies are likely to be associated with a myriad of rare variants, and that for many there is a genetic–environment interaction underlying their epilepsy. It is possible that for the common epilepsies, a small number of key biological pathways will be identified at which drugs can be targeted. Systems biology approaches are currently being used to try and identify such pathways [34].

Finally, the discovery of alternative treatment targets may lead to a repurposing of drugs with existing licenses for other diseases, potentially avoiding the escalating costs of drug development. But even where novel drugs are being developed, improvements in the licensing pathway are important. The European Medicines Agency has introduced the 'Adaptive Pathway', permitting iterative licensing and the incorporation of 'real world' data. With the aim of improving patient access to beneficial drugs, we could be optimistic that pragmatic clinical trials, that usefully inform the clinical treatment decision, would have a greater role in the licensing of medicines in the future.

Key Points

- Thirty percent of patients with epilepsy will fail their first-line ASM and the chance of achieving seizure freedom diminishes with each successive ASM attempt.
- The current evidence base does not inform treatment policy (alternative monotherapy or polytherapy) following first treatment failure and early treatment refractoriness.
- Evidence about the efficacy of 'add-on' ASMs comes from short-term regulatory placebo trials that do not reliably inform everyday decision-making, whilst longer-term uncontrolled observational studies are largely uninterruptable due to a range of important biases.

- Treatment combinations for refractory epilepsy are informed by data from regulatory trials, knowledge about adverse effects, clinical experience and considerations on mechanisms of action.
- Novel ASMs are in development, but a change in treatment paradigm, to address the underlying causes of epilepsy, such as inflammatory and genetic causes, may offer the best chance of achieving measurable progress in the treatment of epilepsy; in addition, the potential repurposing of medications may result in reduced costs and time involved in drug development.

References

1. Stephen LJ, Brodie MJ. Pharmacotherapy of epilepsy: newly approved and developmental agents. *CNS Drugs* 2011;**25**(2):89–107

2. Brodie MJ, Perucca E, Ryvlin P, et al. Comparison of levetiracetam and controlled-release carbamazepine in newly diagnosed epilepsy. *Neurology* 2007;**68**(6):402–408

3. Baulac M, Brodie MJ, Patten A, Segieth J, Giorgi L. Efficacy and tolerability of zonisamide versus controlled-release carbamazepine for newly diagnosed partial epilepsy: a phase 3, randomised, double-blind, non-inferiority trial. *Lancet Neurol* 2012;**11**(7):579–588

4. French JA, Temkin NR, Shneker BF, et al. Lamotrigine XR conversion to monotherapy: first study using a historical control group. *Neurotherapeutics* 2012;**9**(1):176–184

5. SANAD Study Group, Marson AG, Al-Kharusi AM, Alwaidh M, et al. The SANAD study of effectiveness of carbamazepine, gabapentin, lamotrigine, oxcarbazepine, or topiramate for treatment of partial epilepsy: an unblinded randomised controlled trial. *Lancet* 2007;**369**(9566):1000–1015

6. SANAD Study Group, Marson AG, Al-Kharusi AM, Alwaidh M, et al. The SANAD study of effectiveness of valproate, lamotrigine, or topiramate for generalised and unclassifiable epilepsy: an unblinded randomised controlled trial. *Lancet* 2007;**369**(9566):1016–1026

7. Nunes VD, Sawyer L, Neilson J, Sarri G, Cross JH. Diagnosis and management of the epilepsies in adults and children: summary of updated NICE guidance. *BMJ* 2012;**344**:e281

8. ILAE Subcommission on AED Guidelines, Glauser T, Ben-Menachem E, Bourgeois B, et al. Updated ILAE evidence review of antiepileptic drug efficacy and effectiveness as initial monotherapy for epileptic seizures and syndromes. *Epilepsia* 2013;**54**(3):551–563

9. Tomson T, Marson A, Boon P, et al. Valproate in the treatment of epilepsy in girls and women of childbearing potential. *Epilepsia* 2015;**56**(7):1006–1019

10. Voinescu PE, Pennell PB. Management of epilepsy during pregnancy. *Expert Rev Neurother* 2015;**15**(10):1171–1187

11. Karlsson L, Wettermark B, Tomson T. Drug treatment in patients with newly diagnosed unprovoked seizures/epilepsy. *Epilepsy Res* 2014;**108**(5):902–908

12. Bonnett LJ, Tudur Smith C, Smith D, et al. Time to 12-month remission and treatment failure for generalised and unclassified epilepsy. *J Neurol Neurosurg Psychiatry* 2014;**85**(6):603–610

13. Bonnett LJ, Tudur Smith C, Donegan S, Marson AG, et al. Treatment outcome after failure of a first antiepileptic drug. *Neurology* 2014;**83**(6):552–560

14. Kwan P, Brodie MJ. Early identification of refractory epilepsy. *N Engl J Med* 2000;**342**(5):314–319

15. Neligan A, Bell GS, Sander JW, Shorvon SD. How refractory is refractory epilepsy?: patterns of relapse and remission in people with refractory epilepsy. *Epilepsy Res* 2011;**96**(3):225–230

16. Kwan P., Arzimanoglou A, Berg AT, et al. Definition of drug resistant epilepsy: consensus proposal by the ad hoc Task Force of the ILAE Commission on Therapeutic Strategies. *Epilepsia* 2010;**51**(6):1069–1077

17. Callaghan BC, Anand K, Hesdorffer D, Hauser WA, French JA. Likelihood of seizure remission in an adult population with refractory epilepsy. *Ann Neurol* 2007;**62**(4):382–389

18. BASE Study Group, Beghi, E, Gatti G, Tonini C, et al. Adjunctive therapy versus alternative monotherapy in patients with partial epilepsy failing on a single drug: a multicentre, randomised, pragmatic controlled trial. *Epilepsy Res* 2003;**57**(1):1–13

19. Maguire MJ, Hemming K, Hutton JL, Marson AG. Reporting and analysis of open-label extension studies of anti-epileptic drugs. *Epilepsy Res* 2008;**81**(1):24–29

20. Tudur Smith C, Marson AG, Chadwick DW, Williamson PR. Multiple treatment comparisons in epilepsy monotherapy trials. *Trials* 2007;**8**:34

21. Rheims S, Perucca E, Cucherat M, Ryvlin P. Factors determining response to antiepileptic drugs in randomized controlled trials: a systematic review and meta-analysis. *Epilepsia* 2011;**52**(2):219–233

22. Brodie MJ, Yuen AWC. Lamotrigine substitution study: evidence for synergism with sodium valproate? *Epilepsy Res* 1997;**26**(3):423–432

23. St. Louis EK. Truly "rational" polytherapy: maximizing efficacy and minimizing drug interactions, drug load, and adverse effects. *Curr Neuropharmacol* 2009;**7**(2):96–105

24. Hemming K, Maguire MJ, Hutton JL, Marson AG. Vigabatrin for refractory partial epilepsy. *Cochrane Database Sys Rev* 2013;(1):CD007302

25. Beacher NG, Brodie MJ, Goodall C. A case report: retigabine induced oral mucosal dyspigmentation of the hard palate. *BMC Oral Health* 2015;**15**(1):122

26. Tomson T, Battino D, Bonizzoni E, et al. Dose-dependent risk of malformations with antiepileptic drugs: an analysis of data from the EURAP epilepsy and pregnancy registry. *Lancet Neurol* 2011;**10**(7):609–617

27. Löscher W, Schmidt D. Modern antiepileptic drug development has failed to deliver: ways out of the current dilemma. *Epilepsia* 2011;**52**(4):657–678

28. Tan C, Shard C, Ranieri E, et al. Mutations of protocadherin 19 in female epilepsy (PCDH19-FE) lead to allopregnanolone deficiency. *Hum Mol Genet* 2015;**24**(18):5250–5259

29. Porter RJ, Kupferberg HJ, Hessie BJ. Mechanisms of action of anti-seizure drugs and the Anticonvulsant Screening Program of the National Institute of Neurological Disorders and Stroke. *Int J Clin Pharmacol Ther* 2015;**53**(1):9–12

30. Walker L, Sills GJ. Inflammation and epilepsy: the foundations for a new therapeutic approach in epilepsy? *Epilepsy Curr* 2012;**12**(1):8–12

31. Walker LE, Mirza N, Yip VLM, Marson AG, Pirmohamed M. Personalized medicine approaches in epilepsy. *J Int Med* 2015;**277**(2):218–234

32. Mikati MA, Jiang YH, Carboni M, et al. Quinidine in the treatment of KCNT1-positive epilepsies. *Ann Neurol* 2015;**78**(6):995–999

33. Mullen SA, Carney PW, Roten A, et al. Precision therapy for epilepsy due to KCNT1 mutations: a randomized trial of oral quinidine. *Neurology* 2018;**90**(1):e67-e72

34. Mirza N, Appleton R, Burn S, et al. Identifying the biological pathways underlying human focal epilepsy: from complexity to coherence to centrality. *Hum Mol Genet* 2015;**24**(15):4306–4316

Reproductive Health for Women with Medication-Resistant Epilepsy

Jiyeoun Yoo and Cynthia Harden

Introduction

Definition of Refractory Epilepsy

When patients with epilepsy have seizures that are not completely controlled by medications, they are considered to have drug-resistant epilepsy. This condition is also known as medically intractable, medication-resistant, or medication-resistant epilepsy. The International League against Epilepsy defines this condition as the failure of adequate trials of two tolerated, appropriately chosen and administered antiepileptic drugs, whether as monotherapy or in combination, to achieve seizure freedom [1]. An estimated 30% of patients with epilepsy may be medication-resistant.

Women with Medication-Resistant Epilepsy

Women with epilepsy face gender-specific issues, especially during child-bearing age. The problems become more complex for women with refractory epilepsy, as they are often on polytherapy. Therefore, considerations of interactions between anti-seizure medications (ASMs) and reproductive hormones becomes more important. Additional management issues arise for these women when planning and navigating pregnancy. In this chapter, we will discuss the reproductive issues in women with medication-resistant epilepsy with a focus on catamenial seizure exacerbations, ASM polypharmacy and interactions with reproductive hormones, and pregnancy.

Reproductive Hormones and Epilepsy

Reproductive Hormonal Effects on Seizures

Substantial biologic, experimental animal and human clinical studies have demonstrated the influence of female reproductive hormones on seizures; oestrogen being pro-convulsant, while progesterone and its metabolites act as anti-convulsants. Understanding their mechanism of action helps to understand why seizure frequency changes according to their cyclically fluctuating levels across the menstrual cycle, termed catamenial epilepsy. These neurosteroid effects have resulted in attempts at clinical applications using natural progesterone, and both natural hormones and hormonally based synthetic analogues that have anti-epileptic properties.

Oestrogen

There are three biologically active oestrogens; oestradiol is the main oestrogen in fertile women, oestriol is the major oestrogen in pregnancy and oestrone is the main oestrogen post-menopause. Oestradiol exerts direct excitatory effects at the neuronal membrane, by enabling neurons to respond rapidly to the excitatory effect of glutamate, which is primarily mediated by N-methyl-D-aspartate (NMDA) receptors [2]. This effect has been shown to occur within a few seconds, suggesting a direct membrane mechanism rather than a genomic effect. Other mechanisms can occur with a long-latency (hours to days) genomic effect. For example, over time, oestradiol increases the dendritic spine density and alters hippocampal synaptic connectivity via an NMDA-receptor-dependent mechanism [3].

Progesterone

Progesterone, via reduced metabolites such as tetrahydroprogesterone (allopregnanolone), exerts direct membrane-mediated inhibitory effects by potentiating GABA-A-mediated chloride conductance. It also potentiates the action of the endogenous inhibitory substance, adenosine. Long term, progesterone decreases the number of hippocampal CA1 dendritic spines and excitatory synapses faster than the simple withdrawal of oestrogen [4]. Progesterone and allopregnanolone have shown to have neuroprotective effects on hippocampal neurons in kainic-acid-induced seizure models [5].

Reproductive Hormonal Underpinnings of Catamenial Epilepsy

The term catamenial epilepsy refers to cyclic seizure exacerbation in relation to the menstrual cycle. This phenomenon is principally based on three pathophysiologic determinants: (1) the neuroactive properties of reproductive steroids, (2) the variation of neuroactive steroid levels across the menstrual cycle and (3) the susceptibility of the epileptic substrate to neuroactive steroid effects [6,7].

The average menstrual cycle is 28 (range 24–35) days, with day 1 being the first day of menstruation and day 14 being the day of ovulation. The menstrual cycle has two major phases: the follicular phase (days 1–14) and the luteal phase (days 15–28). During the follicular phase, the ovarian follicles grow and the dominant follicle becomes the ovulatory follicle containing the oocyte. On day 14, the oocyte is released (ovulation) and the non-dominant follicles degenerate.

In the luteal phase, the dominant follicle becomes the corpus luteum, which produces progesterone. When there is dysregulation of follicle-stimulating hormone (FSH) secretion, follicles develop poorly, and this leads to lack of ovulation and poor functioning of the corpus luteum. During an anovulatory cycle, there is higher oestrogen-progesterone ratio than an ovulatory cycle. Figure 17.1 shows the fluctuation of oestrogen and progesterone in the normal menstrual cycle, as well as an inadequate luteal-phase cycle with anovulation. The most relevant periods to catamenial epilepsy are: (1) during the beginning of the rapid surge of oestrogen at day 10–13 (periovulation), (2) the rapid decline of progesterone compared to oestrogen on days 26–28 (perimenstruation) and (3) the entire second half of the cycle during an inadequate luteal phase [7]. Anovulatory cycles may be more common in women with epilepsy than in the general population, adding to their risk of catamenial seizure exacerbations [6,8].

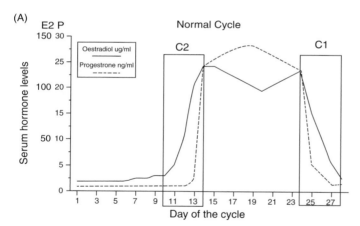

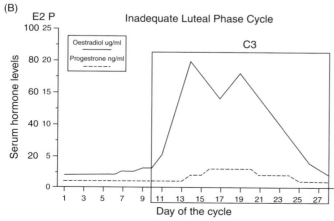

Figure 17.1 Patterns of catamenial epilepsy. (A) Normal cycle with normal ovulation. Exacerbation of seizures occurs in the perimenstrual phase (C1) and periovulatory phase (C2). (B) Inadequate luteal phase cycle with anovulation. Exacerbation of seizures occurs during the entire second half of the cycle (C3). C = catamenial seizure pattern, F = follicular phase, O = periovulatory, L = luteal phase, M = perimenstrual. Reproduced from Herzog and colleagues [7].

Effects of Epilepsy and Anti-Seizure Medications on Reproductive Hormones

Effects of Epilepsy on Reproductive Hormones

Regulation of reproduction involves the hypothalamic–pituitary–gonadal axis. The gonadotropin-releasing hormone (GnRH)-producing neurons, located at the diagonal band of Broca, the vasculosum of the lamina terminalis and the preoptic area of the thalamus, release GnRH, which regulates production and release of leutinizing hormone (LH) and FSH. In animal studies, reduced GnRH fibres were observed following pilocarpine-induced status epilepticus or focal application of kainic acid to the amygdala [9,10].

Hypogonadotropic hypogonadism, a gonadal dysfunction caused by the decreased ability of the hypothalamus to secrete GnRH or of the pituitary gland to secrete LH and FSH, has been reported in patients with epilepsy in both men and women [11,12]. Interestingly, it has been suggested that there is a relationship between laterality in epilepsy and reproductive hormone levels, with more sexual dysfunction in women with right-sided epileptic foci [13].

Effects of Anti-Seizure Medications on Reproductive Hormones

Enzyme-inducing drugs, such as phenobarbital, phenytoin and carbamazepine increase the breakdown and production of sex-hormone-binding globulin (SHBG) and reduce free fractions of steroid hormones. The clinical consequences are unknown so far.

On the other hand, valproate, which inhibits cytochrome p450 isoenzymes 2C9 and 2C19, has adverse effects on the reproduction system. Long-term valproate therapy has been associated with hyperandrogenism and polycystic ovaries in women with epilepsy [14], and this effect seems to be drug specific rather than related to epilepsy, since these findings have also been noted in women treated with valproate for bipolar disorder and in animal studies. In a study using human ovarian follicular cells, valproate was shown to significantly and concentration-dependently decrease basal and FSH-stimulated oestradiol secretion; no such effect was observed with levetiracetam [15]. In this study, both valproate and levetiracetam at higher concentration reduced CYP19 aromatase activity in FSH-stimulated cells, and both drugs were pro-apoptotic to ovarian cells.

Polycystic Ovary Syndrome

In polycystic ovary syndrome (PCOS), there is higher level of LH secretion, with an increased LH to FSH ratio. FSH stimulates ovarian steroidogenesis, and elevated LH/FSH produces numerous and cystic-appearing, immature follicles. These are deficient in aromatase, which is the enzyme that converts testosterone to oestrogen in the ovary. Hence, the PCOS ovarian follicles produce primarily androgens. These are then converted to oestrogen by aromatase in the periphery, which feeds back to the pituitary and deregulates normal LH secretion.

Higher incidence of PCOS in women with epilepsy has been described since early 1980s. Some studies attribute this association to the hypothalamic dysfunction as an effect of epilepsy, while others have attributed it to the use of valproate. In a study comparing women with localization-related epilepsy (LRE), idiopathic generalized epilepsy (IGE), and controls, anovulatory cycles occurred in 14.3% in LRE and 27.1% in IGE, compared to 10.9% in controls. The rate was significantly higher in patients on valproate [16], which could be a confounder. A recent meta-analysis of 11 prospective and controlled studies looking at the incidence of PCOS in women with epilepsy with or without valproate, found approximately 1.95-fold higher incidence of PCOS in women treated with valproate than without valproate [17]. It is possible that both epilepsy and valproate are independent risk factors for the development of PCOS.

Infertility

Infertility is defined as the inability to conceive after 12 months of unprotected regular sexual intercourse. Previous studies have suggested that women with epilepsy may have an increased risk of infertility compared to the general population. Wallace and colleagues, using the General Practice Research Database in the UK, reported a 33% lower rate of fertility in women with epilepsy [18]. Not all studies reported the same result, though. Olafsson and colleagues, using a population-based study in Iceland, found no evidence of a reduced fertility rate in women with epilepsy [19].

In a prospective study of women with epilepsy enrolled in the Kerala Registry of Epilepsy and Pregnancy in India [20], women with ASM exposure had a higher rate of infertility compared to women without ASM exposure, and use of three or more ASMs was associated with a significantly higher rate of infertility, specifically with the use of phenobarbital and phenytoin, which were frequently used in this study population. The higher rate of infertility on polytherapy may be related to the effects of ASMs or more refractory epilepsy itself.

Pregnancy and Epilepsy

Epilepsy is a condition that requires daily medication treatment that is likely to be long term. For women with epilepsy, especially of child-bearing age, questions arise about the safety of pregnancy, the adverse effects of anti-seizure medications on their offspring's long-term cognitive or developmental outcome, birth complications, safety of breastfeeding, etc. Pregnancy is also a period when there is much change in reproductive hormones and body weight, which can affect the serum concentration of the ASMs.

Risks of Seizures during Pregnancy

Studies have found that the most important predictor of seizures during pregnancy is the occurrence of seizures before pregnancy [21,22]. In a study by Thomas and coworkers [22], patients who had seizures in the pre-pregnancy month had 15-times higher risk of seizures during pregnancy compared to those who were seizure-free during the same period, and patients who were on polytherapy had greater risk of seizures than patients on monotherapy. In fact, the majority (80–90%) of women with epilepsy who were seizure-free for 9–12 months before pregnancy were likely to remain so during pregnancy. No higher rates of status epilepticus, increased seizure rate or increased risk of seizure relapse during pregnancy were found for women with epilepsy who were seizure-free [23]. The International Registry of Antiepileptic Drugs and Pregnancy (EURAP) study reported that women with IGE were more likely to remain seizure-free (73.6%) than women with LRE (59.5%), and that patients on lamotrigine and oxcarbazepine were less likely to be seizure-free compared to other monotherapies [21].

Adverse Effects of Seizures on Pregnancy

Specific effects of seizures on the fetus have been studied in both animals and humans. In an animal study using a pilocarpine-induced epilepsy rat model, a significant effect on the development of specific interneurons of hippocampi in the offspring was found. In the same animal model, rats exposed to seizures as a fetus demonstrated deficits in motor coordination and increased immobility in adult life [24,25]. In human studies, identifying an association between seizures and pregnancy outcome in the offspring is often confounded by maternal ASM use. In this respect, a study by Chen et al. [26] is remarkable as this confounder was eliminated. In this retrospective study of two nationwide data sets, many women were untreated and women with epilepsy who were taking medications were excluded from the group used for analysis. They found a significantly increased risk of infants who were small for gestational age (SGA) in women who had seizures during pregnancy compared to women with epilepsy who did not have seizures during pregnancy. This study also compared women with epilepsy to a healthy control group and found that epileptic seizures during pregnancy were independently associated with increased risk of low birth weight, pre-term delivery and SGA. These data provide additional evidence of the adverse effects of seizures on pregnancy outcome and why it is best to control seizures during pregnancy, in addition to protecting the patient and fetus from seizure-related injuries.

Adverse Effects of Anti-Seizure Medications on Pregnancy

For women with refractory epilepsy, the teratogenic risks of polytherapy vs. monotherapy are often a consideration. While polytherapy increases the risk of major congenital malformations (MCMs) in exposed offspring, this increased risk is largely accounted for by the use of valproate in the ASM regimen [27]. Figure 17.2 from the North American AED Pregnancy Registry (NAAEDPR) shows the MCM risks of individual ASM monotherapy in first trimester exposure [27]. Based on this data, which are consistent with worldwide experience, the safest ASMs are probably lamotrigine, carbamazepine, phenytoin and levetiracetam, which all cluster closely around 2–2.5% risk. Compared to the risk of lamotrigine, the risk ratio was fivefold with valproate, threefold with phenobarbital and twofold with topiramate. Valproate was shown to have significantly higher risk than other ASMs in causing MCMs, especially spina bifida and specifically hypospadias at a rate of 6–9%. Phenobarbital had significantly increased risk of mostly cardiac malformations. Topiramate was associated with increased risk of facial clefts (about 1.4% according to

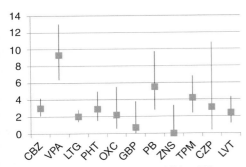

Number of outcomes: CBZ = 1033 VPA = 323
LTG = 1562 PHT= 416 OXC = 182 GBP = 145
PG = 199 ZNS = 99 TPM = 359 CZP = 64 LVT= 450

Figure 17.2 North American AED Pregnancy Registry between 1997 to 2011. Percentage of major congenital malformations and 95% confidence intervals with monotherapy in first trimester exposure. CBZ = carbamazepine, VPA = valproate, LTG = lamotrigine, PHT = phenytoin, OXC = oxcarbazepine, GBP = gabapentin, PB = phenobarbital, ZNS = zonisamide, TPM = topiramate, CZP = clonazepam, LVT = levetiracetam.

the NAAEDPR), which is about a 10-fold increase compared to the control prevalence. This increased risk was also found to be similar in several other studies.

A further consideration for women with refractory epilepsy is that they may be more likely to be taking a robust dose of ASMs, and this also contributes to teratogenic risk. A dose-dependent risk is well demonstrated in the EURAP study [28]. The rate of MCMs was the lowest with less than 300 mg/day of lamotrigine (1.7%) and with less than 400 mg/day of carbamazepine (2%). The risk of valproate at less than 700 mg/day was similar to this risk of lamotrigine or carbamazepine used at higher doses, which is in the range of 4–5%. The risk was greater than 20% when the dose was 1500 mg/day or more. The study showed that the dose-dependent risks were present in all ASMs, although the rate was higher with phenobarbital and valproate in all doses.

If there was a history of MCM in the first pregnancy, the risk was significantly higher to the next offspring if the mother continued to take the same drug (35.7% vs. 3.1%, with an OR 17.6), especially in those taking valproate (57%). In a woman with two or more pregnancies that resulted in ASM-associated malformations, the types were often different [29]. Recently, the EURAP study compared the risk of spontaneous abortions and stillbirth associated with maternal ASM use, and found that the risk was higher in polytherapy vs. monotherapy (RR 1.38) and parental history of MCMs (RR 1.92) [30].

Not only the physical defects, but the cognitive outcome of ASMs in offsprings exposed to ASMs in utero has been recognized in the past decade. The Neurodevelopmental Effects of Antiepileptic Drugs (NEAD) study is an ongoing, prospective, observational and assessor-masked multi-centre study in the USA and the UK [31]. In this study, the primary outcome of IQ at six years of age was investigated in children exposed to carbamazepine, lamotrigine, phenytoin or valproate. A high dose of valproate was negatively associated with IQ, verbal and non-verbal ability, memory and executive function compared to other ASMs. Interestingly, left-handedness was more frequent in the overall study group and verbal abilities were lower than non-verbal abilities for all ASM exposures, which speculated the possibility that ASM exposure may alter the development of cerebral lateralization. As in other studies, higher mean IQ was observed in children exposed to periconceptional folate. An increased risk of autistic spectrum disorder and childhood autism in children exposed to valproate in utero has also been shown in two studies [32,33].

Changes in Serum Levels of Anti-Seizure Medications during Pregnancy

During pregnancy, the pharmacokinetics of medications can be affected at any level from absorption, distribution and metabolism, to elimination. The greatest decline in serum concentration occurs with ASMs that are eliminated by glucuronidation (UGT), in particular lamotrigine. Serum levels of ASMs that are cleared mainly through the kidneys, such as levetiracetam, can also decrease significantly during pregnancy. Some ASMs, such as carbamazepine levels are only marginally affected by pregnancy [34]. Data are lacking for some of the newer medications, such as pregabalin, lacosamide, retigabine and eslicarbazepine acetate.

Obstetric Risks

A recent meta-analysis of women with epilepsy and their obstetric complications found a small but significant increase in the odds of spontaneous miscarriage, ante-partum and post-partum haemorrhage, hypertensive disorders, induction of labour, caesarean section, pre-term birth and fetal growth restriction. The odds of early pre-term birth, gestational diabetes, fetal death or stillbirth, perinatal death or admission to neonatal intensive care unit did not differ [35]. This result suggests that women with epilepsy who are contemplating pregnancy should also be counselled about the increased risks of obstetric complications.

Management

Treatment of Catamenial Epilepsy

The treatment for catamenial epilepsy should be tailored according to the pattern of catamenial seizures and the regularity of the menstruation cycles. A suggested algorithm is shown in Figure 17.3.

The cyclic progesterone treatment is best suited to patients with regular menstrual periods with a C1 pattern, especially when three times more seizures occur during days 25–3 compared to other days of the month [36]. Progesterone lozenges are used to supplement progesterone during the luteal phase, which is gradually withdrawn

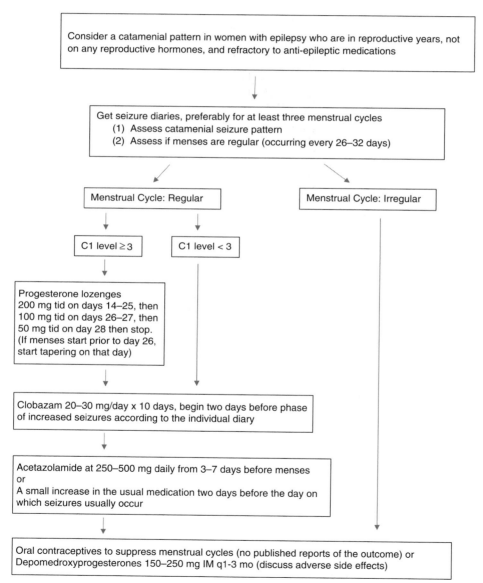

Figure 17.3 Suggested algorithm for evaluation and treatment of catamenial seizures. Modified and adapted from Harden and Pennell [45].

pre-menstrually. Potential adverse effects, such as sedation, depression, breast tenderness, vaginal bleeding, constipation and weight gain, should be discussed and monitored.

While no other benzodiazepines were formally studied for catamenial epilepsy, clobazam has shown to be effective in preventing seizures in catamenial epilepsy in a double-blind, placebo-controlled, cross-over study [37]. In this study, doses of 20–30 mg per day were used for a 10-day treatment period, and most patients had complete seizure control.

If the above measures fail, or if the seizure increase is less than threefold during the perimenstrual period, other less-well-studied therapies can be considered. Acetazolamide, at doses 250–500 mg daily administered from three to seven days before menses, has been reported to be effective [38], although there have been no randomized trials. A small increase in the patient's usual anti-seizure medications two days before the menses can be empirically tried.

In patients with irregular menses, suppressing the menstrual period with oral contraceptive medications or depomedroxyprogesterone can be considered. Their mechanism of action in reducing seizures is presumed to be by cessation of the cyclical oestrogen and progesterone levels. Depomedroxyprogesterone is administered via intra-muscular injection, with a standard dose of 150 mg every 12 weeks. Potential adverse effects include those of natural progesterone, but additionally, after cessation of depomedroxyprogesterone, endogenous hormone concentrates fluctuate substantially and the recovery of regular ovulatory cycles can be delayed up to two years, which could lead to infertility as well as seizure exacerbation during that time.

Management of Neuroendocrine Disorders

Polycystic Ovary Syndrome

During clinic visits, women with epilepsy should be assessed for the presence of abnormal menstrual cycles, hirsutism, male pattern hair loss, acne or increased body mass index. When suspected, testosterone levels can be obtained as a screening measure, and referral to an endocrinologist or gynaecologist should be considered, especially when PCOS is suspected.

Infertility

Physicians should advise about the potential risk of infertility in women with epilepsy and, when patients are suspected for subfertility, a referral for an infertility evaluation and treatment should be made.

Management During Pregnancy

Pre-Pregnancy

The treating physician and patient should have a clear understanding of the foreseeable management plans, potential adverse effects, including physical and cognitive teratogenesis, and obstetric risks from pregnancy. In patients with refractory epilepsy, at least generalized convulsions should be under control before pregnancy is contemplated, because of increased risks to the mother and fetus from convulsive seizures. Patients need to understand the reason why they need to continue taking medication, since compliance can be an issue during pregnancy due to a fear of adverse effects to their offspring. It is also helpful for patients to know that pregnancy itself does not in general increase their seizure frequency, and it is likely to remain similar to their pre-pregnancy seizure control, which is another reason to try to obtain the best seizure control before pregnancy.

Even if there are no immediate plans for pregnancy, switching to safer anti-seizure medications for pregnancy should be discussed with the patient in advance. Changing anti-seizure medications during pregnancy exposes patients to polytherapy, possible allergic reaction and is probably too late, since MCMs develop very early in pregnancy. Prior to pregnancy, two baseline ASM levels should be obtained to assess their effective level and stability.

Further, women with or without epilepsy should take folic acid from 1–4 mg per day pre-pregnancy and throughout pregnancy to reduce the risk of MCMs [39]. It is unclear if higher doses provide more benefit.

During Pregnancy

The visit schedule needs to be tailored based on the stability of the patient's epilepsy, other comorbidities and their ASMs. If possible, it is advised not to use valproate or polytherapy during the first trimester and throughout pregnancy to decrease the risk of MCMs, and to avoid phenytoin and phenobarbital throughout pregnancy to prevent reduced cognitive outcomes [40]. The level of the anti-seizure medications should be checked on a regular basis (recommended monthly), especially for those that are particularly affected during pregnancy, such as lamotrigine or oxcarbazepine (recommended every two weeks at the beginning of the pregnancy). The target level is the pre-determined pre-pregnancy lowest effective level, and dose increases are common in order to maintain this level. Close consultation with the patient's obstetrician is important to address the specific issues, for example, vomiting of ASMs or ultrasound results, etc. When a seizure occurs, it is important to determine if it was typical of the patient's known seizure type, as other problems, such as eclampsia, can provoke seizures.

After Delivery

The dose of the ASMs needs to be decreased within about 10 days to a dose slightly above the pre-pregnancy dose to compensate for post-partum fatigue and sleep deprivation. For lamotrigine, the dose adjustment needs to occur within a couple of days to avoid symptoms of increased serum concentration as clearance of the medication returns to the pre-pregnancy rate.

It is natural for mothers to worry about the potential adverse effects of breast feeding while they are taking ASMs. The concentration of ASM in breast milk is significant for primidone, levetiracetam, gabapentin, lamotrigine and topiramate, but minimal for valproate, phenobarbital, phenytoin and carbamazepine. Recently, the NEAD study published the cognitive outcome of breastfed children who were exposed to lamotrigine, carbamazepine, phenytoin or valproate at age three and six years. This study showed no adverse effects of ASM exposure via breast milk, and at age six, breastfed children exhibited higher IQ and verbal abilities [41].

A recent study revealed that women with epilepsy are at more risk for peripartum depression or anxiety compared to women without epilepsy or other chronic diseases. The rate was higher for those on polytherapy and those with higher doses or levels [42]. Treating physicians should identify these mood issues and take appropriate steps. These management tenets are presented in Figure 17.4.

Epilepsy Surgery and Devices

Epilepsy surgery should be considered in all patients with refractory epilepsy, especially for women of child-bearing age before they become pregnant or contemplate pregnancy.

Epilepsy surgery provides a potential cure for epilepsy, and while most patients who undergo epilepsy surgery do not completely taper off all ASMs, often the doses and number of ASMs can be reduced, and therefore physiologic and cognitive adverse effects to their offspring can be reduced. Furthermore, reducing the burden of seizures provides safety and peace of mind for the mother. Clinicians who are managing women with refractory epilepsy of child-bearing age should not only inform patients about the potential adverse effects of seizures and anti-seizure medications on the mother and fetus before pregnancy, but also about the potential benefits of epilepsy surgery.

For patients who are not resection candidates, neurostimulation can be considered. Vagus nerve stimulation (VNS) was approved by the US Food and Drug Administration (FDA) in 1997 as an adjunctive therapy for reducing the frequency of seizures in patients >12 years with medically refractory partial-onset seizures. The recent guideline from the American Academy of Neurology (AAN) recommends that VNS be also considered for seizures in children, for LGS-associated seizures and for improving mood in adults with epilepsy [43]. Deep brain stimulation (DBS) of bilateral anterior nuclei of thalami is approved in Europe and the United States for adjunctive treatment of epilepsy with focal seizures. The responsive neurostimulator system (RNS) was approved by the US FDA in 2013 as an adjunctive therapy for patients with drug-resistant, partial-onset seizures who have undergone diagnostic testing that localized no more than two epileptogenic foci.

Since its approval in 1997, there have been no reports of VNS causing adverse reactions in the mother or fetus during pregnancy. Although no reports are available on DBS and RNS in pregnancy for patients with epilepsy, patients undergoing DBS for other conditions have reported successful pregnancies [44]. Therefore, the neurostimulation devices appear to be safe during pregnancy and these options should be considered in patients who are not resection candidates.

Conclusion

Women with refractory epilepsy should partner with their neurologist to undertake strategies to achieve seizure freedom. However, they are generally more likely to be taking polytherapy, have catamenial seizure occurrences that persist, even when seizures are otherwise controlled, and face critical decisions about undertaking pregnancy and the risks of pregnancy to both themselves and their offspring.

Prior to planning pregnancy
- Achieve optimal seizure control, in particular, generalized tonic–clonic seizures
- Choose ASMs that have the less teratogenic effects
- Try the lowest effective dose, obtain serum trough levels to assess range of effective levels and to assess stability of levels
- If epilespy is in remission, consider gradual withdrawal of an ASM
- Recommend taking 4 mg of folic acid per day
- If positive history of congenital malformations with previous pregnancy or family history of such, discuss higher risk of malformations and avoid the same ASM that resulted in malformations

During pregnancy
- Avoid changes in ASMs unless necessary due to poor seizure control
- Obtain serum ASM levels at the time of pregnancy confirmation and at regular intervals throughout pregnancy. For lamotrigine, monitor level monthly and increase the dose to restore pre-pregnancy therapeutic level. For phenytoin or valproate, monitor free and total levels
- Monitor for vomiting of ASMs, consider methods to lower vomiting with assistance of an obstetrician
- Follow obstetric outcomes, including ultrasound results
- If seizures occur, determine if the seizure is consistent with the patient's type of epilepsy. Rule out other provoking factors, such as eclampsia or other causes.
- Continue folic acid and pre-natal vitamins throughout pregnancy

After delivery
- If the dose has been increased during pregnancy and the patient is stable, decrease the dose over the first 10 days after delivery to a dose slightly above pre-pregnancy maintenance dose, to compensate for the postpartum sleep deprivation. For lamotrigine, faster adjustment is needed
- Encourage breast feeding
- Identify post-partum depression or anxiety

Figure 17.4 Management of epilepsy during pregnancy. Modified and adapted from Pregnancy and Epilepsy, Harden [46].

Key Points

- The use of valproate is associated with an increased risk of PCOS; while valproate is generally avoided in women of child-bearing potential with epilepsy, it may be the most effective ASM for some women who do not respond to alternative ASM choices.

- There is an increased risk of infertility and early miscarriage for women taking ASM polytherapy; phenobarbital and phenytoin are specifically associated with increased risk of infertility.
- Prior to pregnancy, the ASM regimen should be simplified, if possible, to not include valproate and to decrease ASM doses, aiming for a valproate dose of less than 700 mg per day.

- Pregnancy may not be advisable if generalized tonic–clonic seizures are not controlled, as seizure frequency likely will not change due to pregnancy itself and seizures during pregnancy are associated with a risk to the offspring of being small for gestational age. Every effort, including surgical approaches, should be considered to control seizures prior to pregnancy.

- There are several approaches to suppressing catamenial seizure exacerbations, including hormonal treatments, adjustment of the ASM regimen and cyclic benzodiazepine supplements; the appropriate choice may depend on the exact catamenial pattern documented by the patient.

References

1. Kwan P, Arzimanoglou A, Berg AT, et al., Definition of drug resistant epilepsy: consensus proposal by the ad hoc Task Force of the ILAE Commission on Therapeutic Strategies. *Epilepsia* 2010;51(6):1069–1077

2. Smith SS. Estrogen administration increases neuronal responses to excitatory amino acids as a long-term effect. *Brain Res* 1989;503(2):354–357

3. Woolley CS, McEwen BS. Estradiol regulates hippocampal dendritic spine density via an N-methyl-D-aspartate receptor-dependent mechanism. *J Neurosci* 1994;14(12):7680–7687

4. Woolley CS, McEwen BS. Roles of estradiol and progesterone in regulation of hippocampal dendritic spine density during the estrous cycle in the rat. *J Comp Neurol* 1993;336(2):293–306

5. Frye CA. The neurosteroid 3 alpha, 5 apha-THP has antiseizure and possible neuroprotective effects in an animal model of epilepsy. *Brain Res* 1995;696 (1–2):113–120

6. Herzog AG. Catamenial epilepsy: definition, prevalence pathophysiology and treatment. *Seizure* 2008;17 (2):151–159

7. Herzog AG, Klein P, Ransil BJ. Three patterns of catamenial epilepsy. *Epilepsia* 1997;38(10):1082–1088

8. Cummings LN, Giudice L, Morrell MJ. Ovulatory function in epilepsy. *Epilepsia* 1995;36(4):355–359

9. Friedman MN, Geula C, Holmes GL, Herzog AG. GnRH-immunoreactive fiber changes with unilateral amygdala-kindled seizures. *Epilepsy Res* 2002;52 (2):73–77

10. Amado D, Cavalheiro EA, Bentivoglio M. Epilepsy and hormonal regulation: the patterns of GnRH and galanin immunoreactivity in the hypothalamus of epileptic female rats. *Epilepsy Res* 1993;14(2):149–159

11. Herzog AG, Seibel MM, Schomer DL, Vaitukaitis JL, Geschwind N. Reproductive endocrine disorders in men with partial seizures of temporal lobe origin. *Arch Neurol* 1986;43(4):347–350

12. Herzog AG, Seibel MM, Schomer DL, Vaitukaitis JL, Geschwind N. Reproductive endocrine disorders in women with partial seizures of temporal lobe origin. *Arch Neurol* 1986;43(4):341–346

13. Herzog AG, Coleman AE, Jacobs AR, et al. Relationship of sexual dysfunction to epilepsy laterality and reproductive hormone levels in women. *Epilepsy Behav* 2003;4(4):407–413

14. Isojarvi JI, Laatikainen TJ, Pakarinen AJ, Juntunen KT, Myllylä VV. Polycystic ovaries and hyperandrogenism in women taking valproate for epilepsy. *N Engl J Med* 1993;329(19):1383–1388

15. Taubøll E, Gregoraszczuk EL, Wojtowicz AK, Milewicz T. Effects of levetiracetam and valproate on reproductive endocrine function studied in human ovarian follicular cells. *Epilepsia* 2009;50(8):1868–1874

16. Morrell MJ, Giudice L, Flynn KL, et al. Predictors of ovulatory failure in women with epilepsy. *Ann Neurol* 2002;52(6):704–711

17. Hu X, Wang J, Dong W, et al. A meta-analysis of polycystic ovary syndrome in women taking valproate for epilepsy. *Epilepsy Res* 2011;97(1–2):73–82

18. Wallace H, Shorvon S, Tallis R. Age-specific incidence and prevalence rates of treated epilepsy in an unselected population of 2,052,922 and age-specific fertility rates of women with epilepsy. *Lancet* 1998;352 (9145):1970–1973

19. Olafsson E, Hauser WA, Gudmundsson G. Fertility in patients with epilepsy: a population-based study. *Neurology* 1998;51(1):71–73

20. Sukumaran SC, Sarma PS, Thomas SV. Polytherapy increases the risk of infertility in women with epilepsy. *Neurology* 2010;75(15):1351–1355

21. Battino D, Tomson T, Bonizzoni E, et al., Seizure control and treatment changes in pregnancy: observations from the EURAP epilepsy pregnancy registry. *Epilepsia* 2013;54(9):1621–1627

22. Thomas SV, Syam U, Devi JS. Predictors of seizures during pregnancy in women with epilepsy. *Epilepsia* 2012;53(5):e85-e88

23. Harden CL, Hopp J, Ting TY, et al. Practice parameter update. Management issues for women with epilepsy – focus on pregnancy (an evidence-based review): obstetrical complications and change in seizure frequency. Report of the Quality Standards Subcommittee and Therapeutics and Technology Assessment Subcommittee of the American Academy of Neurology and American Epilepsy Society. *Neurology* 2009;73(2):126–132

24. Do Vale TG, Da Silva AV, Lima DC, et al. Seizures during pregnancy modify the development of hippocampal interneurons of the offspring. *Epilepsy Behav* 2010;**19**(1):20–25

25. Lima DC, Vale TG, Argañãraz GA, et al. Behavioral evaluation of adult rats exposed in utero to maternal epileptic seizures. *Epilepsy Behav* 2010;**18**(1–2):45–49

26. Chen YH, Chiou HY, Lin HC, Lin HL. Affect of seizures during gestation on pregnancy outcomes in women with epilepsy. *Arch Neurol* 2009;**66**(8):979–984

27. Hernandez-Diaz S, Smith CR, Shen A. Comparative safety of antiepileptic drugs during pregnancy. *Neurology* 2012;**78**(21):1692–1699

28. Tomson, T, Battino D, Bonizzoni E, et al. Dose-dependent risk of malformations with antiepileptic drugs: an analysis of data from the EURAP epilepsy and pregnancy registry. *Lancet Neurol* 2011;**10** (7):609–617

29. Vajda FJ, O'Brien TJ, Lander CM, et al. Teratogenesis in repeated pregnancies in antiepileptic drug-treated women. *Epilepsia* 2013;**54**(1):181–186

30. Tomson T, Battino D, Bonizzoni E, et al. Antiepileptic drugs and intrauterine death: a prospective observational study from EURAP. *Neurology* 2015;**85**(7):580–588

31. NEAD Study Group, Meador KJ, Baker GA, Browning N, et al. Fetal antiepileptic drug exposure and cognitive outcomes at age 6 years (NEAD study): a prospective observational study. *Lancet Neurol* 2013;**12**(3):244–252

32. Liverpool and Manchester Neurodevelopment Group, Bromley RL, Mawer G, Clayton-Smith J, Baker GA. Autism spectrum disorders following in utero exposure to antiepileptic drugs. *Neurology* 2008;**71** (23):1923–1924

33. Christensen J, Grønborg TK, Sørensen MJ, et al. Prenatal valproate exposure and risk of autism spectrum disorders and childhood autism. *J Am Med Assoc* 2013;**309**(16):1696–1703

34. Tomson T, Landmark CJ, Battino D, et al. Antiepileptic drug treatment in pregnancy: changes in drug disposition and their clinical implications. *Epilepsia* 2013;**54**(3):405–414

35. EBM CONNECT Collaboration, Viale L, Allotey J, Cheong-See F, et al. Epilepsy in pregnancy and reproductive outcomes: a systematic review and meta-analysis. *Lancet* 2015;**386**(10006):1845–1852

36. Progesterone Trial Study Group, Herzog AG, Fowler KM, Smithson SD, et al. Progesterone vs placebo therapy for women with epilepsy: A randomized clinical trial. *Neurology* 2012;**78** (24):1959–1966

37. Feely M, Calvert R, Gibson J. Clobazam in catamenial epilepsy: a model for evaluating anticonvulsants. *Lancet* 1982;**2**(8289):71–73

38. Poser CH. Letter: modification of therapy for exacerbation of seizures during menstruation. *J Pediatr* 1974;**84**(5):779–780

39. American Academy of Neurology, American Epilepsy Society, Harden CL, Pennell PB, Koppel BS, et al. Practice parameter update. Management issues for women with epilepsy–focus on pregnancy (an evidence-based review): vitamin K, folic acid, blood levels, and breastfeeding. Report of the Quality Standards Subcommittee and Therapeutics and Technology Assessment Subcommittee of the American Academy of Neurology and American Epilepsy Society. *Neurology* 2009;**73**(2):142–149

40. American Academy of Neurology, American Epilepsy Society, Harden CL, Meador KJ, Pennell PB, et al. Practice parameter update. Management issues for women with epilepsy–focus on pregnancy (an evidence-based review): teratogenesis and perinatal outcomes. Report of the Quality Standards Subcommittee and Therapeutics and Technology Assessment Subcommittee of the American Academy of Neurology and American Epilepsy Society. *Neurology* 2009;**73**(2):133–141

41. Neurodevelopmental Effects of Antiepileptic Drugs (NEAD) Study Group, Meador, KJ, Baker GA, Browning N, et al. Breastfeeding in children of women taking antiepileptic drugs: cognitive outcomes at age 6 years. *JAMA Pediatr* 2014;**168**(8):729–736

42. Bjork MH, Veiby G, Reiter SC, et al. Depression and anxiety in women with epilepsy during pregnancy and after delivery: a prospective population-based cohort study on frequency, risk factors, medication, and prognosis. *Epilepsia* 2015;**56**(1):28–39

43. Morris GL, 3rd, Gloss D, Buchhalter J, et al. Evidence-based guideline update: vagus nerve stimulation for the treatment of epilepsy. Report of the Guideline Development Subcommittee of the American Academy of Neurology. *Neurology* 2013;**81** (16):1453–1459

44. Scelzo E, Mehrkens JH, Bötzel K, et al. Deep brain stimulation during pregnancy and delivery: experience from a series of "DBS Babies". *Front Neurol* 2015;**6**:191

45. Harden CL, Pennell PB. Neuroendocrine considerations in the treatment of men and women with epilepsy. *Lancet Neurol* 2013;**12**(1):72–83

46. Harden CL. Pregnancy and epilepsy. *Continuum (Minneap Minn)* 2014;**20**(1 Neurology of Pregnancy):60–79

Chapter 18

Resective Surgery for Medication-Resistant Epilepsy

Barbara C. Jobst and Krzyszof A. Bujarski

Resective epilepsy surgery is to date the most effective treatment for focal medication-resistant epilepsy. In multiple retrospective studies the median percentage for remaining seizure-free is approximately 60–65%, depending on the epilepsy syndrome [1]. Surgery for epilepsy was pioneered by Penfield in the first part of the twentieth century and has been refined since, with advanced imaging and neurophysiologic recordings [2]. Despite the obvious success, surgery remains underutilized [1,3]. If seizures are focal in onset and medication resistant, which is defined by the ILAE as having failed two anti-epileptic medications at standard doses, surgical evaluation at a specialized centre is indicated [4].

Localization of the Surgical Target

The Concept of Focal Epilepsy vs. Epileptic Networks

Epilepsy surgery is based on the concept that seizures begin in a focal area with distinct pathology and subsequently propagate to other areas of the brain. Removing the focal area will eliminate the pathology and, therefore, cure the epilepsy. Within this framework the area that is responsible for causing the epilepsy is termed the epileptogenic zone (EZ). The epileptogenic zone is the area that, if removed, renders the patient seizure-free. It is the epileptologist's task to identify the epileptogenic zone and assess whether it is functionally safe to remove it. However, current diagnostic capabilities sometimes fall short of exactly identifying the underlying abnormality, especially in non-lesional (MRI-negative) epilepsy. The seizure-onset zone (SOZ) is the area that can be defined by intra-cranial EEG as being the earliest area involved in the seizure. The symptomatogenic zone (SZ) is the area that determines the clinical manifestation of the seizures (Figure 18.1). This focal model of epilepsy is based on the long-standing

success of epilepsy surgery, which remains the most successful treatment option to date.

An alternative model is based on excitation of neuronal network nodes that entrain seizures by synchronizing with each other, with multiple parts being required to initiate and maintain pathological ictal activity. However, in this model, it remains unclear, from an epilepsy surgery point of view, which nodes of the network need to be removed and which can remain [5].

Identifying the Seizure-Onset Zone

To identify the seizure-onset zone, the clinical presentation of seizures, the history of the patient's epilepsy and the identification of the patient's epilepsy syndrome remain the most important clinical tools, in addition to MRI imaging. Video-EEG monitoring is essential to lateralize and localize the seizure-onset zone. For correlation of clinical symptomatology to cortical areas see Figure 18.1.

MRI imaging identifies lesions that can be epileptogenic. It is now state-of-art to perform 3 tesla (3 T) imaging that includes sagittal and coronal whole-volume T1 thin cuts, coronal and axial T2-weighted imaging and FLAIR imaging angulated along the axis of the hippocampus [6]. Imaging at 3 T has advantages in identifying lesions as compared to 1.5 T imaging [7]. Currently human imaging at 7 T is being investigated, but still needs to be assessed for its clinical value [8]. MRI lesions have to be carefully correlated to the clinical and video-EEG findings, as they may not represent the actual epileptogenic zone or could represent incidental findings. Lesional epilepsy is easier to approach surgically, as it is likely that the identified abnormality is concurrent with the epileptogenic zone. For a list of common lesions associated with medication-resistant epilepsy see Table 18.1.

Lesional and non-lesional focal epilepsies require varying surgical approaches (Figure 18.2). In non-

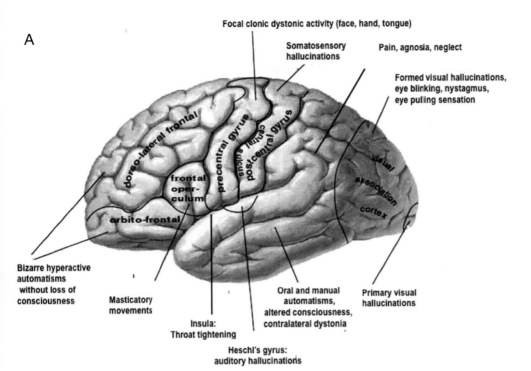

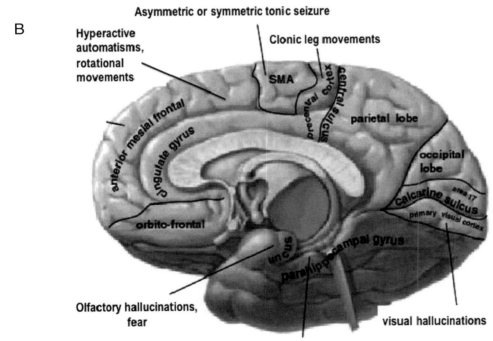

Figure 18.1 Symptomatogenic zones during epileptic seizures: (A) lateral cortical areas and their seizure manifestations, (B) medial cortical and medial temporal areas and their respective seizure manifestations.

Table 18.1 List of epileptogenic lesions frequently associated with medication-resistant epilepsy and apparent on routine MRI imaging

- **Intra-cerebral tumours:**
  - Low-grade gliomas (astrocytomas and oligodendrogliomas)
  - Hamartoma (including hypothalamic hamartoma)
  - Gangliogliomas
  - DNETs
  - Tubers

- **Malformations of cortical development:**
  - Focal cortical dysplasia
  - Polymicrogyria
  - Periventricular and other heterotopia
  - Schizencephaly
  - Pachygyria

- **Mesial temporal sclerosis**

- **Encephalomalacia and gliosis:**
  - Post-traumatic
  - s/p Haemorrhage
  - s/p Infection
  - s/p Hypoxia
  - Post-surgical
  - Ulegyria

- **Vascular malformations:**
  - Cavernomas
  - Sturge–Weber Syndrome
  - AVM
  - Dural arteriovenous fistula

- **Other:**
  - Rasmussen encephalitis
  - Infectious: tuberculoma, neurocysticercosis

- **Not considered epileptogenic:**
  - Small deep, white matter imaging abnormalities (ischaemic or demyelinating)
  - Vascular: teleangiectasias, cerebellar and brain stem cavernomas
  - Cerebellar or brain stem lesions
  - Extradural or abnormalities in the subarachnoid space without significant mass effect
  - Incidental meningioma in a location not consistent with seizure semiology
  - Choroidal fissure and hippocampal sulcus remnant cysts

lesional epilepsy more extensive ancillary testing may be necessary to identify the seizure-onset zone. This includes ictal single-photon emission computed tomography (SPECT), positron emmision tomography (PET) and magnetencephalography (MEG).

Inter-ictal and ictal SPECT are metabolic perfusion tests to identify the seizure-onset zone. Inter-ictal SPECT can be helpful in identifying the seizure-onset zone and has been reported to be concordant with the intra-cranial seizure-onset zone in 29% and has lateralizing value in non-lesional epilepsy [9]. Ictal SPECT is a resource-intensive test that requires injection of the radioactive tracer within seconds of seizure onset. Post-ictal injections are of limited value [10]. Subtraction of inter-ictal from ictal images and coregistration to MRI imaging (SISCOM: subtraction ictal–inter-ictal SPECT coregistered with MRI) are helpful tools to identify the seizure-onset zone and are concordant with the intra-cranial EEG seizure-onset zone in 52–67% [9,11]. Statistical parametric mapping of the imaging data may improve accuracy further [12,13]. SISCOM and MRI are most likely to identify the seizure-onset zone, compared to other non-invasive imaging studies, but the retrospective nature and variability of reported imaging studies in epilepsy makes this a difficult assessment [13–15]. Ictal SPECT has a greater sensitivity than inter-ictal PET (87% vs. 56%) [16]. Inter-ictal PET can also be helpful in identifying the seizure-onset zone, especially in non-lesional epilepsy [11,16,17]. PET has greater sensitivity in mesial temporal lobe epilepsy than in neocortical epilepsy [13].

MEG and magnet source imaging (MSI, a technique to coregister magnetic dipoles with MRI) are additional tools to identify the seizure-onset zone. MEG and MSI measure inter-ictal activity. Both techniques have value in non-lesional epilepsy and especially if focal cortical dysplasias are suspected [18,19]. In a systematic review mean sensitivity and specificity is estimated to be 84% and 54%, respectively [19].

Resective epilepsy surgery does not only have the benefit of eliminating seizures, but also has the risk of acquiring an additional deficit. Of special concern are language, motor and cognitive deficits. Neuropsychological testing gives an estimate of overall cognitive function and specific deficits. Other imaging techniques such as functional MRI (fMRI) and intra-carotid amytal testing determine language and memory dominance. fMRI can also localize motor areas. Visual field testing may be helpful if occipital lobe epilepsy or posterior temporal lobe epilepsy is suspected. Findings with these diagnostic tests may not only help in estimating the risk of resection, but can also be helpful in diagnosing the seizure-onset zone. For example, severely impaired unilateral memory function on intra-carotid amytal testing may indicate onset in the respective mesial temporal region. Specific deficits on neuropsychological testing can also provide evidence for suspected seizure-onset zones.

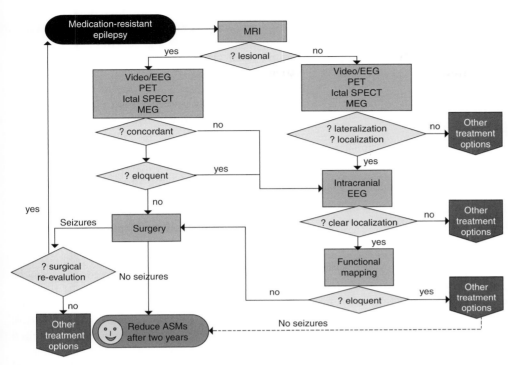

Figure 18.2 Algorithm of how to approach a patient with medication-resistant epilepsy surgically.

The type of pre-surgical work-up necessary is based on the patient's clinical and imaging findings and tailored to the individual patient. In non-lesional epilepsy certainly more exploratory diagnostic testing such as ictal SPECT and PET can be necessary. For an algorithmic approach to epilepsy surgery see Figure 18.2.

Determining Surgical Margins

After all non-invasive testing is obtained and a reasonable hypothesis about the seizure-onset zone is formulated, more invasive testing such as intra-cranial EEG may be required to localize the seizure onset further. In the case of lesional epilepsy, resection may be performed without intra-cranial EEG (Figure 18.2). In most surgical epilepsy centres patients are discussed in multi-disciplinary conferences, as intra-cranial EEG and surgical approaches are highly individualized.

Lesional Epilepsy

In patients with unequivocal lesions on MRI, further testing with intra-cranial EEG recordings may not be necessary if the scalp video-EEG monitoring, the clinical presentation of the seizure and epilepsy,

and other non-invasive testing is concordant with the lesion (Figure 18.2). Resecting the lesion has a high likelihood of eliminating the epilepsy [20]. It has been demonstrated that the lesion itself may not be the seizure-onset zone, but the surrounding brain tissue [21]. Resection of the lesion only has been shown to be less successful in eliminating seizures compared to resection of the lesion with the surrounding cortical margins or with a complete hippocampectomy if the lesion involves the mesial temporal structures [22]. In the case of cavernomas it is still discussed whether a lesionectomy alone is sufficient to treat seizures or whether additional resection of the hemosiderin ring is required [23]. Although single studies have reported improved seizure outcomes with extensive resection of the hemosiderin ring, a meta-analysis did not identify a benefit [23,24].

If pre-surgical diagnostic testing reveals highly discordant data about the seizure-onset zone and the visible lesion on MRI, or if the lesion is in areas close to functional eloquent brain areas (Figure 18.2), intra-cranial EEG may be required to obtain further clarity about the seizure-onset zone and/or enable functional mapping to identify eloquent cortex [25]. Motor, language and visual function are the main areas of concern. Alternatively, functional mapping can also be obtained intra-operatively [25]. However, intra-operative language mapping requires awake surgery and is limited in length in the operating room.

Non-Lesional Epilepsy

In most patients with MRI-negative non-lesional epilepsy, intra-cranial EEG is required. There is discussion as to whether non-lesional temporal lobe epilepsy with concordant pre-surgical data requires intra-cranial EEG, especially if MRI is normal and PET shows hypometabolism in the temporal areas [17,26].

The purpose of intra-cranial EEG is to determine the electrical seizure-onset zone, determine the resection margins and perform functional mapping to identify eloquent cortex. There are several ways intra-cranial EEG can be recorded. In the USA the traditional method has utilized subdural grid and strip electrodes that cover larger areas of the cortex, but this has changed over recent years toward greater use of depth electrodes (Figure 18.3A and B). Grid electrodes are larger electrode arrays with multiple electrodes in multiple rows. Grid electrodes require a craniotomy. Strip electrodes are electrode arrays with one row of electrodes that can also be placed through smaller burr holes without requiring craniotomy. Grid and strip electrodes allow for sampling and mapping of larger cortical areas. Currently available grid and strip electrodes have a disk diameter of 4 mm and are frequently spaced 1 cm apart.

Depth electrodes are electrodes that are stereotactically placed in deeper brain regions. Depth electrodes are frequently used to sample the mesial temporal regions, including the hippocampus. Depth electrodes in the mesial temporal structures can either be placed from a lateral approach (Figure 18.3D) or in an occipito-temporal approach (Figure 18.3C). Commercially available depth electrodes have a diameter of 1.1 mm. Depth and strip electrodes can be combined and a craniotomy may not be required if no grids are used (Figure 18.3C). Any combination of electrodes may be used, and most intra-cranial EEG is tailored to the specific patient.

Since the 1950s, a surgically similar but conceptionally alternative method, stereo-EEG (S-EEG) has been utilized in Europe by placing multiple depth electrodes anchored to the skull into cortical and deeper brain regions (Figure 18.3D) [27]. Initially conventional angiography was required to avoid haemorrhages by puncturing functionally important brain vessels. This now has been replaced by more advanced MR-angiographic and frameless robotic placement techniques, which do not require conventional angiography and make the placement procedure less time-intensive. This approach has now increased in popularity in North America [28]. Currently commercially available S-EEG electrodes are slightly thinner than conventional depth electrodes, having a diameter of 0.86 mm. S-EEG does not require a craniotomy and requires only small burr holes (Figure 18.3). Sphenoidal electrodes, foramen ovale, peg and epidural electrodes are less invasive approaches to obtain intra-cranial EEG recordings, but are limited in spatial resolution [29].

EEG findings on intra-cranial recordings can be quite varied [30]. Hippocampal and mesial temporal seizures may have a different electrophysiological signature from cortical seizures (Figures 18.4 and 18.5). Typical seizures of hippocampal origin are characterized on intra-cranial EEG by pre-ictal periodic spiking, a high-amplitude sharp transient, possibly followed by irregular polyspikes and electrodecrement until a synchronized theta rhythm establishes and propagates further to temporal neocortical structures or contralateral (Figure 18.4) [31]. A meta-analysis of intra-cranial EEG of ictal onset patterns acknowledges that it is difficult to make final conclusions from the heterogeneity of studies that are reported, but concluded that mesial temporal lobe patterns with low-frequency ictal spiking (Figure 18.4) are the onset patterns that are associated with the best surgical outcome. Sinusoidal and delta patterns seem to indicate seizure spread [30]. Others reported that fast ictal activity (>8 Hz) in temporal lobe epilepsy is more commonly associated with a good outcome compared to slower rhythmic activity or attenuation of the background activity [32].

In neocortical epilepsy, seizure onsets with fast-frequency, low-amplitude activity has been shown to be most frequently associated with a seizure-free outcome in some but not all studies (Figure 18.5) [30,33]. Rhythmic theta activity is also frequently noted, as well as rhythmic delta activity. However, patients with delta onsets are less frequently seizure-free than patients with high-frequency seizure onsets [30]. Regional seizure onsets are less likely to result in a seizure-free outcome. Seizures with rapid EEG spread to other structures also indicate a less favourable outcome [33]. Seizure

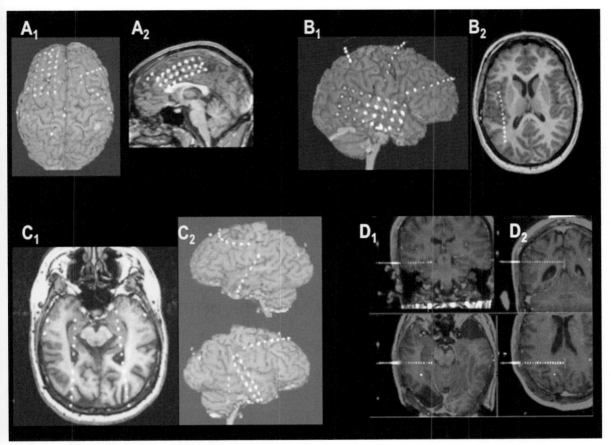

Figure 18.3 Various approaches to intra-cranial EEG recordings in four different patients (A–D). (A) 1: Placement of a grid electrode (4×8) over the R frontal cortex and some strip electrodes over the left frontal cortex. 2: The use of double-sided inter-hemispheric grids to sample the mesial cortical areas. This electrode array is useful for suspected supplementary motor or frontal lobe seizures. (B) 1: Placement of a lateral temporal 4×8 grid electrode and two additional strip electrodes over the frontal lateral cortex. 2: This was combined with depth electrodes in insular placed from posterior and the hippocampus (not shown). (C) 1: Bilateral sampling of the hippocampus and amygdala in an occipito-temporal approach. 2: This was combined with the placement of additional strip electrodes over the left frontal and temporal (top) and the right frontal and temporal cortex (bottom). This patient did not require a craniotomy for electrode placement. (D) 1: S-EEG with placement in the hippocampal structures from a lateral approach. The patient already had a previous left anterior temporal resection and a right-sided occipital resection. 2: Placement of S-EEG electrode in the posterior temporal and medial occipital cortex. (S-EEG illustrations, courtesy of Dr Arnaud Biraben, University of Rennes, France).

propagation patterns later in the seizure can also provide important information about the initial seizure-onset zone [34].

The relationship of inter-ictal spikes to the seizure-onset zone has been debated and is not necessarily linear [35–37]. Nevertheless, inter-ictal activity can contribute important information for seizure-onset lateralization and localization [35–37]. However, exact quantification of inter-ictal spiking activity requires automated detection of inter-ictal activity and long-term recordings [36,37].

Lately, high-frequency oscillations (HFOs, fast ripples) have been shown to correlate with the seizure-onset zone [38]. Retrospective review of HFOs has shown that oscillations over 250 Hz are more frequently observed in the seizure-onset zone, as compared to areas not involved at seizure onset [39]. Oscillations below 250 Hz are of lesser importance [38]. However, identification and quantification of HFO remains time-consuming and so far remains only semi-automated [40]. Integration of HFO identification into clinical practice has been progressing slowly [41].

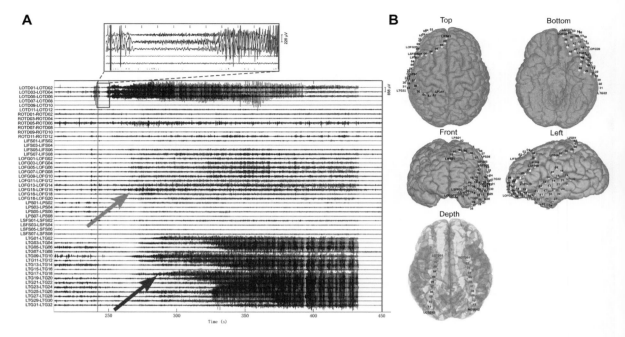

Figure 18.4 Example of intra-cranial EEG with onset in the hippocampus. (A) Intra-cranial EEG with earliest seizure onset at electrodes LOTD 1–6 (red line). The seizure shows a typical pattern with a high-amplitude transient followed by some polyspiking, electrodecrement and then rhythmic theta activity (blue frame). The seizure shows an initial spread pattern to the ipsilateral orbito-frontal area (green arrow) and then to the ipsilateral temporal neocortex. (B) Coregistration of the patient's electrodes with the MRI to demonstrate electrode placement. LOTD = left occipito-temporal (hippocampal) depth electrode, ROTD = right occipito-temporal (hippocampal) depth electrode, LIFS = left inferior frontal strip, LOFG = left orbito-frontal grid, LPS = left parietal strip, LSFS = left superior frontal strip, LTG = left temporal grid.

Identifying Functional Tissue Included in the Seizure-Onset Zone (Functional Mapping)

Pre-surgically obtained information, such as f-MRI mapping, neuropsychological testing, intra-carotid amytal testing and mapping for functional area with MEG/MSI, can help identify functionally relevant cortex [19]. However, in some cortical areas of the brain, electrical stimulation mapping of the areas may be required. Functional mapping is usually performed with electrical stimulation at 50 Hz [42]. Current ranges between 0.5–15 mA, stimulus duration 2–5 seconds with a pulse width of 300–500 microseconds. Electrical stimulation of the brain can induce after-discharges (AD) and ultimately can induce seizures. If after-discharges occur, shorter pulses of stimulation at the same frequency can abort them [43]. Mapping procedures at lower frequencies are less likely to produce after-discharges but require higher currents [42]. Motor activity can be mapped with shorter stimuli than 5 seconds; language mapping requires stimuli of 5 seconds to present items to the patient to be named.

If eloquent and functionally important cortex is included in the seizure-onset zone, the extent of resective surgery may be limited or cannot be performed at all.

Surgical Procedures and Outcome After Surgery

A meta-analysis of thousands of patients reported an average of 62% chance to become seizure-free after resective epilepsy surgery [1]. This is far superior to any outcomes of add-on medication or stimulation trials that usually report a mean reduction in seizure frequency or the percentage of patients who have 50% less seizures (responder rate) [44]. Two randomized controlled trials have clearly demonstrated that surgical therapy in temporal lobe epilepsy is superior to medical therapy in terms of seizure outcome [45,46]; 58% became seizure-free after surgery compared to 17% after optimization of medical therapy [45]. A smaller trial studying surgery within two years of seizure onset similarly showed the superiority of surgery [46]. Quality of life also clearly improved in both trials.

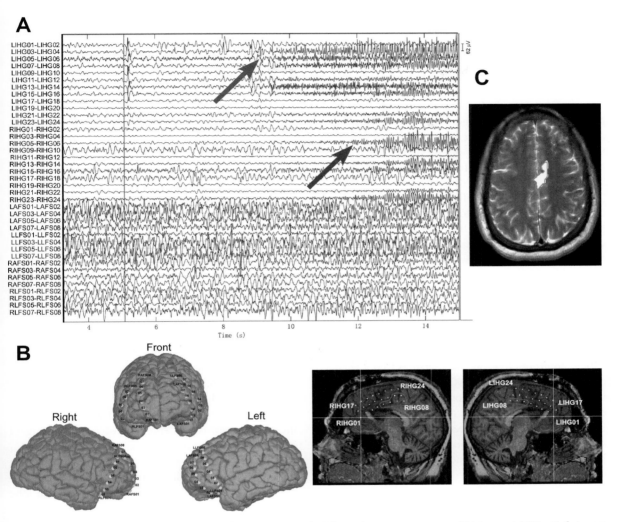

Figure 18.5 Intra-cranial recording of a patient with seizure onset in the left supplementary motor area. (A) Intra-cranial EEG with first onset seen with a sharp transient (red line). Later, rhythmic fast activity develops over the left supplementary motor area (LIHG 5–8, red arrow) and then spreads to the RIHG (blue arrow). There is little change in any activity over the lateral frontal cortex (LAF, LLFS, RAF, RLF). (B) Coregistration of the electrodes visualized on CT scan to reconstructions of the MRI. RIHG = right inter-hemispheric grid, LIHG = left inter-hemispheric grid (double-sided), LAFS =left anterior frontal strip, LLFS = left lateral frontal strip, RAFS = right anterior frontal strip, RLFS = right lateral frontal strip. The red outline on the inter-hemispheric grid shows the results of functional mapping. Complex motor responses in the upper and lower extremities could be elicited, indicating location of the supplementary motor area. (C) SISCOM (ictal SPECT) of the same patient, with clear hyperperfusion in the medial frontal area. The patient underwent a resection of the left supplementary motor area.

Temporal lobe epilepsy surgery can be performed utilizing various procedures. The most commonly performed procedure is a complete resection of the anterior temporal pole, the lateral temporal neocortex and the mesial (or medial) temporal structures [1]. On the left the length of the resection is limited by language function, as compared to right-sided procedures, in which the resection can be carried out further posteriorly [1]. Resection of the dominant

temporal lobe can result in significant deficits of verbal memory and confrontation naming [47].

Selective amygdalo-hippocampectomy is a procedure where only the mesial temporal structures (hippocampus, amygdala and parahippocampal gyrus) are resected. Access can be gained through the middle temporal gyrus, the sylvian fissure or the anterior temporal pole [1,48]. A complete temporal lobectomy is slightly superior in terms of becoming seizure-free after surgery, but may also be associated with a slightly higher risk of memory impairment after surgery [48–50].

Outcome of neocortical epilepsy has not been studied in randomized controlled trials, but retrospective studies clearly demonstrate the efficacy of resective epilepsy surgery [1]. Lesional epilepsy has a better outcome than non-lesional neocortical epilepsy [20]. Neocortical epilepsy surgery has a less favourable outcome than mesial temporal epilepsy surgery. Seizure-free rates vary widely depending on the study. A meta-analysis of frontal lobe epilepsy reports seizure-free rates of 20–78%, with a median of 45% [51]. Patient selection, differing surgical approaches and the use of various outcome measures account for the wide range [1]. Nevertheless, the chance of being seizure free is far superior to other approaches such as continued medication changes or stimulation.

Seizures are not the only relevant outcomes after epilepsy surgery. Quality of life is a more comprehensive outcome measure, but may be influenced greatly by other factors, such as depression [52]. Quality of life improves after epilepsy surgery, if the patient remains seizure-free [1,45,53,54]. However, if the patient continues to experience seizures [55], the effect on quality of life may be less, even if seizures improve in frequency [55]. Other outcomes to consider are employment and psychosocial factors, such as driving. Employment gains have been reported after epilepsy surgery, but warrant more systematic assessment [1,56]. Driving ability also increased after surgery [57].

Trade-Offs when Considering Surgery

When epilepsy surgery is considered, the risks and benefits of the procedure call for extensive discussion with the patient. The risk of epilepsy surgery is comparable to other intra-cranial surgery. The mortality was estimated in a meta-analysis at 0.4%. This has to be weighed against the overall risk of sudden unexpected death in epilepsy (SUDEP), the incidence of which has been estimated to be significant, 2.2–10:1000, in the medication-resistant population [58]. However, studies could not demonstrate a definite advantage of epilepsy surgery in terms of mortality [59].

The morbidity of epilepsy surgery overall is low, with 1.5% serious complications. Minor complications are reported in 5.1% [60]. This includes neurologic deficits such as superior quadrantanopia, which is frequently observed after temporal lobe resection due to resection of Meyer's loop, and expected. Intra-cranial

EEG alone is associated with a risk of major complications of 0.6% and 7.7% for minor complications [60].

The risk of epilepsy surgery on cognitive function is more difficult to predict [61]. Resection of the dominant temporal lobe can have an impact on verbal memory deficits and confrontation naming, but memory loss is variable and not consistent. Memory may also improve after surgery if seizures are eliminated. Although epilepsy surgery may worsen memory outcomes, it has been shown that it merely anticipates the memory loss that would occur if seizures continued. Ten-year memory outcomes have been shown to not differ whether the patients continued medical treatment or received surgery [62]. However, this study was neither prospective nor randomized [61,62]. Subjective memory may also vary from objective memory measures in epileptic patients, which further complicates cognitive outcomes after surgery [61,63]. In addition, memory complaints are highly correlated with depression [63].

After temporal lobectomy patients may experience difficulties adjusting to sudden alleviation of chronic disease. This has been described as 'burden of normalcy' [64]. The phenomenon seems transient, but should be recognized. Mood changes such as depression also need to be acknowledged, but are difficult to address as they are prevalent in the epilepsy population. The overall incidence of new-onset depression after epilepsy surgery is low, but has been reported [65].

Extratemporal resections can be associated with other adverse events, dependent on the location of the resection. For example, resection of the occipital lobe results in contralateral hemianopia or may worsen pre-existing deficits. This can be tolerable for patients as trade-off for seizure freedom, but before proceeding to surgery this warrants detailed discussion. Even if there is a pre-existing complete hemianopia, changes in motion detection can further worsen visual perception [66].

Resection of the supplementary motor area (SMA) may result in a transient motor deficit with difficulties initiating motor movement [67]. This is reversible and should not preclude resection of the SMA [67]. Large frontal lobe resections can result in deficits in motivation and personality.

In conclusion, resective epilepsy surgery remains to date the mainstay of treating medication-resistant focal epilepsy. Resection has to be carefully planned to achieve optimal outcomes, but in many cases epilepsy surgery leads to sustained seizure freedom.

Key Points

- Epilepsy surgery remains the most successful treatment to date, eliminating seizures in approximately 60–65% of patients.
- Clinical observation of seizures, EEG and MRI imaging are the most helpful techniques to identify the seizure-onset zone.
- Intra-cranial EEG may be necessary to define the seizure-onset zone, especially in patients with MRI-negative epilepsy.
- Resective epilepsy surgery can be limited if the seizure-onset zone involves eloquent cortex.
- The most commonly performed procedures are temporal lobectomies for mesial temporal epilepsy, which has a more favourable outcome than neocortical resections.

Acknowledgements

We thank Yinchen Song, PhD for the help with illustrations and electrode coregistration.

References

1. Jobst BC, Cascino GD. Resective epilepsy surgery for drug-resistant focal epilepsy: a review. *J Am Med Assoc* 2015;**313**(3):285–293

2. Penfield W, Jasper H *Epilepsy and the Functional Anatomy of the Human Brain*. Boston: Little, Brown & Co., 1954.

3. Haneef Z, Stern J, Dewar S, Engel J, Jr. Referral pattern for epilepsy surgery after evidence-based recommendations: a retrospective study. *Neurology* 2010;**75**(8):699–704

4. Kwan P, Arzimanoglou A, Berg AT, et al. Definition of drug resistant epilepsy: consensus proposal by the ad hoc Task Force of the ILAE Commission on Therapeutic Strategies. *Epilepsia* 2010;**51**(6):1069–1077

5. McGonigal A, Bartolomei F, Regis J, et al. Stereo electroencephalography in presurgical assessment of MRI-negative epilepsy. *Brain* 2007;**130**(Pt 12):3169–3183

6. Steinhoff BJ, Bacher M, Bucurenciu I, et al. The impact of guidelines on the quality of MRI diagnostics in adult patients referred to a tertiary epilepsy centre. *J Neurol* 2013;**260**(12):3174–3175

7. Phal PM, Usmanov A, Nesbit GM, et al. Qualitative comparison of 3-T and 1.5-T MRI in the evaluation of epilepsy. *Am J Roentgenol* 2008;**191**(3):890–895

8. De Ciantis A, Barba C, Tassi L, et al. 7T MRI in focal epilepsy with unrevealing conventional field strength imaging. *Epilepsia* 2016;**57**(3):445–454

9. Thadani VM, Siegel A, Lewis P, et al. Validation of ictal single photon emission computed tomography with depth encephalography and epilepsy surgery. *Neurosurg Rev* 2004;**27**(1):27–33

10. Spanaki MV, Spencer SS, Corsi M, et al. Sensitivity and specificity of quantitative difference SPECT analysis in seizure localization. *J Nucl Med* 1999;**40**(5):730–736

11. Perissinotti A, Setoain X, Aparicio J, et al. Clinical role of subtraction ictal SPECT coregistered to MR imaging and (18)F-FDG PET in pediatric epilepsy. *J Nucl Med* 2014;**55**(7):1099–1105

12. Sulc V, Stykel S, Hanson DP, et al. Statistical SPECT processing in MRI-negative epilepsy surgery. *Neurology* 2014;**82**(11):932–939

13. Knowlton RC. The role of FDG-PET, ictal SPECT, and MEG in the epilepsy surgery evaluation. *Epilepsy Beha* 2006;**8**(1):91–101

14. Whiting P, Gupta R, Burch J, et al. A systematic review of the effectiveness and cost-effectiveness of neuroimaging assessments used to visualise the seizure focus in people with refractory epilepsy being considered for surgery. *Health Technol Assess* 2006;**10**(4):1–250

15. Task Force on Practice Parameter Imaging Guidelines for International League Against Epilepsy, Commission for Diagnostics, Gaillard WD, Cross JH, Duncan JS, Stefan H, Theodore WH. Epilepsy imaging study guideline criteria: commentary on diagnostic testing study guidelines and practice parameters. *Epilepsia* 2011;**52**(9):1750–1756

16. Desai A, Bekelis K, Thadani VM, et al. Interictal PET and ictal subtraction SPECT: sensitivity in the detection of seizure foci in patients with medically intractable epilepsy. *Epilepsia* 2013;**54**(2):341–350

17. LoPinto-Khoury C, Sperling MR, Skidmore C, et al. Surgical outcome in PET-positive, MRI-negative patients with temporal lobe epilepsy. *Epilepsia* 2012;**53**(2):342–348

18. Bagic A. Look back to leap forward: the emerging new role of magnetoencephalography (MEG) in nonlesional epilepsy. *Clin Neurophysiol* 2016;**127**(1):60–66

19. Lau M, Yam D, Burneo JG. A systematic review on MEG and its use in the presurgical evaluation of localization-related epilepsy. *Epilepsy Res* 2008;**79**(2–3):97–104

20. Tellez-Zenteno JF, Hernandez Ronquillo L, Moien-Afshari F, Wiebe S. Surgical outcomes in lesional and non-lesional epilepsy: a systematic review and meta-analysis. *Epilepsy Res* 2010;**89**(2–3):310–318

21. Mittal S, Barkmeier D, Hua J, et al. Intracranial EEG analysis in tumor-related epilepsy: evidence of distant epileptic abnormalities. *Clin Neurophysiol* 2016;**127**(1):238–244

22. Englot DJ, Han SJ, Berger MS, Barbaro NM, Chang EF. Extent of surgical resection predicts seizure freedom in low-grade temporal lobe brain tumors. *Neurosurgery* 2012;**70**(4):921–928;discussion 928

23. Surgical Task Force Commission on Therapeutic Strategies of the ILAE, Rosenow F, Alonso-Vanegas MA, Baumgartner C, et al. Cavernoma-related epilepsy: review and recommendations for management–report of the Surgical Task Force of the ILAE Commission on Therapeutic Strategies. *Epilepsia* 2013;**54**(12):2025–2035

24. Englot DJ, Han SJ, Lawton MT, Chang EF. Predictors of seizure freedom in the surgical treatment of supratentorial cavernous malformations. *J Neurosurg* 2011;**115**(6):1169–1174

25. Duffau H. Brain mapping in tumors: intraoperative or extraoperative? *Epilepsia* 2013;**54**(Suppl 9):79–83

26. Yang PF, Pei JS, Zhang HJ, et al. Long-term epilepsy surgery outcomes in patients with PET-positive, MRI-negative temporal lobe epilepsy. *Epilepsy Behav* 2014;**41**:91–97

27. Schijns OE, Hoogland G, Kubben PL, Koehler PJ. The start and development of epilepsy surgery in Europe: a historical review. *Neurosurg Rev* 2015;**38**(3):447–461

28. Serletis D, Bulacio J, Bingaman W, Najm I, Gonzalez-Martinez J. The stereotactic approach for mapping epileptic networks: a prospective study of 200 patients. *J Neurosurg* 2014;**121**(5):1239–1246

29. Sperling MR, Guina L. The necessity for sphenoidal electrodes in the presurgical evaluation of temporal lobe epilepsy: pro position. *Clin Neurophysiol* 2003;**20** (5):299–304

30. Singh S, Sandy S, Wiebe S. Ictal onset on intracranial EEG: do we know it when we see it? State of the evidence. *Epilepsia* 2015;**56**(10):1629–1638

31. Pacia SV, Ebersole JS. Intracranial EEG substrates of scalp ictal patterns from temporal lobe foci. *Epilepsia* 1997;**38**(6):642–654

32. Dolezalova I, Brazdil M, Hermanova M, et al. Intracranial EEG seizure onset patterns in unilateral temporal lobe epilepsy and their relationship to other variables. *Clin Neurophysiol* 2013;**124** (6):1079–1088

33. Holtkamp M, Sharan A, Sperling MR. Intracranial EEG in predicting surgical outcome in frontal lobe epilepsy. *Epilepsia* 2012;**53**(10):1739–1745

34. Jenssen S, Roberts CM, Gracely EJ, Dlugos DJ, Sperling MR. Focal seizure propagation in the intracranial EEG. *Epilepsy Res* 2011;**93**(1):25–32

35. Goncharova, II, Spencer SS, Duckrow RB, et al. Intracranially recorded interictal spikes: relation to seizure onset area and effect of medication and time of day. *Clin Neurophysiol* 2013;**124**(11):2119–2128

36. Marsh ED, Peltzer B, Brown MW, 3rd, et al. Interictal EEG spikes identify the region of electrographic seizure onset in some, but not all, pediatric epilepsy patients. *Epilepsia* 2010;**51**(4):592–601

37. Bourien J, Bartolomei F, Bellanger JJ, et al. A method to identify reproducible subsets of co-activated structures during interictal spikes: application to intracerebral EEG in temporal lobe epilepsy. *Clin Neurophysiol* 2005;**116**(2):443–455

38. Engel J, Jr, da Silva FL. High-frequency oscillations – where we are and where we need to go. *Prog Neurobiol* 2012;**98**(3):316–318

39. Jacobs J, Zijlmans M, Zelmann R, et al. High-frequency electroencephalographic oscillations correlate with outcome of epilepsy surgery. *Ann Neurol* 2010;**67** (2):209–220

40. Dumpelmann M, Jacobs J, Schulze-Bonhage A. Temporal and spatial characteristics of high frequency oscillations as a new biomarker in epilepsy. *Epilepsia* 2015;**56**(2):197–206

41. Jobst BC, Engel J, Jr. Is it time to replace epileptic spikes with fast ripples? *Neurology* 2015;**85**(2):114–115

42. Zangaladze A, Sharan A, Evans J, et al. The effectiveness of low-frequency stimulation for mapping cortical function. *Epilepsia* 2008;**49**(3):481–487

43. Lesser RP, Kim SH, Beyderman L, et al. Brief bursts of pulse stimulation terminate afterdischarges caused by cortical stimulation. *Neurology* 1999;**53** (9):2073–2081

44. Wheeler M, De Herdt V, Vonck K, et al. Efficacy of vagus nerve stimulation for refractory epilepsy among patient subgroups: a re-analysis using the Engel classification. *Seizure* 2011;**20**(4):331–335

45. Wiebe S, Blume WT, Girvin JP, Eliasziw M. A randomized, controlled trial of surgery for temporal-lobe epilepsy. *N Engl J Med* 2001;**345**(5):311–318

46. Engel J, Jr, McDermott MP, Wiebe S, et al. Early surgical therapy for drug-resistant temporal lobe epilepsy: a randomized trial. *J Am Med Assoc* 2012;**307** (9):922–930

47. Bell B, Lin JJ, Seidenberg M, Hermann B. The neurobiology of cognitive disorders in temporal lobe epilepsy. *Nat Rev Neurol* 2011;**7**(3):154–164

48. Josephson CB, Dykeman J, Fiest KM, et al. Systematic review and meta-analysis of standard vs selective temporal lobe epilepsy surgery. *Neurology* 2013;**80** (18):1669–1676

49. Bujarski KA, Hirashima F, Roberts DW, et al. Long-term seizure, cognitive, and psychiatric outcome following trans-middle temporal gyrus amygdalohippocampectomy and standard temporal lobectomy. *J Neurosurg* 2013;**119**(1):16–23

50. Helmstaedter C. Cognitive outcomes of different surgical approaches in temporal lobe epilepsy. *Epileptic Disord* 2013;**15**(3):221–239

51. Englot DJ, Wang DD, Rolston JD, et al. Rates and predictors of long-term seizure freedom after frontal lobe epilepsy surgery: a systematic review and meta-analysis. *J Neurosurg* 2012;**116**(5):1042–1048

52. Hamid H, Blackmon K, Cong X, et al. Mood, anxiety, and incomplete seizure control affect quality of life after epilepsy surgery. *Neurology* 2014;**82**(10):887–894

53. Early Randomized Surgical Epilepsy Trial (ERSET) Study Group, Engel J, Jr, McDermott MP, Wiebe S, et al. Early surgical therapy for drug-resistant temporal lobe epilepsy: a randomized trial. *J Am Med Assoc* 2012;**307**(9):922–930

54. Seiam AH, Dhaliwal H, Wiebe S. Determinants of quality of life after epilepsy surgery: systematic review and evidence summary. *Epilepsy Behav* 2011;**21**(4):441–445

55. Birbeck GL, Hays RD, Cui X, Vickrey BG. Seizure reduction and quality of life improvements in people with epilepsy. *Epilepsia* 2002;**43**(5):535–538

56. Chin PS, Berg AT, Spencer SS, et al. Employment outcomes following resective epilepsy surgery. *Epilepsia* 2007;**48**(12):2253–2257

57. Hamiwka L, Macrodimitris S, Tellez-Zenteno JF, et al. Social outcomes after temporal or extratemporal epilepsy surgery: a systematic review. *Epilepsia* 2011;**52**(5):870–879

58. Tellez-Zenteno JF, Ronquillo LH and Wiebe S. Sudden unexpected death in epilepsy: evidence-based analysis of incidence and risk factors. *Epilepsy Res* 2005;**65**(1–2):101–115

59. Ryvlin P, Montavont A, Kahane P. The impact of epilepsy surgery on mortality. *Epileptic Disord* 2005;**7**(Suppl 1):S39–S46

60. Hader WJ, Tellez-Zenteno J, Metcalfe A, et al. Complications of epilepsy surgery: a systematic review of focal surgical resections and invasive EEG monitoring. *Epilepsia* 2013;**54**(5):840–847

61. Sherman EM, Wiebe S, Fay-McClymont TB, et al. Neuropsychological outcomes after epilepsy surgery: systematic review and pooled estimates. *Epilepsia* 2011;**52**(5):857–869

62. Helmstaedter C, Kurthen M, Lux S, Reuber M, Elger CE. Chronic epilepsy and cognition: a longitudinal study in temporal lobe epilepsy. *Ann Neurol* 2003;**54**(4):425–432

63. Rayner G, Wrench JM, Wilson SJ. Differential contributions of objective memory and mood to subjective memory complaints in refractory focal epilepsy. *Epilepsy Behav* 2010;**19**(3):359–364

64. Wilson SJ, Bladin PF, Saling MM, McIntosh AM, Lawrence JA. The longitudinal course of adjustment after seizure surgery. *Seizure* 2001;**10**(3):165–172

65. Cleary RA, Baxendale SA, Thompson PJ, Foong J. Predicting and preventing psychopathology following temporal lobe epilepsy surgery. *Epilepsy Behav* 2013;**26**(3):322–334

66. Jobst BC, Williamson PD, Thadani VM, et al. Intractable occipital lobe epilepsy: clinical characteristics and surgical treatment. *Epilepsia* 2010;**51**(11):2334–2337

67. Zentner J, Hufnagel A, Pechstein U, Wolf HK, Schramm J. Functional results after resective procedures involving the supplementary motor area. *J Neurosurg* 1996;**85**(4):542–549

Chapter 19

Ablative Surgery for Medication-Resistant Epilepsy

Christian Hoelscher, Kofi-Buaku Atsina,
Chengyuan Wu and Ashwini Sharan

Medication-resistant epilepsy continues to be a challenging condition, but numerous medical as well as surgical treatment options developed over the years have added significantly to the therapeutic arsenal of both neurologists and neurosurgeons. One such approach to epileptic patients focuses around physically disrupting their epileptogenic circuitry, with relevant modalities including traditional open surgical resection and radiosurgery, as well as ablation via radiofrequency, cryotherapy or laser interstitial thermal therapy [1–10]. The interest in less-invasive methods for control of medication-resistant epilepsy has been motivated by several factors, including: reducing perioperative morbidity, decreasing length of stay and associated complications/costs, and offering treatments for patients that are otherwise not eligible for traditional surgical resections, be it for reasons related to medical comorbidities or factors inherent to their epileptic pathology. Additionally, the perceived risks of open craniotomy may play a role in limiting both the number of patients referred to tertiary epilepsy centres by primary care physicians, as well as the number of patients willing to undergo traditional open resection, even in the face of significant evidence in support of the safe role of surgery in refractory epilepsy [11]. Stereotactic laser ablation (SLA) is among the most relevant surgical advances in the treatment of drug-resistant epilepsy, offering the benefit of high rates of seizure control in epileptic patients with varying underlying seizure aetiologies, combined with minimization of the amount of normal cerebral tissue disrupted due to the advent of real-time image-guided feedback [3,4,5,8,10,12].

Hardware and Procedural Details

Stereotactic laser ablation systems are available in two commercial forms (Visualase, Medtronic, Houston, Texas; and NeuroBlate, Monteris, Plymouth, Minnesota). Both systems consist of two main components: (1) The laser probe (15 W, 980 nm diode laser for the Visualase system; 12 W, 1064 nm yttrium aluminum garnet laser for the NeuroBlate system) and cooling component (saline for the Visualase system; CO_2 for the NeuroBlate system) are inserted intra-cranially through a stereotactically placed twist drill and anchor bolt. The device is advanced to the target tissue through a rigidly fixed anchor bolt or platform and the entire system is secured in place. An MRI subsequently confirms probe placement, after which the ablation procedure may begin. (2) The workstation, whose software provides a means for planning, controlling and monitoring the ablation procedure and controls the cooling system to prevent eschar development, which can disrupt the delivered laser energy (Figure 19.1) [13,14]. Energy is transmitted through the laser applicator, constructed of a silicone fibreoptic core with a light-diffusing tip, which yields either a cylindrical field of light energy in line with the axis of the electrode or a directional delivery of heat. This light energy is absorbed, transmitted or reflected based on the properties of the tissue being targeted. Absorption of this light energy releases heat, with irreversible cell damage occurring at temperatures greater than ~45 °C in a time-dependent fashion [11,15].

Both SLA systems are compatible with all major MRI scanners, and contain multi-planar imaging software for purposes of preoperative planning as well as real-time monitoring of the ablation as it is occurring via thermal maps. These maps are created using magnetic resonance (MR) thermometry, generated by comparing the phase shift at the proton resonance frequency in gradient-recalled echo phase images performed at body temperature and after the delivery of an energy pulse [15]. Such methods are capable of detecting temperature changes of less than 1 °C during repeated assessment for such temperature changes. The system has shown precision to approximately 1 mm or less in relatively homogeneous tissues, such as the

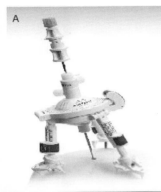
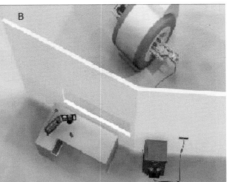
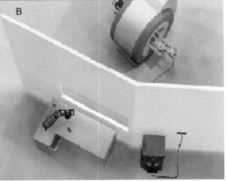
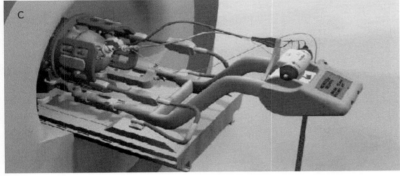

Figure 19.1 (A) The Monteris anchoring device through which the heating and cooling probes are inserted and directed toward the target via a twist-drill burrhole. (B) The ablation is executed and monitored in the adjacent workroom with the aid of specially designed SLA software. (C) Close-up view of the anchoring device and probes attached to the MRI-compatible control system. Images courtesy of www.monteris.com.

amygdalohippocampal complex [13]. An additional feature of some SLA software is the ability to place 'safety markers' around key anatomic structures and pathways. When such markers are heated beyond a specified non-lethal temperature (eg. 45 °C), the heating laser shuts down immediately. Once the procedure has been completed, post-operative MR imaging allows for confirmation not only of the successful ablation, but of an abrupt transition into unaffected surrounding tissue [13].

Obvious benefits of SLA for epilepsy involve the reduced tissue disruption compared to traditional craniotomy for open resection. SLA procedures involve only small incisions; enough to accommodate a single twist drill and anchor bolt insertion. Hair clipping, as well as skin and subcutaneous tissue suturing, is minimal. Patients do not necessarily require an intensive care unit (ICU) stay post-operatively and they are most often discharged the next day. These features of SLA offer benefits over craniotomy in terms of perioperative risks and complications, and access to patients that are hesitant to undergo open resection, as well as the potential for cost-savings, given the reduced length of stay and avoidance of an ICU admission. Finally, the advantage of SLA over radiofrequency-related ablations include the ability to radiographically identify

the delivery of the probe to the intended target structure, as well as monitor tissue heating, both adjacent to the probe tip and distant surrounding tissue, in real time with MR thermography (Figure 19.2).

Background and Clinical Data

SLA has been studied and validated extensively in early animal studies as well as multiple human clinical trials. The details of such early studies are beyond the scope of this chapter; however, they have provided vital information that would form the basis of the use of SLA for a variety of lesions in clinical practice today, including: confirmation of the ability of SLA to destroy target tissue, the efficacy of 'safety markers' in the SLA software, and the expected post-operative evolution of the ablation zone, perilesional enhancement and surrounding oedema on post-operative imaging. This information is key to both planning an ablation procedure, and post-operative follow-up and monitoring, as well as counselling patients regarding expected side effects or possible risks and complications [16].

SLA was first performed intra-cranially in humans in France in 2006, in the treatment of metastatic tumours [14], and was first approved for use in the

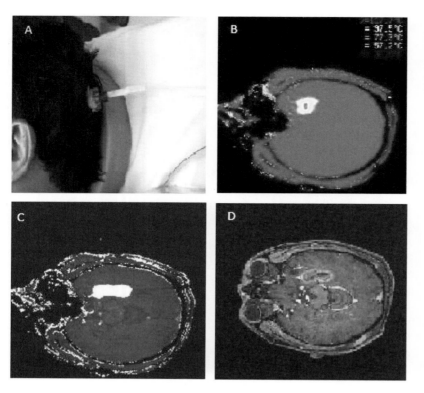

Figure 19.2 (A) Medtronic Visualase anchoring device through which the heating and cooling probes are inserted. Example of an MR thermography map showing details of tissue (B) heating and (C) ablation. (D) Post-contrast MRI immediately post-op.

United States in 2007, with the initial procedures again performed in the setting of neoplastic disease. SLA was first used as a means of treating medically refractory epilepsy in 2010 in a patient with tuberous sclerosis [6] and was subsequently reported in a variety of studies that encompassed several underlying aetiologies for epilepsy, including hypothalamic hamartoma, focal cortical dysplasia, tuberous sclerosis and mesial temporal sclerosis, as well as mass lesions causing seizures, such as cavernomas and tumours [5,13,15,17].

Hypothalamic Hamartoma

While rare, hypothalamic hamartomas represent a neurosurgical challenge given the density of critical surrounding structures and pathways. Patients often present with gelastic seizures, with or without other seizure semiology. Traditional surgical treatment modalities, including both open and endoscopic neurosurgery, as well as radiosurgery, are associated with significant morbidity due to damage to structures including the optic nerves/chiasm/radiations, fornix, mammillary bodies and pituitary stalk. The resulting complications include visual field deficits, loss of memory, and a variety of endocrinopathies, including diabetes insipidus and precocious puberty, among others. Further, seizure control rates using multi-modality therapy including the aforementioned surgical interventions range broadly [18–20]. Due to its minimally invasive approach, SLA has recently been employed as a means of disconnecting epileptic hamartomas from surrounding brain tissue. In a recent series of hypothalamic hamartoma treated with SLA, Wilfong et al. reported achieving a 79% seizure-freedom rate at nine-month follow-up. This success rate improved to 86% after one patient had a second ablation and subsequently also achieved seizure freedom. In terms of complications, the authors reported only a subclinical subarachnoid haemorrhage, which required no intervention. There were no permanent neurologic deficits or significant endocrinopathies reported [4]. Another more recent study presented two cases of patients with hypothalamic hamartomas with persistent seizures after radiosurgery who were treated with SLA and remained Engel class I at five- and seven-month follow-up, respectively, without significant complications [19].

Focal Cortical Dysplasia

SLA for focal cortical dysplasia (FCD) is especially useful because diagnostic adjunctive procedures can often be performed through the same twist drill hole required for placement of an ablation catheter. For example, stereotactic placement of depth electrodes to assess the epileptogenicity of adjacent tissue, as well as stereotactic needle biopsy to evaluate for a non-enhancing tumour have both been reported [3,12]. The utility of SLA for FCD has been described recently, including a case report of a patient with bilateral occipital FCD and refractory epilepsy, treated with SLA without complication who remained Engel class I at eight-month follow-up [21]. Another review of 19 patients treated with SLA for predominantly FCD showed a 47% rate of Engel class I or II outcome at mean follow-up of 16 months [22]. Similar to open surgery, the success rate of SLA for FCD depends on several factors, including accurate mapping of the epileptogenic zone and its careful and precise elimination. The less invasive nature of SLA vs. traditional surgical options offers the benefit of potential seizure freedom with lower risk of damage to surrounding critical structures and/or eloquent cortex.

Tuberous Sclerosis

Tubers with associated perilesional hyper-excitable cortex can be treated via SLA. Similarly, other tuberous-sclerosis-associated lesions, including subependymal giant cell astrocytoma, have been targeted using SLA with subsequent adequate seizure control [5]. Similar to FCD, adjunctive diagnostic procedures, including stereotactic biopsy and/or depth electrode monitoring for perilesional epileptic circuits can be achieved through the same twist drill hole used for placement of the ablation catheter.

Mesial Temporal Lobe Epilepsy

One of the most frequent pathologic processes targeted with SLA is medial temporal lobe epilepsy (MTLE) (Figure 19.3). Recently reported series [8,10,17,23] have shown efficacy rates similar to historical figures often quoted with open temporal lobectomies or more selective amygdalohippocampectomy procedures. Willie et al. noted an efficacy rate of 77% Engel class I–III status (54% Engel class I, 23% Engel class III and 23% Engel class IV) at median 14-month follow-up in 13 patients. Morbidity in this series included one subdural haematoma requiring craniotomy for evacuation without any permanent deficit, and one patient who

suffered from a homonymous hemianopsia [8]. In their recent review of SLA for MTLE, Gross et al. documented a 61.5% seizure-freedom rate at 12 months post-operatively from their initial series of 13 patients, with a similar success rate in their expanded series of 32 patients [24]. Complication rates were similar to other studies of SLA for MTLE, with visual field deficits being the most commonly noted events, but importantly occurring at rates below those seen with standard open resections [24–26]. Waseem et al. reviewed a series of 14 consecutive patients with MTLE over the age of 50 treated with either anterior temporal lobectomy (ATL) (n = 7) or SLA (n = 7), and noted no significant differences in seizure outcome, complications or neurocognitive changes [27].

One recent study, however, documented a modestly lower seizure-freedom rate when compared to established ATL values. Kang et al. reported on 20 patients treated with SLA for MTLE, 19 of whom had MRI-confirmed medial temporal structural abnormalities, and documented seizure-freedom rates of 53%, 36% and 60% at 6, 12 and 24 months respectively [10]. Of the treatment failures, four underwent ATL, of whom three enjoyed subsequent seizure freedom. Complication rates were minimal and similar to other studies. The authors postulated that the somewhat lower seizure-freedom rate compared to historical open resection baselines may have been due to sampling error from having long-term follow-up only for a subset of patients, undiagnosed dual pathology or failure of the ablation volume to include the entirety of the mesial temporal epileptic circuitry. Regardless, this study did confirm SLA as a safe alternative to open resection for patients with MTLE.

Imaging Features and the Role of Ablation Volume

Given the increasing use of SLA for the treatment of medication-resistant epilepsy, an understanding of the expected imaging findings, particularly MRI evolution of laser ablation lesions, as well as the relationship between ablation volume and seizure control, are important parameters to consider. A retrospective review of MRI scans from 26 patients from our institution currently pending publication who underwent SLA for refractory epilepsy generated a description of four discrete timeframes after ablation: immediate (post-operative day 0), subacute (up to ~4 weeks post-operatively), transitional (up to ~ 8 weeks post-operatively) and chronic. The notable

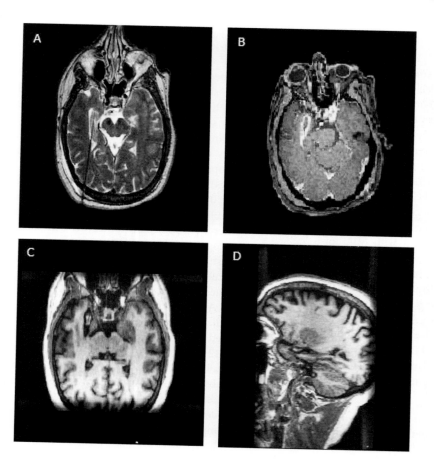

Figure 19.3 Example of an SLA procedure for a patient with right-sided MTLE. (A) T2 MRI confirming placement of the probe in the intended target. (B) Immediate post-op T1+c sequence showing the ablation zone. (C) and (D) 6-month post-op T1 sequences showing the ablation cavity.

trends included initial ring-enhancement of the ablation site on immediate and subacute imaging that subsequently faded, a period of perilesional oedema that peaked in the subacute phase before decreasing as the lesions became chronic and the development of gliotic cavities in the chronic phase (Figure 19.4). Additionally, we noted that punctate areas of intra-parenchymal or intra-ventricular haemorrhage were not uncommon, as was temporary increased enhancement of the ipsilateral choroid plexus. These radiographic findings were not associated with adverse events.

The relationship between ablation volume and the attainment of enduring seizure freedom has not been as consistent as the aforementioned temporal evolution of ablative lesions. As with any surgical procedure, evaluation of perioperative imaging is an important means of evaluating the intervention in question. However, evaluating the volume of successfully resected medial temporal structures, and the relationship of the percentage of ablated vs. total mesial temporal lobe volume, is

challenging. At our institution, we have created a standardized, modular approach to volumetric analysis of mesial temporal lobe resection (Figure 19.5). By subjecting pre-operative MR images to automatic anatomic segmentation using publicly available software and overlaying coregistered post-ablation MR images, volumetric assessment of the degree of ablation of the various mesial temporal lobe structures can be clearly quantified. Such analysis has also been used to facilitate optimization of laser probe trajectories to maximize the efficiency of mesial temporal ablation volumes, as well as to analyze the relationship between ablation volume and outcomes.

With regards to SLA for epilepsy, the exact relationship between ablation volume and seizure freedom is currently unclear. Various studies over the past 30 years have attempted to correlate extent of resection of mesial temporal structures with seizure outcome, with varied results. Recently, Willie et al., in their analysis of 13 patients treated with SLA for MTLE, noted a roughly 60% average ablation volume without

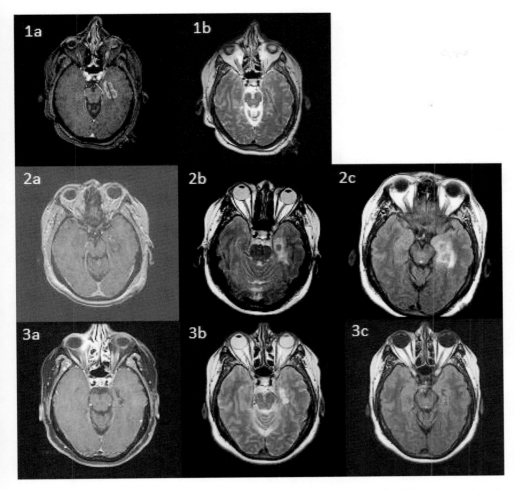

Figure 19.4 Temporal evolution of SLA on MRI. (1a and 1b) Immediately post-op T1+C and T2 sequences show ring-enhancement and mild oedema. (2a–c) At three months, enhancement has decreased significantly, while perilesional oedema remains on T2 and FLAIR sequences.(3a–c) At 10 months post-op, enhancement and oedema have both faded.

a dose-dependency between ablation volume and seizure outcome, suggesting the possibility of acceptable outcomes with subtotal ablation [8]. Kang et al. echoed this possibility, noting, in their review of 20 MTLE patients treated with SLA, that there was no relationship between ablation volume and seizure freedom [10]. Although the exact relationship between mesial temporal ablation/resection and seizure freedom is not clear, it appears likely that elimination of the offending aberrant circuitry is possible with subtotal mesial temporal ablation. Further research in this area will be necessary to help streamline SLA trajectories to optimize clinical outcomes while limiting the amount of tissue destroyed.

Neurocognitive Outcomes

In addition to documented safety and efficacy, perhaps one of the most important factors supporting the use of SLA for MTLE is the decreased neurocognitive side effects associated with this procedure vs. standard open resections [23–26]. Studies of MTLE reported significant improvement post-SLA compared to ATL in this regard with similar rates of post-operative seizure control. This suggested the possibility of 'collateral damage' to more anterolaterally located extrahippocampal temporal lobe structures and white matter tracts that are important for preserving neurocognitive function [24–26]. Importantly, these structures appear to be at risk during both traditional ATL as well as more

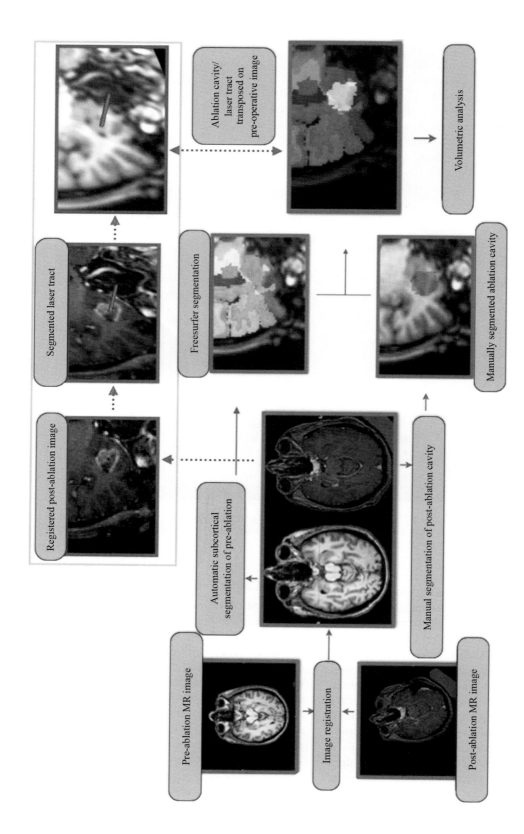

Figure 19.5 Workflow for volumetric analysis of the ablation site. Pre- and post-ablative MRI sequences are coregistered, followed by automatic anatomic segmentation of pre-ablation sequences to facilitate an analysis of the volume of the targeted lesion that was successfully treated.

selective amygdalohippocampectomies. The dissection corridor required for SLA is a small amount of white matter tract from an occipital-temporal approach [7], whereas a standard MTLE surgical corridor for open resection would be through the temporal lobe tissue. Drane et al. prospectively compared 58 patients undergoing surgical treatment for temporal lobe epilepsy, 39 with standard surgical resections and 19 with SLA. They noted similar rates of seizure control; however, no patients undergoing SLA showed performance decline in neurocognitive measures, while 95% of open resections on the dominant temporal lobe resulted in significant deficits in naming and 65% of open resections on the non-dominant temporal lobe resulted in significant deficits in object/face recognition [26]. These neurocognitive benefits of SLA force one to critically re-evaluate the often-presumed unique role of the medial temporal lobe in naming and memory. Given the ability of SLA to access the medial temporal lobe without damage to surrounding anterolateral temporal structures, combined with the neurocognitive protection afforded by this modality, the future of MTLE interventions may favour preservation of these anterolateral structures as a means of preserving patients' neurocognitive baseline.

Specific Complications

The complications associated with SLA are similar to other stereotactic procedures. Commonly cited risks include haemorrhage, neurological deficit, cerebral oedema and failure to control seizures. Recent studies have confirmed the relatively low adverse event profile of SLA. Kang et al. noted that 17 out of 20 patients were discharged on post-operative day 1, with the remaining 3 patients discharged on post-operative day 2. They noted one serious adverse event, a 3×2 cm intraparenchymal haematoma adjacent to the ablation site that did not expand or require evacuation, but did result in a persistent superior quadrantanopsia. Additionally, one patient with documented pre-operative depression and continued seizures post-operatively, committed suicide four months after SLA [10]. This highlights the importance of neuropsychological evaluation in the pre-operative setting. Other reported minor complications included insomnia (5%), scalp numbness (5%) and transient fourth nerve palsy (5%). Gross et al., in a review of 49 cases of SLA for mesial temporal epilepsy, reported complications, including haemorrhage (4%), visual field deficit (8%) and cranial nerve deficit (4%) [24]. Other studies have shown similarly low complication profiles for laser ablation procedures performed for epilepsy [4,8,19,23]. However, as with any invasive procedure, there is inherent risk. One recent case report profiled a high-functioning patient treated with laser ablation of a hypothalamic hamartoma who developed a severely disabling post-operative amnestic syndrome, with imaging revealing evidence of thermal damage to the bilateral mammillary bodies [28].

There have been very few reported complications due to malfunction of the laser ablation software and/or hardware, with the only published events including one episode of cooling catheter malfunction and one patient in whom the laser probe broke off and was ultimately left in situ [22]. Further, given the reduced length of both ICU and hospital stays afforded by laser ablation, common inpatient complications such as pneumonia, deep venous thrombosis, pulmonary embolus, etc. are often reduced compared to more traditional surgical procedures.

Conclusions

The emergence of SLA has offered epileptologists and neurosurgeons a new therapeutic strategy to offer patients suffering from chronic seizures. Similar preliminary outcomes combined with a less-invasive profile and reduced complication rates compared to traditional craniotomy have made SLA an attractive treatment option for physician and patient alike. Potential additional benefits include cost-savings, as well as increased access to potentially curative therapy for epileptic patients who are either not candidates for traditional open resection or are unwilling to accept the associated perioperative morbidities thereof. Additional work will be needed to fully evaluate the scope and therapeutic potential of SLA in regard to medically refractory epilepsy. However, the preliminary evidence suggests that SLA will likely play an ever-increasing role in the multidisciplinary management of complex epilepsy patients.

Key Points

- Stereotactic laser ablation serves as a new minimally invasive therapeutic option for patients suffering from medication-resistant epilepsy.
- Evidence to date consists of promising clinical outcomes with regards to seizure freedom and overall complications.
- Further studies are required to better understand how factors of patient selection and nuances of the ablation technique affect clinical outcomes.

References

1. Liscak R, Malikova H, Kalina M, et al. Stereotactic radiofrequency amygdalohippocampectomy in the treatment of mesial temporal lobe epilepsy. *Acta Neurochir* 2010;**152**(8):1291–1298

2. Chkhenkeli SA, Šramka M, Rakviashvili TN, et al. Bitemporal intractable epilepsy: could it be surgically treatable? *Stereotact Funct Neurosurg* 2013;**91**(2):104–112

3. Gonzalez-Martinez J, Vadera S, Mullin J, et al. Robot-assisted stereotactic laser ablation in medically intractable epilepsy: operative technique. *Neurosurgery* 2014;**10**(suppl 2):167–172

4. Wilfong AA, Curry DJ. Hypothalamic hamartomas: optimal approach to clinical evaluation and diagnosis. *Epilepsia* 2013;**54**(Suppl 9):109–114

5. Tovar-Spinoza Z, Carter D, Ferrone D, et al. The use of MRI-guided laser-induced thermal ablation for epilepsy. *Childs Nerv Syst* 2013;**29**(11):2089–2094

6. Curry DJ, Gowda A, McNichols RJ, et al. MR-guided stereotactic laser ablation of epileptogenic foci in children. *Epilepsy Behav* 2012;**24**(4):408–414

7. Wu C, Lariviere MJ, Laxpati N, et al. Extraventricular long-axis cannulation of the hippocampus: technical considerations. *Neurosurgery* 2014;**10**(Suppl 2):325–332

8. Willie JT, Laxpati NG, Drane DL, et al. Real-time magnetic resonance-guided stereotactic laser amygdalohippocampotomy for mesial temporal lobe epilepsy. *Neurosurgery* 2014;**74**(6):569–584

9. Quigg M, Rolston J, Barbaro NM. Radiosurgery for epilepsy: clinical experience and potential antiepileptic mechanisms. *Epilepsia* 2012;**53**(1):7–15

10. Kang JY, Wu C, Tracy J, et al. Laser interstitial thermal therapy for medically intractable mesial temporal lobe epilepsy. *Epilepsia* 2016;**57**(2):325–334

11. Bandt KS, Leuthardt EC. Minimally invasive neurosurgery for epilepsy using stereotactic MRI guidance. *Neurosurg Clin N Am* 2016;**27**(1):51–58

12. Esquenazi Y, Kalamangalam GP, Slater JD, et al. Stereotactic laser ablation of epileptogenic periventricular nodular heterotopia. *Epilepsy Res* 2014;**108**(3):547–554

13. Quigg M, Harden C. Minimally invasive techniques for epilepsy surgery: stereotactic radiosurgery and other technologies. *J Neurosurg* 2014;**121**(Suppl):232–240

14. Carpentier A, McNichols RJ, Stafford RJ, et al. Real-time magnetic resonance-guided laser thermal therapy for focal metastatic brain tumors. *Neurosurgery* 2008;**63**(1):21–29

15. Medvid R, Ruiz A, Komotar RJ, et al. Current applications of MRI-guided laser interstitial thermal therapy in the treatment of brain neoplasma and epilepsy: a radiologic and neurosurgical overview. *Am J Neuroradiol* 2015;**36**(11):1998–2006

16. Kangasniemi M, McNichols RJ, Bankson JA, et al. Thermal therapy of canine cerebral tumor using a 980 nm diode laser with MR temperature-sensitive imaging feedback. *Lasers Surg Med* 2004;**35**(1):41–50

17. Gross RE, Willie JT, Mehta AD, et al. Multicenter experience with minimally invasive stereotactic laser thermal amygdalohippocampotomy for mesial temporal lobe epilepsy. Abstract and Platform Presentation, American Association of Neurological Surgeons, New Orleans, 2013.

18. Abla A, Shetter AG, Chang SW, et al. Gamma Knife surgery for hypothalamic hamartomas and epilepsy: patient selection and outcomes. *J Neurosurg* 2010;**113** (Suppl):207–214

19. Rolston JD, Chang EF. Stereotactic laser ablation for hypothalamic hamartoma. *Neurosurg Clin N Am* 2016;**27**(1):59–67

20. Rosenfeld JV, Feiz-Erfan I. Hypothalamic hamartoma treatment: surgical resection with the transcallosal approach. *Semin Pediatr Neurol* 2007;**14**(2):88–98

21. Clarke DF, Tindall K, Lee M, et al. Bilateral occipital dysplasia, seizure identification, and ablation: a novel surgical technique. *Epileptic Discord* 2014;**16** (2):238–243

22. Lewis EC, Weil AG, Duchowny M, et al. MR-guided laser interstitial thermal therapy for pediatric drug-resistant lesional epilepsy. *Epilepsia* 2015;**56**(10):1590–1598

23. Buckley R, Estronza-Ojeda S, Ojemann JG. Laser ablation in pediatric epilepsy. *Neurosurg Clin N Am* 2016;**27**(1):69–78

24. Gross RE, Willie JT, Drane DL. The role of stereotactic laser amygdalohippocampotomy in mesial temporal lobe epilepsy. *Neurosurg Clin N Am* 2016;**27**(1):37–50

25. Gross RE, Mahmoudi B, Riley JP. Less is more: novel less-invasive surgical techniques for mesial temporal lobe epilepsy that minimize cognitive impairment. *Curr Opin Neurol* 2015;**28**(2):182–191

26. Drane DL, Loring DW, Voets NL, et al. Better object recognition and naming outcome with MRI-guided stereotactic laser amygdalohippocampotomy for temporal lobe epilepsy. *Epilepsia* 2015;**56**(1):101–113

27. Waseem H, Osborn KE, Schoenberg MR, et al. Laser ablation therapy: an alternative treatment for medically resistant mesial temporal lobe epilepsy after age 50. *Epilepsy Behav* 2015;**51**:152–157

28. Zubkov S, Del Bene VA, MacAllister WS, et al. Disabling amnestic syndrome following stereotactic laser ablation of a hypothalamic hamartoma in a patient with a prior temporal lobectomy. *Epilepsy Behav Case Rep* 2015;**10**(4):60–62

Stimulation Treatment for Medication-Resistant Epilepsy

1. Vagus and Trigeminal Nerve Stimulation

George Nune and Christianne Heck

Vagus Nerve Stimulation

Vagus Nerve Functions

The vagus nerve performs many different functions in the human body. Understanding these functions helps inform the potential side effects of vagus nerve stimulation (VNS). The nerve consists of 80% afferent fibres [1,2]. These include visceral sensory and taste fibres which travel primarily to the nucleus of the tractus solitarius, as well as cutaneous sensation fibres from the external auditory meatus which project to the spinal nucleus of the trigeminal nerve. The efferent component includes branchial motor fibres from the nucleus ambiguus, parasympathetic fibres primarily from the dorsal nucleus of the vagus and parasympathetic fibres from the nucleus ambiguus to the heart. The motor fibres innervate skeletal muscles in the head and neck involved in speech production and swallowing, while the parasympathetic fibres innervate most of the viscera serving to control heart rate, respiration, gastrointestinal motility and many other autonomic functions. The majority of fibres in the vagus nerve consist of unmyelinated C fibres, but commensurate with its wide variety of functions, it also contains larger and faster-conducting A- and B-type fibres. The brainstem nuclei that receive vagal inputs integrate homeostatic information, provide commensurate adjustments to autonomic functions and also send this information to other brainstem nuclei projecting widely throughout the brain.

Mechanism of Action

The mechanism of action of vagal nerve stimulation remains to be fully elucidated. The typical stimulation intensities used in humans are only sufficient to recruit the larger A- and B-type nerve fibres [1]. This is confirmed by the fact that lesioning of C-fibres in rats does not attenuate the seizure reduction produced by VNS [3]. Afferent VNS signals ascend through the nucleus of the solitary tract to a variety of brainstem nuclei, including the locus cerruleus, reticular formation and raphe nucleus, thereby affecting widespread cortical areas [4]. The locus cerruleus is particularly important for the function of VNS and its lesioning in rats also attenuates the effects of VNS [5]. The end-effect of vagal nerve stimulation ascending through the aforementioned brainstem nuclei is a decrease in cortical hyperexcitability. This was demonstrated in humans as a decrease in the rate of inter-ictal epileptiform discharges during active stimulation and for a period of time thereafter [6]. Furthermore, the degree of reduction in inter-ictal discharges in response to VNS was particularly significant in patients who reported a more than 50% reduction in seizures using the device and in those who reported that magnet use helps terminate their seizures.

Efficacy

The efficacy of vagal nerve stimulation was initially established in two pivotal randomized controlled studies (see [7–9] for further reviews of efficacy trials). These included a total of 314 patients in whom high-intensity therapeutic stimulation was compared to low-intensity subtherapeutic but still subjectively detectable stimulation over the course of 14 weeks. The therapeutic stimulation groups had a median seizure reduction of 23%. While the efficacy difference between the treatment and subtherapeutic stimulation groups was small, it was statistically significant.

One of the most interesting aspects of VNS is that efficacy continues to improve over time. Morris and colleagues performed a three-year open-label long-term follow-up study of the 454 patients in the regulatory study trials, E01 through E05 [9]. They demonstrated that the median seizure reduction continued to improve up to 44% with a 72% patient retention rate. A longer-term, retrospective, open-label study of 85 patients showed a 56% mean seizure reduction at five years of follow-up[10]. This study is likely to be biased in that patient retention will be skewed towards those who had a good response, but it still suggests sustained improvement. Another retrospective review of patients with more than 10 years of VNS therapy suffered from the same biases, but demonstrated a 75.5% mean seizure reduction at the last time point [11].

Patient Selection

The VNS system is generally reserved as an adjunctive therapy for patients with medication-resistant epilepsy, meaning that they have continued seizures despite adequate trials of at least two medications. These patients are unlikely to become seizure-free with additional medications and side effects often become limiting. In patients with focal medication-resistant epilepsy, resective surgery is preferred as it confers the best chance of seizure freedom. VNS is used in those patients who either are not candidates for potentially curative surgery, refuse surgery or have continued seizures despite surgery. Individuals may not be surgical candidates due to having a seizure focus within eloquent cortex, a non-localizable seizure focus or multiple unresectable seizure foci, such as in bilateral temporal lobe epilepsy. The majority of patients in the initial VNS clinical studies suffered from focal epilepsy, also called partial-onset epilepsy.

In the United States, the VNS system is FDA approved for focal epilepsy, although in Canada, Europe, Japan and many other parts of the world it has regulatory approval for generalized epilepsy as well. One clinical trial included 25 patients with generalized seizures who demonstrated an excellent response, with a 46.6% median seizure reduction at the end of the three-month trial period [8]. A number of subsequent studies have also confirmed the efficacy of VNS in specific types of generalized epilepsy. A pooled analysis of 113 paediatric patients with Lennox–Gastaut syndrome from four separate studies showed that more than 55% of patients were able to achieve a seizure reduction of more than 50% [12]. A retrospective review from New York University with an average follow-up of 22 months found that of 14 patients with idiopathic generalized epilepsy 57% had a seizure reduction of 50% or more [13]. Another study including 16 patients with symptomatic or idiopathic generalized epilepsy demonstrated a 43% median seizure reduction after 12–21 months of follow-up [14].

Regulatory approval for VNS in the United States is also limited to patients aged 4 years and over, but it has been used 'off-label' at younger ages, and much regulatory agencies have different restrictions. An AAN evidence-based practice guideline included 14 Class III studies with a pooled analysis of 481 paediatric patients demonstrating a 50%-responder rate of 55% [15].

Other factors may also play into the decision to employ the VNS system. For example, it has also demonstrated efficacy in the treatment of depression [12], which is a common comorbidity in patients with epilepsy.

Device Description and Practical Considerations

The VNS system consists of a helical electrode connected to a pulse generator. The electrode is wrapped around the vagus nerve within the carotid sheath at the fifth or sixth cervical level. It is tunnelled under the skin and connects to the pulse generator, which is usually placed subcutaneously in the left chest. The newer model has tachycardia detection for use as an indicator of seizure occurrence and requires a pre-operative assessment using an electrocardiogram (ECG) machine in order to ensure the device position allows for accurate heart rate detection.

Battery life is typically between three and eight years, but is highly dependent on the intensity of stimulation and percentage of time it is delivered, also called the duty cycle. When the battery is depleted, the generator is replaced and connected to existing leads. Complete explanting of the VNS system is not always possible due to fibrous encapsulation, which prevents lead separation from the nerve without injury. In such cases, the lead is often left in place. The VNS system is MRI compatible, using transmit and receive coils for the head or extremities with up to 3 tesla scanners, provided that the device is turned off prior to imaging. The newer VNS systems do not require the use of transmit and receive coils, so checking the VNS model and current MRI guidelines is recommended.

It should also be noted that non-invasive transcutaneous vagus nerve stimulation (tVNS) devices have also become available. These consist of an externally worn pulse generator delivering transcutaneous stimulation to the skin of the outer ear and thereby stimulating the auricular branch of the vagus nerve.

Stimulation Parameters

Stimulation parameters are often separated into those for standard programmed cycling function, described as 'normal mode', those for stimulation in response to moving a hand-held magnet over the device, named 'magnet mode', and, in newer models, on-demand stimulation in response to rapid heart rate increases, which is called 'auto-stim mode'. Table 20.1 shows the safe range and typical stimulation parameters for normal mode stimulation. Stimulation consists of a square wave pulse. The charge density delivered is equal to the amplitude, or current output, multiplied by the pulse width over time. The duty cycle is the ratio of time the patient is receiving stimulation. It is calculated as the ON time plus 2 seconds for the ramp-up time and 2 seconds for the ramp-down time divided by the sum of the ON time and the OFF time. The duty cycle should not exceed 50% due to concerns over nerve injury, based on animal studies. The magnet mode allows patients to activate the device when they feel a seizure or aura, and magnet current output is generally set to 0.25 mA above the normal mode. The auto-stim mode parameters include settings to configure accurate detection of tachycardia correlated with seizure activity and the intensity of stimulation to be delivered. Tachycardia-triggered stimulation is ideally used in selected patients who have demonstrated ictal tachycardia on pre-implantation testing.

Programming Recommendations

Although VNS has the longest track record of any neuromodulation therapy, few human studies have

systematically investigated optimal stimulation parameters. In most VNS clinical studies, stimulation parameters were allowed to vary based on the preference of the treating physicians. From these studies, we know the general range of stimulation parameters that have demonstrated efficacy [16]. In one study, the mean output current was 1.1 mA at the end of the three-month controlled phase and 1.7 mA at the end of one year. The output current is generally increased in 0.25 mA steps, as tolerated, to a target of 1 to 2 mA. Side effects including cough, throat tightness and voice changes may increase along with increasing output current. These symptoms may be minimized, generally without loss of efficacy, by decreasing the output current by 0.25 mA, the pulse width from 500 to 250 µs or the frequency from 30 to 20 or 25 Hz.

Patients are often started with an ON time of 30 seconds and an OFF time of 5 minutes. However, a number of studies have suggested that increasing the duty cycle by decreasing the OFF time may be more effective in certain patients. One of the largest trials investigating VNS parameter settings involved 154 patients from a randomized controlled VNS efficacy trial who were subsequently enrolled in a long-term follow-up trial [17]. Patients in the therapeutic stimulation group were programmed at 30 seconds ON and 5 minutes OFF and individual physicians were allowed to vary stimulus parameters until the 12-month point. While all stimulation parameters were significantly different between 3 months and 12 months, the most significant differences were in current and OFF time. None of the individual parameter changes were correlated with reduced seizure frequency. However, a subgroup of 26 patients who had a poor response to VNS at three months and had a reduction in the OFF time to less than 1.1 minutes by 12 months showed a statistically significant improvement in the median seizure reduction from 21% to 39%. This suggests that non-responders may benefit from an increase in the duty cycle, although it may not be necessary for all patients. A randomized controlled trial of stimulation parameters in 64 patients over three months of VNS treatment failed to identify a significant difference in efficacy between standard stimulation parameters (30 seconds ON, 3 minutes OFF), increased duty cycle (30 seconds ON, 0.5 minutes OFF), and rapid cycling (7 seconds ON, 18 seconds OFF) [18]. However, it should be noted that the duration of this study was limited and that other parameters besides duty cycle also varied

Table 20.1 Vagus nerve stimulation parameters

Parameters	Safe range	Typical settings
Output current (mA)	0–3.5	1–2
Frequency (Hz)	1–30	20–30
Pulse width (µs)	130–1000	250–500
ON time (s)	7–60	30
OFF time (min)	0.2–180	0.5–5

between the groups. Other studies have not been able to confirm an increase in efficacy with increases in the duty cycle or rapid cycling [19,20]. Despite these studies, the possibility remains that some patients who do not respond to standard cycling parameters may benefit from increases in the duty cycle. A trial of an increased duty cycle up to 50% may be warranted in patients who do not respond to standard cycling.

Adverse Effects

We now have a considerable amount of data on device safety. Adverse effects are usually directly related to active stimulation and can be minimized by decreasing the current output, pulse width or frequency of stimulation. Based on clinical experience, it also seems that patients habituate to stimulation, and tolerance improves over time. This was demonstrated in an open-label long-term follow-up study of 454 patients from two studies. The most frequent side effects were hoarseness, cough, paraesthesia and shortness of breath. While hoarseness occurred most frequently at year one with 29% of the population affected, each of these symptoms occurred less frequently over time. By three years of follow-up, each of these side effects were present in less than 3.2% of patients [9].

Trigeminal Nerve Stimulation

Trigeminal nerve stimulation (TNS) is a newer non-invasive epilepsy treatment modality that is approved for use in Europe and many other parts of the world, but not yet in the United States. It consists of an external pulse generator delivering electrical stimulation transcutaneously through disposable adhesive electrodes to the ophthalmic branches of the trigeminal nerve bilaterally. Thus, it is a non-invasive therapy which may be worn at night with a pre-set stimulation algorithm eliminating the need for programming.

The mechanism of action of external TNS (eTNS) is thought to be similar to that of VNS in that it modulates the activity of brain regions implicated in epilepsy utilizing the direct connections of the trigeminal nerve to the brainstem. It is known that the trigeminal system projects to the thalamus and subsequently the cortex, allowing it to affect the electrical activity of these structures. Studies in the rat pentylenetetrazole seizure model have demonstrated optimal anti-seizure effects using high-frequency stimulation (>100 Hz) and bilateral as opposed to unilateral stimulation [21].

The largest randomized double-blind clinical trial of eTNS in the United States involved 50 patients with medication-resistant epilepsy who underwent an 18-week trial of therapeutic vs. active control stimulation followed by open-label stimulation for up to one year. Therapy was delivered for a minimum of 12 hours per day, typically during sleep. The treatment group responder rate (>50% reduction in seizure frequency) improved from 17.8% at 6 weeks to 40.5% at 18 weeks. The between-group responder rate comparison of treatment to active control at 18 weeks was 40.5% and 15.6%, respectively [22]. Further long-term efficacy data has demonstrated sustained effects of treatment to 12 months of eTNS therapy [23]. Additionally, significant positive effects on mood were demonstrated in this cohort, as evidenced by Beck Depression Inventory (BDI) changes at six weeks of treatment and persisting throughout the trial. The treatment group mean change in BDI was 8.13 in the negative direction (improved) compared to active control mean improvement of 3.95. These changes were observed independent of seizure improvement.

eTNS was very well tolerated with the most significant adverse effect being mild skin irritation at the site of the adhesive electrode placement. It remains to be shown whether such an external neuromodulatory device might be predictive of the efficacy of an implantable device, but such a role may be an important one, as devices for neuromodulation in epilepsy become commonplace.

Key Points

- Vagus nerve stimulation (VNS) has shown efficacy in the treatment of drug-resistant epilepsy due to a variety of causes.
- As with other neuromodulation devices, efficacy appears to improve over time.
- The mechanism of action of VNS relies on broadly projecting brainstem nuclei.
- Trigeminal nerve stimulation (TNS) may elicit similar effects via transcutaneous stimulation using an external device.

References

1. Krahl SE. Vagus nerve stimulation for epilepsy : a review of the peripheral mechanisms. *Surg Neurol Int* 2012;3:47–52

2. Yuan H, Silberstein SD. Vagus Nerve and vagus nerve stimulation, a comprehensive review. *Headache* 2016; **56**(1):71–78

3. Krahl SE, Senanayake SS, Handforth A. Destruction of peripheral c-fibers does not alter subsequent vagus nerve stimulation-induced seizure suppression in rats. *Epilepsia* 2001;**42**(5):586–589

4. Krahl SE, Clark KB. Vagus nerve stimulation for epilepsy: a review of central mechanisms. *Surg Neurol Int* 2012;**3**(Suppl 4):S255-S259

5. Krahl SE, Clark KB, Smith DC, Browning RA. Locus coeruleus lesions suppress the seizure-attenuating effects of vagus nerve stimulation. *Epilepsia* 1998;**39** (7):709–714

6. Kuba R, Guzaninova M, Brazdil M, et al. Effect of chronic vagal nerve stimulation on interictal epileptiform discharges. *Epilepsia* 2002;**43** (10):1181–1188

7. Panebianco M, Rigby A, Weston J, Marson AG. Vagus nerve stimulation for partial seizures. *Cochrane Database Syst Rev* 2015;(4)CD002896

8. Cyberonics *VNS Therapy® System Physician's Manual*, 2015.

9. Morris GL, Mueller WM. Long-term treatment with vagus nerve stimulation in patients with refractory epilepsy: the Vagus Nerve Stimulation Study Group E01–E05. *Neurology* 1999;**53**(8):1731–1735

10. Kuba R, Brázdil M, Kalina M, et al. Vagus nerve stimulation: longitudinal follow-up of patients treated for 5 years. *Seizure* 2009;**18**(4):269–274

11. Elliott RE, Morsi A, Kalhorn SP, et al. Vagus nerve stimulation in 436 consecutive patients with treatment-resistant epilepsy: long-term outcomes and predictors of response. *Epilepsy Behav* 2011;**20** (1):57–63

12. Morris GL, Gloss D, Buchhalter J, et al. Evidence-based guideline update: vagus nerve stimulation for the treatment of epilepsy. Report of the guideline development subcommittee of the American Academy of Neurology. *Neurology* 2013;**81**(16):1453–1459

13. Ng M, Devinsky O. Vagus nerve stimulation for refractory idiopathic generalised epilepsy. *Seizure* 2004;**13**(3):176–178

14. Holmes MD, Silbergeld DL, Drouhard D, Wilensky AJ, Ojemann LM. Effect of vagus nerve stimulation on adults with pharmacoresistant generalized epilepsy syndromes. *Seizure* 2004;**13**(5):340–345

15. Morris GL, Gloss D, Buchhalter J, et al. Evidence-based guideline update: vagus nerve stimulation for the treatment of epilepsy. Report of the guideline development subcommittee of the American Academy of Neurology. *Epilepsy Curr* 2013;**13** (6):297–303

16. Heck C, Helmers SL, DeGiorgio CM. Vagus nerve stimulation therapy, epilepsy, and device parameters: scientific basis and recommendations for use. *Neurology* 2002;**59**(6 Suppl 4):S31–S37

17. Degiorgio CM, Thompson J, Lewis P, et al. Vagus nerve stimulation: analysis of device parameters in 154 patients during the long-term XE5 study. *Epilepsia* 2001;**42**(8):1017–1020

18. DeGiorgio C, Heck C, Bunch S, et al. Vagus nerve stimulation for epilepsy: randomized comparison of three stimulation paradigms. *Neurology* 2005;**65**(2 Suppl 1):317–319

19. Scherrmann J, Hoppe C, Kral T, Schramm J, Elger CE. Vagus nerve stimulation clinical experience in a large patient series. *J Clin Neurophysiol* 2001;**18**(5):408–414

20. Labar D. Vagus nerve stimulation for 1 year in 269 patients on unchanged antiepileptic drugs. *Seizure* 2004:392–398

21. Fanselow EE, Reid AP, Nicolelis MA. Reduction of pentylenetetrazole-induced seizure activity in awake rats by seizure-triggered trigeminal nerve stimulation. *J Neurosci* 2000;**20**(21):8160–8168

22. DeGiorgio CM, Soss J, Cook IA, et al. Randomized controlled trial of trigeminal nerve stimulation for drug-resistant epilepsy. *Neurology* 2013;**80** (9):786–791

23. Soss J, Heck C, Murray D, et al. A prospective long-term study of external trigeminal nerve stimulation for drug-resistant epilepsy. *Epilepsy Behav* 2015;**42**:44–47

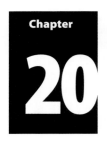

Chapter

20

2. Stimulation of the Anterior Nucleus of the Thalamus

Mohamad Z. Koubeissi and Amr Ewida

Introduction

Despite the plethora of newer generation anti-seizure medications (ASMs), medication-resistant seizures continue to occur in 20% of individuals with generalized epilepsy and 40% of those with focal epilepsy [1]. Surgical resection of the seizure focus is superior to continued medical therapy once medical refractoriness has been established [2], but epilepsy surgery is highly underutilized [3], and only half of the patients evaluated for epilepsy surgery prove to be good surgical candidates [4,5]. Therefore, there is a great need for alternative treatments such as diet therapies and targeted electrical stimulation. Deep brain stimulation (DBS) has been established as an effective treatment for medically refractory Parkinson's disease, dystonia and some psychiatric conditions [6]. Many attempts have been made over the past several decades to find an optimal target for DBS in medication-resistant epilepsy. Investigated targets have included the vagus nerve, cerebellum, subthalamic nucleus, centromedian nucleus, anterior thalamic nucleus, hippocampus, seizure focus and caudate nucleus, among others. Among these regions, the anterior nucleus of the thalamus (ANT) was subjected to a controlled trial [7], and long-term follow-up of implanted patients has become available [8].

Anatomy of the Anterior Nucleus of the Thalamus

The ANT represents a group of nuclei within the medial diencephalon at the rostral end of the thalamus (Figure 20.1). It is composed of three nuclei: the anterodorsal, anteroventral and anteromedial. However, some authors consider including the lateral dorsal thalamic nucleus as part of the ANT, considering its functional similarity and limbic connections [9]. The ANT has complex and extensive cortical, subcortical and limbic connections that make it an attractive target for electrical stimulation. In general,

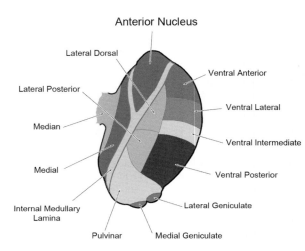

Figure 20.1 Drawing of the lateral-superior view of the right thalamus. The anterior thalamic nucleus is bordered by the bifurcated internal medullary lamina, which also separates the rest of the thalamic nuclei into lateral and medial groups.

most of the ANT connections are bidirectional. These connections widely extend to prefrontal, cingulate, insular, hippocampal and temporal neocortex [10]. In addition to the wide anatomical connections of the ANT, there is a histological differentiation among the three main nuclei. A separate cellular architecture is distinguished for each nucleus, as well as different degrees of immunoreactivity to acetylcholinesterase and other calcium-binding proteins [9]. Figure 20.2 summarizes that main afferent and efferent connections of the anteromedial, anterodorsal and anteroventral nuclei of the ANT. This widespread connectivity suggests that ANT stimulation may help reduce seizures regardless of their area of origin.

Importantly, the ANT is part of the Papez circuit, which is important for episodic memory and control of emotional expression [10]. A portion of ANT neurons participate in the rhythmical theta firing of the thalamus [11], which is vital to the synaptic plasticity of the hippocampal circuitry. Episodic memory

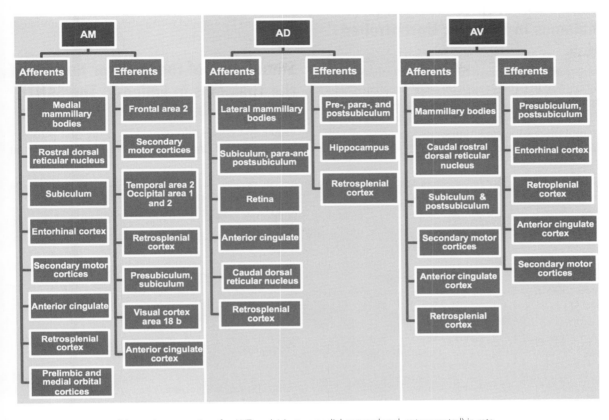

Figure 20.2 Diagram of the main connections for ANT nuclei (anteromedial, anterodorsal, anteroventral) in rats.

deficits can result from damage of the ANT or its afferent projections from the mammillary bodies, such as in Korsakoff syndrome and thalamic strokes [12]. This connectivity probably explains the efficacy of ANT stimulation in reducing medial temporal lobe seizures.

Pre-Clinical Studies of ANT Stimulation

Pre-clinical studies that assessed the role of the ANT in epilepsy were performed using lesion interventions or electrical stimulation in animal models of both focal and generalized seizures. In experimental focal epilepsy in cats and rhesus monkeys, lesioning the ANT resulted in significant seizure reduction [13]. In addition, bilateral interruption of the mammil-lothalamic tract in guinea pigs resulted in prevention of pentylenetetrazol (PTZ)-induced seizures [14]. Moreover, PTZ injection into the thalamus, sparing the mammillary bodies (MB), resulted in facilitation of electrographic seizures and the convulsant effect of

systemically injected PTZ, suggesting a regulatory role for the ANT in seizure propagation [15]. Later reports confirmed that disconnecting the mammil-lothalamic tract from the ANT resulted in a protective anti-seizure effect against PTZ-induced generalized seizures in guinea pigs [16]. Therefore, the mammil-lothalamic tracts and other structures in mid-dience-phalic regions might contribute to a major role in seizure propagation that could be prevented by lesion-ing these areas [14].

The effect of ANT stimulation in rats was studied later. High-frequency stimulation (100 Hz) of the ANT did not affect PTZ-induced electrographic sei-zures, but increased the threshold for clonic seizures compared with control animals [17,18]. In addition, high-frequency, low-voltage stimulation reduced the frequency of electrographic seizures and status epi-lepticus in the pilocarpine model [19–21]. Similarly, an anti-seizure effect was produced by ANT stimula-tion in rats kindled by stimulation of the amygdala [22,23].

Stimulation of Anterior Nucleus of Thalamus in Humans: Uncontrolled Trials

Cooper and colleagues were the first to attempt ANT stimulation in patients with intractable epilepsy. They reported seizure reduction exceeding 60% in four of six implanted patients [24,25]. Multiple uncontrolled attempts at ANT stimulation were done in small samples that are listed in Table 20.2. These studies reported benefit and called for a controlled trial to assess the efficacy and tolerability of ANT stimulation in intractable epilepsy.

Stimulation of the Anterior Nucleus of the Thalamus in Epilepsy: The SANTE Trial

Fisher and collaborators published the first prospective, controlled, double-blinded multi-centre clinical

Table 20.2 List of uncontrolled trials of electrical stimulation of the anterior nucleus of the thalamus (CPS, complex partial (currently classified as focal impaired awareness) seizure; GTCS, generalized tonic-clonic seizure; SPS, simple partial (currently classified as focal aware) seizure)

Trial	N	Seizure type	Follow-up time	Results	Complications
Upton and Cooper [32]	6	All patients had CPS	24–36 months	Four out of the six patients had a statistically and clinically significant seizure reduction	None
Sussman [35]	5	Four patients had CPS and one had secondarily GTCS	12–24 months	A preliminary abstract reported three of the five experiencing improvement with resolution of GTCS and drop attacks in one patient. Absence and CPS did not resolve	None
Hodaie [36]	5	Two patients had GTCS, one had atonic seizures, staring spells, and GTCS, and two had SPS, CPS and GTCS	10–20 months	Bipolar unilateral stimulation of (2–10 Hz, 0.5–10 V, and 330–450 ms pulse duration) resulted in a statistically significant decrease in seizure frequency by 54%, and two patients had >75% seizure reduction	One patient has skin erosions over DBS site
Kerrigan [34]	5	Two patients had SPS, CPS, and GTCS; 2 had CPS with secondarily GTCS; and one had SPS and CPS	6–36 months	100 Hz; pulse width, 90 µs; stimulation voltages ≤5V. Clinical improvement occurred in four out of five with statistically significant decrease in frequency of CPS and GTCS. One patient had significant overall reduction in seizure frequency	None
Andrade [33]	6	Most of the patients with partial epilepsy	5–6 years	Five patients had 50% seizure reduction. Suggested delayed benefit of stimulation. Electrode implantations induced seizure reduction suggesting microthalamotomy effect	None
Osorio [37]	4	Four patients had bi-temporal mesial epilepsy with CPS and secondarily GTCS in three patients	6–36 months	Closed loop, higher frequency stimulation 145–175 Hz; 4.1 V; 90 µs; 1 min ON, 5 min OFF. Mean reduction in seizure frequency of 75.6% ($t = -8.24$; $p \le 0.01$) (range: 92% to 53%) with efficacy in patients with MTLE	None
Lim [38]	4	One patient with generalized seizure, and three had partial seizure with secondary generalization into GTCS	24 months	Bipolar high-frequency stimulation rate of 90-110 Hz, standard pulse width of 60-90 µs. mean seizure reduction rate was 49.6 %. Microthalamotomy effect was questioned as factor responsible for seizure reduction	One patient had ICH, and another had an allergic reaction

trial for stimulation of ANT in 2010 [7]. They recruited 110 patients (18–65 years old) with refractory seizures defined as failure of three or more ASMs to produce seizure freedom. After electrode implantation, the subjects were randomized to either 0 V or 5 V for a three-month blinded phase. Unblinded stimulation ensued for nine months during which medications were also unchanged. Over the three-month blinded phase (Figure 20.3), the stimulated group had a significant mean seizure reduction of 40.5%, compared with 14.5% for the 0 V group. A greater seizure reduction was observed in patients with temporal lobe epilepsy: 44% in the treated group, vs. 22% in the 0 V group (p = 0.025). Significant reduction was noticed in both focal and secondarily generalized seizures. Upon follow-up at 25 months post-implantation, 56% reduction in median seizure frequency was reported, and the responder rate (percentage of subjects experiencing at least 50% seizure reduction) was 54%. Additionally, seizure freedom was reported in 14 patients for at least six months.

The reported adverse events included depression and memory impairment, with no overall changes in neurocognitive outcome between the treatment and control groups. Two subjects had stimulation-related status epilepticus, and two had sudden unexpected death in epilepsy (SUDEP), but that was within the average recognized range of SUDEP occurrence in the study population.

A five-year follow-up reported 69% reduction of the median frequency [26] (Table 20.3). This was associated with a significant improvement in quality of life. Meanwhile, the patients were undergoing alterations of the stimulation parameters and of their ASM regimens, and lacosamide, for example, had been added in almost half of the subjects. However, seizure reduction was similar in subjects with or without addition of ASMs. Serious adverse events at five years of follow-up occurred in 34% of the subjects. The most significant adverse effects included depression in 37.3%, memory impairment in 27.3% and status epilepticus in 6.4%, as well as SUDEP in four cases.

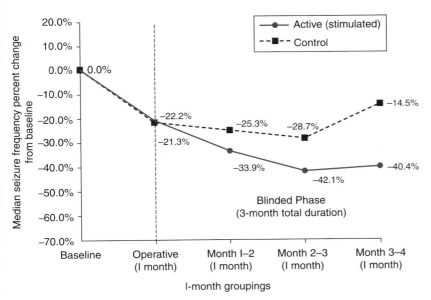

Figure 20.3 DBS of ANT results during the blinded phase (from [7]).

Table 20.3 ANT stimulation study: results upon one-, two-, and five-year follow-up

SANTE study	One year	Two years	Five years
Median seizure reduction	41%	56%	69%
The responder rate (≥50% reduction in seizure frequency)	43%	54%	68%
Seizure-freedom for at least six months	2%	13%	16%
Serious device-related adverse events	+	+ (29.5)	+ (34%)

The five-year ANT stimulation data, representing class IV evidence of 69% reduction in median seizure frequency, are similar to the results of other stimulation modalities: 50% for VNS and 44% for RNS at one year [26,27]. The side effects are also similar, although ANT stimulation may result in relatively higher rates of depression and subjective memory impairment [28]. Like the VNS and RNS, ANT stimulation is now approved in the European Union for treatment of intractable epilepsy. The US Food and Drug Administration approved its indication in 2018 for epilepsy with focal onset seizures that has been resistant to three or more anti-seizure medications.

Mechanism of Action of Electrical Stimulation

Although the exact mechanism of action is not fully understood, it is clear that DBS results in alteration of neural networks [29]. Direct electrical stimulation of neurons can result in either excitation or inhibition, depending on multiple factors, including the stimulation parameters and the nature of stimulated neurons. Low-voltage, high-frequency stimulation in general causes inhibitory neural response or increased threshold potential (hyperpolarization) due to accumulation of the extracellular potassium [29,30]. Another possible mechanism could be through a desynchronizing effect that limits the building up and propagation of epileptic activity.

The specific mechanism of remote anti-seizure effect caused by ANT stimulation is unknown. One hypothesized mechanism is that of modification of neural plasticity of the epileptogenic network as a result of ANT stimulation through its cortical connections [31]. This may also explain the common phenomenon that occurs in nearly all stimulation modalities resulting in a more desirable effect upon extended periods of stimulation. The heteropathogenicity of epilepsy may explain why a specific neuromodulation intervention may help one patient but not another.

Technique of ANT Surgical Approach

All patients evaluated for DBS of ANT undergo stereotactic frame placement followed by MRI. Direct targeting of the ANT is usually performed using standard stereotactic planning software in a lateral position [32]. ANT is identified by the orientation of the anatomy of the lateral ventricle and the sagittal mammillothalamic tract. Implantation of the intra-cranial electrodes is usually done with postoperative recording that usually shows high-frequency bursts that vary among different anterior thalamic nuclei. Scalp EEG recording during ANT stimulation shows a driving-like response that is maximally seen in the fronto-polar electrodes of the bipolar montage in almost all patients [33].

Key Points

- Deep brain stimulation (DBS) of the anterior nucleus of the thalamus (ANT) can reduce seizures in patients with medically refractory epilepsy.
- Long-term follow-up suggests the possibility of continued seizure reduction years after implantation of ANT-DBS.
- Adverse events of ANT-DBS include depression and memory impairment.

References

1. Kwan P, Schachter SC, Brodie MJ. Drug-resistant epilepsy. *N Engl J Med* 2011;**365**(10):919–926

2. Wiebe S. Epilepsy: outcome patterns in epilepsy surgery – the long-term view. *Nat Rev Neurol* 2012;**8** (3):123–124

3. Englot DJ, Chang EF. Rates and predictors of seizure freedom in resective epilepsy surgery: an update. *Neurosurg Rev* 2014;**37**(3):389–405

4. Bergey GK. Neurostimulation in the treatment of epilepsy. *Exp Neurol* 2013;**244**:87–95

5. Duncan JS. Selecting patients for epilepsy surgery: synthesis of data. *Epilepsy Behav* 2011;**20**(2):230–232

6. Sironi VA. Origin and evolution of deep brain stimulation. *Front Integr Neurosci* 2011;**5**:42

7. Fisher R, Salanova V, Witt T, et al. Electrical stimulation of the anterior nucleus of thalamus for treatment of refractory epilepsy. *Epilepsia* 2010;**51** (5):899–908

8. Salanova V, Witt T, Worth R, et al. Long-term efficacy and safety of thalamic stimulation for drug-resistant partial epilepsy. *Neurology* 2015;**84** (10):1017–1025

9. Morel A, Magnin M, Jeanmonod D. Multiarchitectonic and stereotactic atlas of the human thalamus. *J Comp Neurol* 1997;**387**(4):588–630

10. Jankowski MM, Ronnqvist KC, Tsanov M, et al. The anterior thalamus provides a subcortical circuit supporting memory and spatial navigation. *Front Syst Neurosci* 2013;**7**:45

11. Vertes RP, Albo Z, Di Prisco GV. Theta-rhythmically firing neurons in the anterior thalamus: implications for mnemonic functions of Papez's circuit. *Neuroscience* 2001;**104**(3):619–625

12. Child ND, Benarroch EE. Anterior nucleus of the thalamus: functional organization and clinical implications. *Neurology* 2013;**81**(21):1869–1876

13. Kusske JA, Ojemann GA, Ward AA. Effects of lesions in ventral anterior thalamus on experimental focal epilepsy. *Exp Neurol* 1972;**34**(2):279–90

14. Mirski MA, Ferrendelli JA. Interruption of the mammillothalamic tract prevents seizures in guinea pigs. *Science* 1984;**226**(4670):72–74

15. Mirski MA, Ferrendelli JA. Anterior thalamic mediation of generalized pentylenetetrazol seizures. *Brain Res* 1986;**399**(2):212–223

16. Mirski MA, Ferrendelli JA. Interruption of the connections of the mammillary bodies protects against generalized pentylenetetrazol seizures in guinea pigs. *J Neurosci* 1987;**7**(3):662–670

17. Mirski MA, Rossell LA, Terry JB, Fisher RS. Anticonvulsant effect of anterior thalamic high frequency electrical stimulation in the rat. *Epilepsy Research* 1997;**28**(2):89–100

18. Mirski MA, Ferrendelli JA. Anterior thalamic mediation of generalized pentylenetetrazol seizures. *Brain Res* 1986;**399**(2):212–223

19. Hamani C, Ewerton FIS, Bonilha SM, et al. Bilateral anterior thalamic nucleus lesions and high-frequency stimulation are protective against pilocarpine-induced seizures and status epilepticus. *Neurosurgery* 2003;**54**(1):191–195

20. Covolan L, de Almeida AC, Amorim B, et al. Effects of anterior thalamic nucleus deep brain stimulation in chronic epileptic rats. *PLoS ONE* 2014;**9**(6):e97618

21. Jou SB, Kao IF, Yi PL, Chang FC. Electrical stimulation of left anterior thalamic nucleus with high-frequency and low-intensity currents reduces the rate of pilocarpine-induced epilepsy in rats. *Seizure* 2013;**22**(3):221–229

22. Zhang Q, Wu ZC, Yu JT, et al. Mode-dependent effect of high-frequency electrical stimulation of the anterior thalamic nucleus on amygdala-kindled seizures in rats. *Neuroscience* 2012;**217**:113–122

23. Zhang Q, Wu ZC, Yu JT, et al. Anticonvulsant effect of unilateral anterior thalamic high frequency electrical stimulation on amygdala-kindled seizures in rats. *Brain Res Bull* 2012;**87**(2–3):221–226

24. Upton AR, Cooper IS, Springman M, Amin I. Suppression of seizures and psychosis of limbic system origin by chronic stimulation of anterior nucleus of the thalamus. *Int J Neurol* 1985–1986;**19–20**:223–230

25. Cooper IS, Upton AR. Therapeutic implications of modulation of metabolism and functional activity of cerebral cortex by chronic stimulation of cerebellum and thalamus. *Biol Psychiatry* 1985;**20**(7):811–813

26. Elliott RE, Rodgers SD, Bassani L, et al. Vagus nerve stimulation for children with treatment-resistant epilepsy: a consecutive series of 141 cases. *J Neurosurg Pediatr* 2011;**7**(5):491–500

27. Bergey GK, Morrell MJ, Mizrahi EM, et al. Long-term treatment with responsive brain stimulation in adults with refractory partial seizures. *Neurology* 2015;**84**(8):810–817

28. Sprengers M, Vonck K, Carrette E, Marson AG, Boon P. *Deep Brain and Cortical Stimulation for Epilepsy*, Boon P, (ed.) Chichester, UK: John Wiley & Sons, Ltd; 1996.

29. Park EH, Barreto E, Gluckman BJ, Schiff SJ, So P. A model of the effects of applied electric fields on neuronal synchronization. *J Comput Neurosci* 2005;**19**(1):53–70

30. Bikson M, Lian J, Hahn PJ, et al. Suppression of epileptiform activity by high frequency sinusoidal fields in rat hippocampal slices. *J Physiol* 2004;**531**(1):181–191

31. Koubeissi MZ. Between the pulse generator and the anterior thalamic nucleus: the light at the end of the tunnel. *Epilepsy Curr* 2015;**15**(4):183–184

32. Upton AR, Amin I, Garnett S, et al. Evoked metabolic responses in the limbic-striate system produced by stimulation of anterior thalamic nucleus in man. *Pacing Clin Electrophysiol* 1987;**10**(1 Pt 2):217–225

33. Andrade DM, Zumsteg D, Hamani C, et al. Long-term follow-up of patients with thalamic deep brain stimulation for epilepsy. *Neurology* 2006;**66**(10):1571–1573

34. Kerrigan JF, Litt B, Fisher RS, et al. Electrical stimulation of the anterior nucleus of the thalamus for the treatment of intractable epilepsy. *Epilepsia* 2004;**45**(4):346–354

35. Sussman NM GHJR, Goldman HW SNJR. Anterior thalamus stimulation in medically intractable epilepsy, part II: preliminary clinical results. *Epilepsia* 1988;**29**:677

36. Hodaie M, Wennberg RA, Dostrovsky JO, Lozano AM. Chronic anterior thalamus stimulation for intractable epilepsy. *Epilepsia* 2002;**43**(6):603–608

37. Osorio I, Overman J, Giftakis J, Wilkinson SB. High frequency thalamic stimulation for inoperable mesial temporal epilepsy. *Epilepsia* 2007;**48**(8):1561–1571

38. Lim SN, Lee ST, Tsai YT, et al. Electrical stimulation of the anterior nucleus of the thalamus for intractable epilepsy: a long-term follow-up study. *Epilepsia* 2007;**48**(2):342–347

3. Responsive Neurostimulation of the Brain

Ritu Kapur and Martha J. Morrell

Introduction and History of Brain Responsive Neurostimulation

For patients with medication-resistant epilepsy, surgical resection is an option only if the epileptogenic zone can be identified and resected without undue risk to cognitive or eloquent cortical function. However, a substantial portion of patients are not candidates for surgical resection, and these may receive meaningful improvements in quality of life and reductions in seizure burden from brain stimulation.

Closed-loop, or 'responsive' neurostimulation systems deliver stimulation in response to epileptiform activity detected with electrodes implanted in the brain. The majority of clinical experience with responsive neurostimulation to date has been with systems that detect and stimulate in cortical areas, at the presumed seizure focus (Figure 20.4).

In the future this technology could lend itself to detection and stimulation in subcortical regions, or to detection in one brain region and responsive stimulation in another, though the effectiveness and safety profiles of these paradigms is currently investigational.

In 1954, Penfield and Jasper [5] asserted that, '… stimulation has as its primary purpose the analysis of the site of origin of seizures and the identification of functional areas so that excision may be safe and effective'. Since that time, brain stimulation has emerged as a treatment for epilepsy. Initial observations on the effects of cortical stimulation for seizure control came from experiments performed in patients undergoing intracranial monitoring for localization of the seizure focus. Lesser reported that brief pulses of cortical stimulation decreased the duration of stimulus-induced after-discharges, and proposed that electrical stimulation applied at the seizure onset could abort seizures in humans.[6]

Velasco described the anti-epileptic effects of sub-acute and chronic hippocampal stimulation in patients with medically intractable seizures [1]. Acute stimulation abolished clinical seizures and significantly decreased EEG spiking, and chronic stimulation had therapeutic effects lasting three to four months. Furthermore, there were no adverse effects on short-term memory, and analysis of the resected tissue confirmed that short-term stimulation did not cause additional damage. Motamedi observed that brief pulses of stimulation were more likely to terminate after-discharges at electrodes placed in the epileptogenic zone and when the stimulus pulse was delivered 'early' (within the first 5 seconds) [7]. Subsequently, the advent of algorithms and systems capable of real-time automated seizure detection [2,8] made it possible for non-implanted systems to sample neural signals from the seizure focus and deliver cortical stimulation early in the seizure.

A multi-centre study of an external responsive neurostimulator (eRNS, NeuroPace, Mountain View, CA) was undertaken as the first step in investigating whether a future, implantable device with automated seizure detection and responsive stimulation capabilities could reduce or abort seizures. The authors observed terminations of electrographic seizure activity after contingent stimulation [9].

Brain responsive stimulation was demonstrated to be safe and effective as a treatment for medically intractable partial onset seizures in a randomized, controlled, double-blinded trial leading to US FDA approval (RNS System, NeuroPace, Mountain View); 191 adults with partial onset seizures arising from one or two foci were evaluated at 32 centres [3]. During the blinded evaluation period, the mean reduction in seizure frequency was significantly greater in patients receiving responsive stimulation than in patients receiving sham stimulation, while there was no difference in adverse event rates [3]. Open-label long-term follow-up showed acceptable safety and improving efficacy [4]. The

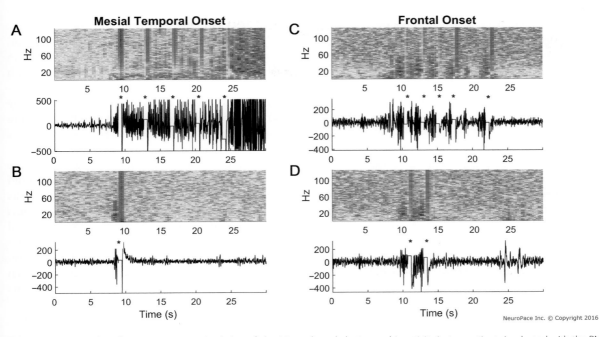

Figure 20.4 Examples of responsive neurostimulation of physician-selected electrographic activity in two patients implanted with the RNS system. Spectrograms plot the power of the ECoG signal at given frequencies over time and time-series data for the ECoG are shown below each spectrogram. Asterisks indicate time points at which responsive stimulation was delivered. Panels (A) and (B) are from a 59-year-old male patient with a history of infection and sclerosis. The patient had generalized tonic–clonic seizures and complex partial seizures characterized by oral automatisms and had failed to achieve adequate seizure control with three anti-epileptic medications, including phenytoin, zonisamide and lorazepam. Intra-cranial EEG monitoring suggested independent bilateral mesial temporal seizures. The patient was implanted using an occipital approach and two depth leads were targeted at the hippocampi. (A) shows an example in which stimulation delivered in response to the detection of epileptiform activity did not prevent the subsequent evolution of an electrographic seizure in the left hippocampus. (B) shows an instance in which the same detector was used and the same stimulus was delivered, but in which responsive stimulation was not followed by an electrographic seizure. The patient was a responder and reported an 87% reduction in disabling seizures during the most recent three months in a last observation carried forward (LOCF) analysis. Panels (C) and (D) are from a 33-year-old female patient with simple partial motor seizures of idiopathic origin characterized by posturing. She failed to achieve seizure control with lamotrigine, clonazepam, diazepam, and lorazepam, as well as with a vagus nerve stimulator. An intra-cranial EEG study suggested two foci in the left frontal lobe, one medial and one lateral. The patient was implanted with four subdural strip leads, two of which were connected to the neurostimulator and used for recording and stimulation. One lead was implanted in the inter-hemispheric fissure and the other was positioned along the superior aspect of the frontal and parietal lobes. (C) shows an instance in which stimulation was delivered in response to epileptiform activity detected on the inter-hemispheric lead but did not prevent the subsequent evolution of an electrographic seizure. (D) depicts an instance in which there was no subsequent electrographic event. As with the first patient, it is not possible to know whether this epileptiform activity would have evolved into a seizure if left untreated. This patient reported a 95% reduction in disabling seizures in the most recent three months of a LOCF analysis. These events are representative for each of these patients and occurred in an inter-leaved fashion throughout the course of treatment. Data cutoff was on 11/01/2014.

median percentage reduction in seizures at one year was 44% and by the sixth year of treatment it was 66% [4]. Rates of haemorrhage and infection were within the range expected with other chronically implanted neurostimulation devices, such as deep brain stimulation for movement disorders and for epilepsy [10]. Patients reported clinically meaningful improvements in quality of life, and mood remained stable [11]. There were no cognitive side effects, and there were indications of moderate improvements in naming and memory that were associated with the region of the brain receiving stimulation [12].

Observations from Long-Term Electrocorticographic Monitoring

The delivery of responsive stimulation is based on an incoming electrocorticographic (ECoG) signal, and these signals have been recorded and analyzed with the intention that information therein will enhance the understanding of epilepsy and help optimize therapeutic strategies. Early on, Peters [2] captured detection-triggered snapshots of ECoG and used these to generate reports on seizure intensity and duration, the aim of which was to provide feedback for epileptologists in assessing the effectiveness of a particular stimulation protocol for the individual patient being treated.

Long-term ECoG data captured during clinical trials of a brain responsive neurostimulator [3,4] and a seizure prediction device [13] suggest that patients with epilepsy have frequent electrographic seizures that do not have clinical correlates. Over two years of continuous recording in 15 patients, Cook [13] reported that there were clinically silent electrocorticographic events that were identical to the electrocorticographic activity that occurred during clinical seizures. Similarly, the authors of a study in a canine model of epilepsy noted that inter-ictal epileptiform bursts often bore a 'pronounced similarity to seizure onsets', though they were more prevalent and occurred with greater regularity [14].

An example of clinically evident and clinically silent electrographic seizures from one patient treated with the RNS system is provided in Figure 20.5. Patients implanted with the RNS system and their caregivers are provided with a magnet, which they swipe over the neurostimulator in the event of a seizure. The example shown illustrates that electrographically similar events are sometimes clinical seizures and are at other times clinically silent. It is an open question whether successful treatment with responsive neurostimulation requires that these subclinical events be treated, and the impact of having this type of persistent epileptiform activity occurring in the brain is not well understood from a cognitive or behavioural standpoint.

This also raises the possibility that therapeutic devices that record electrocorticographic data could provide objective measures to help epileptologists better evaluate disease activity and the effectiveness of therapeutic interventions. Accurate recognition and recording of seizures is a challenge due to poor memory in this patient population and the nature of the seizures themselves, which can occur during sleep and often involve loss of awareness [15]. Electrocorticographic data could provide a more objective measure. When experts performed a visual inspection of more than

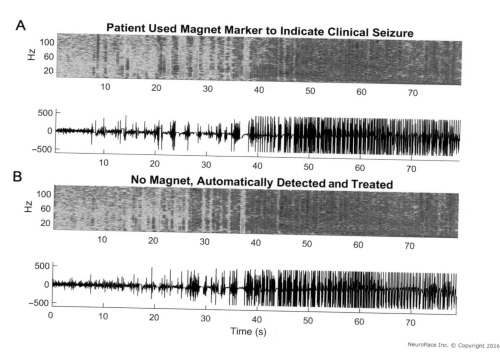

NeuroPace Inc. © Copyright 2016

Figure 20.5 Example of clinical and subclinical events with similar electrocorticographic signatures. Data are from a 49-year-old female with medically intractable seizures resulting from an anoxic event and characterized by epigastric sensation, oral automatism, urinary incontinence and loss of consciousness. Intra-cranial EEG revealed bilateral mesial temporal onsets, and the patient was implanted with the RNS system and bilateral hippocampal depth leads using an occipital approach. This patient used a magnet swipe over the neurostimulator to denote a clinical seizure, and an example of an ECoG associated with this is presented in (A). An electrographically similar event is shown in (B). The device detected and treated an average of 300 of these electrographic events per month, though the patient reported on average two clinical seizures per month during this time period, suggesting that many of these events, though electrographically similar, were subclinical. This patient's most recent assessment showed a 75% reduction in disabling seizures.

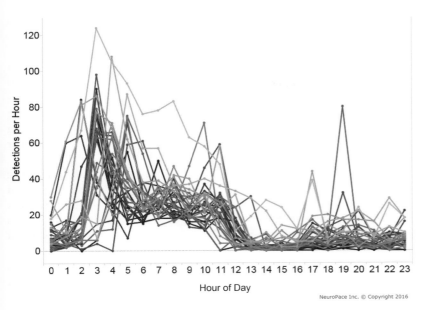

Figure 20.6 Circadian pattern of detection events in one patient: one month of daily detections by hour. Each line represents one day of data. Data are from the same patient presented in Figure 20.4 A and B. The events depicted in Figure 20.4 A and B would both be counted as detections by the device, and because therapy is responsive, an increase in these types of epileptiform events would result in an increase in the number of stimulations delivered.

NeuroPace Inc. © Copyright 2016

7000 ECoG recordings from 128 patients being treated with responsive neurostimulation, detected events were reliably interpreted as either electrographic seizures or non-ictal epileptiform activity in the majority of patients [16].

Long-term ECoG monitoring in a naturalistic setting has made previously inaccessible information available to clinicians. The question remains whether and how this information will effect a shift in treatment paradigms. From a pharmacologic and behavioural standpoint, event detection data could be useful in determining the timing and dosage of ASMs, and for behavioural counselling such as time of sleep and daytime schedules. It has been observed that there are circadian patterns of seizure [17] and inter-ictal activity [18]. An example of the strong circadian influence on detection rates is presented in Figure 20.6.

It may also be possible to screen the effects of therapeutic interventions, such as a change in ASMs, by observing the electrographic effects of the intervention. Figure 20.7 illustrates the association between a change in an ASM and changes in detection and seizure rates. This relationship has been observed anecdotally in several patients, and studies are underway to examine it more closely. This raises the possibility that epileptologists could adjust ASM, behavioural and stimulation therapies by using detection biomarkers as a read out rather than relying solely on self-reported seizure counts, which are often inaccurate and that can only be obtained over a long timeline.

About 35% of patients do not have good outcomes after resections for focal-onset epilepsy [19]. One possibility for failed epilepsy resective surgeries is that the seizure focus was not adequately localized using the standard diagnostic approach of one to two weeks of video-EEG monitoring with scalp or intra-cranial electrodes. Because seizures are dynamic, it is clear that localization of the seizure focus is more confident with greater temporal sampling [20]. This has been demonstrated in patients with mesial temporal lobe epilepsy who were evaluated with long-term ECoG monitoring in order to determine whether seizure onsets were unilateral or bilateral. All patients had intra-cranial electrodes placed in right and left mesial temporal lobes. In 20% of the patients, the ultimate localization of the seizure focus was different from what was supposed before long-term ECoG monitoring. In those patients who were shown to have left and right mesial temporal seizure onsets, the length of time needed to record a bilateral seizure was greater than five weeks on average, which exceeds the typical length of admission for video-EEG monitoring [21].

Long-term ECoG monitoring in a naturalistic setting may identify patients who can benefit from other types of treatment. For example, in one case series, recordings from a chronically implanted responsive neurostimulator were used to revisit the possibility of resective surgery in four patients thought to have more than one seizure focus [22]. Based on the long-

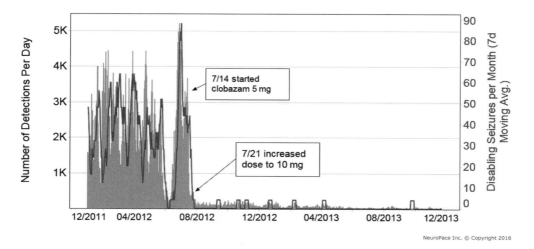

Figure 20.7 Detection rates vary with clinical seizure rates and change in response to a change in anti-seizure medication. RNS system detection data (light grey bars) for an individual patient overlaid with that patient's clinical seizure counts (dark grey line). There is a noticeable difference in both immediately after the patient started taking clobazam. There were no changes in device detection or stimulation settings during the time when clobazam was introduced.

term monitoring, it was determined that while two patients had bilateral MTL seizures, seizures on one side were controlled with medication. Recordings helped localize seizures to a focal source on interhemispheric leads in another patient, and the final patient with suspected mesial temporal and occipital onsets had seizures from occipital focus only. The patients achieved seizure freedom after surgery, and two of the four continued to be treated with responsive neurostimulation.

Open Questions and Conclusions

Observations that brain stimulation has both an acute and a delayed effect suggest that there are multiple mechanisms of action [23]. The acute effects of stimulation may be mediated by local cellular inhibition and/or excitation [24]. Cellular effects could differ, depending on whether stimulation is high or low frequency. High-frequency stimulation (≥ 100 Hz) produces a local axonal block of both afferent and efferent fibres [25] that creates a functional disconnection. Lower stimulation frequencies can drive axonal projections which may be excitatory or inhibitory [26]. Acute effects could be related to changes in cerebral blood flow and in release of neurotransmitters from axons and bordering astrocytes, while later therapeutic effects could be related to changes in synaptic plasticity, neurogenesis or cortical reorganization [23]. Responsive stimulation can adapt to these

dynamic physiological changes, which might offer an advantage over non-responsive, scheduled or continuous stimulation.

A randomized controlled trial demonstrated that brain responsive stimulation can reduce the frequency of medically intractable partial-onset seizures in adults, and further study will determine whether patients with other types of epilepsy will derive similar benefits. Future investigation will assess the relative efficacy of particular stimulation parameters, of stimulation applied directly to or remotely from the seizure focus, and of combining different stimulation approaches (e.g. combined scheduled and responsive stimulation).

Brain responsive neurostimulation is effective in reducing seizures, is well tolerated by patients and has a long-term safety profile indicating that surgical and cognitive risks are well within an acceptable range [3,4]. In addition, early observations suggest that systems that record long-term ECoG data can provide objective measures that can be combined with clinical reports of seizures to help assess the effectiveness of therapeutic interventions.

Key Points

- Brain responsive neurostimulation is effective in reducing seizures in adults with medication-resistant partial-onset seizures.
- Brain responsive neurostimulation is well tolerated, has an acceptable long-term safety

profile and does not pose a risk to cognitive function, including memory.

- Electrocorticographic data collected over the long term in a naturalistic setting could be used to optimize surgical outcomes and pharmacological interventions.

References

1. Velasco AL, Velasco M, Velasco F et al. Subacute and chronic electrical stimulation of the hippocampus on intractable temporal lobe seizures: preliminary report. *Arch Med Res* 2000;**31**:316–328

2. Peters TE, Bhavaraju NC, Frei MG, et al. Network system for automated seizure detection and contingent delivery of therapy. *J Clin Neurophysiol* 2001;**18**:545–549

3. RNS System in Epilepsy Study Group, Morrell MJ. Responsive cortical stimulation for the treatment of medically intractable partial epilepsy. *Neurology* 2011;**77**:1295–1304

4. Bergey GK, Morrell MJ, Mizrahi EM, et al. Long-term treatment with responsive brain stimulation in adults with refractory partial seizures. *Neurology* 2015;**84**:810–817

5. Penfield W, Jasper H. *Epilepsy and the Functional Anatomy of the Human Brain*. Boston, MA: Little, Brown and Company, 1954:239.

6. Lesser RP, Kim SH, Beyderman L et al. Brief bursts of pulse stimulation terminate afterdischarges caused by cortical stimulation. *Neurology* 1999;**53**:2073–2081

7. Motamedi GK, Lesser RP, Miglioretti DL, et al. Optimizing parameters for terminating cortical afterdischarges with pulse stimulation. *Epilepsia* 2002;**43**:836–846

8. Harding GW. An automated seizure monitoring system for patients with indwelling recording electrodes. *Electroencephalogr Clin Neurophysiol* 1993;**86**:428–437

9. Kossoff EH, Ritzl EK, Politsky JM, et al. Effect of an external responsive neurostimulator on seizures and electrographic discharges during subdural electrode monitoring. *Epilepsia* 2004;**45**:1560–1567

10. Fisher R, Salanova V, Witt T, et al. Electrical stimulation of the anterior nucleus of thalamus for treatment of refractory epilepsy. *Epilepsia* 2010;**51**:899–908

11. Meador KJ, Kapur R, Loring DW, et al. Quality of life and mood in patients with medically intractable epilepsy treated with targeted responsive neurostimulation. *Epilepsy Behav* 2015;**45**:242–247

12. Loring DW, Kapur R, Meador KJ, et al. Differential neuropsychological outcomes following targeted responsive neurostimulation for partial-onset epilepsy. *Epilepsia* 2015;**56**:1836–1844

13. Cook MJ, Karoly PJ, Freestone DR, et al. Human focal seizures are characterized by populations of fixed duration and interval. *Epilepsia* 2016;**57**(3):359–368

14. Davis KA, Ung H, Wulsin D, et al. Mining continuous intracranial EEG in focal canine epilepsy: relating interictal bursts to seizure onsets. *Epilepsia* 2016;**57**:89–98

15. Fisher RS, Blum DE, DiVentura B, et al. Seizure diaries for clinical research and practice: limitations and future prospects. *Epilepsy Behav* 2012;**24**:304–310

16. Quigg M, Sun F, Fountain NB, et al. Interrater reliability in interpretation of electrocorticographic seizure detections of the responsive neurostimulator. *Epilepsia* 2015;**56**:968–971

17. Durazzo TS, Spencer SS, Duckrow RB, et al. Temporal distributions of seizure occurrence from various epileptogenic regions. *Neurology* 2008;**70**:1265–1271

18. Anderson CT, Tcheng TK, Sun FT, et al. Day-night patterns of epileptiform activity in 65 patients with long-term ambulatory electrocorticography. *J Clin Neurophysiol* 2015;**32**:406–412

19. Engel J, Jr, Wiebe S, French J, et al. Practice parameter: temporal lobe and localized neocortical resections for epilepsy. Report of the Quality Standards Subcommittee of the American Academy of Neurology, in association with the American Epilepsy Society and the American Association of Neurological Surgeons. *Neurology* 2003;**60**:538–547

20. Struck AF, Cole AJ, Cash SS, et al. The number of seizures needed in the EMU. *Epilepsia* 2015;**56**:1753–1759

21. King-Stephens D, Mirro E, Weber PB, et al. Lateralization of mesial temporal lobe epilepsy with chronic ambulatory electrocorticography. *Epilepsia* 2015;**56**:959–967

22. DiLorenzo DJ, Mangubat EZ, Rossi MA, et al. Chronic unlimited recording electrocorticography-guided resective epilepsy surgery: technology-enabled enhanced fidelity in seizure focus localization with improved surgical efficacy. *J Neurosurg* 2014;**120**:1402–1414

23. Lozano AM, Lipsman N. Probing and regulating dysfunctional circuits using deep brain stimulation. *Neuron* 2013;**77**:406–424

24. Hess CW, Vaillancourt DE, Okun MS. The temporal pattern of stimulation may be important to the mechanism of deep brain stimulation. *Exp Neurol* 2013; **247**:296–302

25. Jensen AL, Durand DM. High frequency stimulation can block axonal conduction. *Exp Neurol* 2009;**220**:57–70

26. McIntyre CC, Hahn PJ. Network perspectives on the mechanisms of deep brain stimulation. *Neurobiol Dis* 2010;**38**:329–337

Chapter 20

4. Transcranial Magnetic Stimulation

Lara M. Schrader

Introduction

For over one and a half decades, investigators have been exploring the therapeutic potential of transcranial magnetic stimulation (TMS) in epilepsy. Transcranial magnetic stimulation is a type of non-invasive brain stimulation performed using an encased wire coil placed on the scalp (Figure 20.8). An electrical pulse through the coil creates a brief magnetic field. This rapidly changing magnetic field then creates an electrical current in the brain tissue underlying the coil. Various shapes and sizes of coils influence the depth and extent of current induction. Stimulation is generally well tolerated and creates the sensation of a tap on the head, although it can become uncomfortable at higher intensities or when stimulation is near the frontalis or temporalis muscles, due to stimulation-induced muscle contractions.

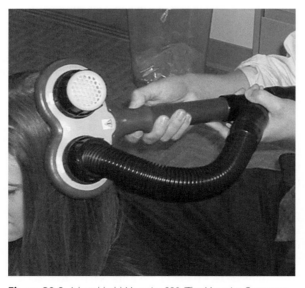

Figure 20.8 A hand-held Magstim 220 (The Magstim Company Ltd., Wales, UK) stimulator with a 70 mm air-cooled figure-of-eight coil positioned over the scalp.

When TMS stimulations are delivered at a fixed repetition rate (repetitive TMS or rTMS), excitability of the underlying cortical tissue can be increased when performed at high frequencies (>1 Hz) or decreased when performed at low frequencies (≤1 Hz). Because low frequency rTMS (LF-rTMS) can reduce cortical excitability, it has been studied as a therapy for epilepsy. In this section, the literature on TMS as a therapy for epilepsy will be reviewed.

Mechanism of Action

The effects of high- and low-frequency rTMS on cortical excitability have been demonstrated by assessing the influence of rTMS directed at hand motor cortex on contralateral hand motor-evoked potential (MEP) amplitude. High-frequency rTMS (HF-rTMS) causes an increase and LF-rTMS causes a decrease in MEP amplitude [1]. Changes in cortical excitability after rTMS have been reported to last from minutes to hours to days [1]. The frequencies of high- and low-frequency rTMS that produce such changes are similar to the frequencies of high- and low-frequency repetitive electrical stimulation that produce long-term potentiation (LTP) and long-term depression (LTD), respectively, in the basic science literature. Therefore, a main hypothesis is that high- and low-frequency rTMS may exert their effects on cortical excitability through LTP- and LTD-like mechanisms, respectively [1]. Another proposed mechanism is that rTMS may exert its effects by modulation of spontaneous oscillatory rhythms in cortical networks [1].

LF-rTMS for Medication-Resistant Epilepsy

The first clinical trial of LF-rTMS for epilepsy was published in 1999 [2]. Since then, numerous reports on the efficacy of LF-rTMS for epilepsy have been published. These reports have used varying LF-rTMS methodologies, tended to have small sample sizes and included various types of epilepsy (both across and within studies). These factors are hypothesized to be reasons that reports on efficacy in epilepsy have had differing outcomes [1]. A recent meta-analysis [3] and recent published guidelines [1] have carefully and systematically examined this literature in an attempt to make sense of the range of existing data.

A 2011 meta-analysis [3] on the anti-epileptic effects of LF-rTMS covered findings in 11 journal articles comprising a total of 164 research subjects. To be included in the analysis, articles needed to focus on the effect of rTMS on seizure frequency or EEG spike number and have a sample size of at least four subjects receiving active rTMS. Regarding seizure frequency, a statistically significant pooled effect size of 0.34 was revealed (95% confidence interval 0.10–0.57, $p < 0.05$). There were many differences among the studies, such as differences in types of epilepsy included, duration of LF-rTMS ranging from one session to up to three months of sessions, and LF-rTMS stimulus frequency ranging from 0.3 to 1.0 Hz. Therefore, three potential moderators were analyzed: (1) LF-rTMS duration (<1 week vs. >1 week), (2) LF-rTMS frequency (<1 Hz vs. 1 Hz) and (3) underlying aetiology (cortical dysplasia or neocortical epilepsy vs. other epileptic disorders). The only moderator variable that was significant and believed to explain varied results of different studies was aetiology of epilepsy. The subgroup mean effect size was 0.71 for cortical dysplasia or neocortical epilepsy (95% confidence interval 0.30–1.12, $p = 0.001$) compared to 0.22 for other epileptic disorders (95% confidence interval 0.05–0.39, $p < 0.05$). The authors concluded that LF-rTMS has a favourable effect on seizure frequency, especially in patients with neocortical epilepsy or cortical dysplasia [3].

Three years later, a group of European experts was commissioned to establish evidence-based guidelines on the therapeutic use of rTMS from evidence published through March 2014 for several neurological and psychiatric disorders, including epilepsy [1]. While a literature search identified 102 papers, only five were original placebo-controlled trials with ≥10 epilepsy patients who received active TMS [4–8]. Together these five reports included 165 patients, with efficacy of LF-rTMS ranging from no significant reduction in seizure frequency [4,5] to significant improvement [6,7]. The experts concluded that 'given the heterogeneity and limitations of the reported studies, recommendations for the use of rTMS in epilepsy do not exceed Level C recommendation (possible efficacy)' for 'focal LF-rTMS of the epileptic focus' with 'no recommendation for non-focal LF-rTMS at the vertex' with 'no recommendation' meaning absence of sufficient evidence to date, and not evidence for an absence of effect [1].

In the published guidelines [1], the authors noted some general methodological limitations within the LF-rTMS epilepsy literature. One obvious limitation was the issue of small sample sizes, resulting in low statistical power. The authors [1] noted that only five rTMS studies included more than 20 subjects with epilepsy [4–7,9]. In addition, there was absence of a control arm in most studies [1]. Of five studies comparing active and sham TMS [4–8], two showed a significant therapeutic effect in the active group [6,7], two showed a trend toward improvement [4,8] and one showed an improvement in EEG abnormalities but no effect on seizures [5].

The authors of the guidelines also noted methodological issues specific to TMS and epilepsy that made the literature difficult to meaningfully interpret [1]. In most studies, subjects had various epilepsy syndromes, aetiologies and localizations of epileptic foci. Therefore, analyzing the data across such a heterogeneous group has the potential to mask a therapeutic response that could have been present in certain subgroups. For example, the first controlled trial of LF-rTMS in epilepsy published in 2002 did not show a significant response for patients overall, but did show a trend towards improvement in patients with neocortical epileptic foci compared to those with deeper mesial temporal foci [4]. Therefore, it has been long suspected that more superficial neocortical epileptic foci may be more responsive to LF-rTMS. The 2011 meta-analysis supported this hypothesis [3]. The brain region stimulated with LF-rTMS has also differed among studies, with some studies stimulating with a circular coil (less focal stimulation) over the vertex and other studies using a figure-of-eight coil (more focal stimulation) directed at the epileptogenic focus. A 2011 analysis [10] of 87 subjects from three placebo-controlled trials [4–6] indicated that targeting the epileptic focus (figure-of-eight coil positioned over the seizure focus [4]) resulted in significantly higher responder rates compared to sham rTMS while non-targeted LF-rTMS (figure-of-eight [6] or round coil [5] positioned over the vertex) did not differ significantly from sham rTMS. Overall, these findings suggest that lowering excitability of the epileptic focus with targeted LF-rTMS has therapeutic potential, and that optimal candidates have an epileptic focus that near the cerebral convexity, where it is more accessible to the TMS delivered across the scalp/skull.

LF-rTMS and Status Epilepticus

LF-rTMS may be beneficial in status epilepticus. A 2015 systematic review of this literature identified 11 original articles, all case series or case reports, describing 21 patients (13 adult and 8 paediatric) [11]. Of 21 patients, 18 (86%) had seizures classified as focal status epilepticus (FSE) or focal refractory status epilepticus (FRSE), while two had generalized refractory status epilepticus (GRSE) and one had undefined SE. Aetiologies were varied and included primary epilepsy, stroke, hypoglycaemia, Rasmussen's encephalitis, Dravet's syndrome, focal cortical dysplasia, lipofuscinosis, post-anoxic encephalopathy, post-vascular malformation resection, herpes simplex encephalitis, Alpert's disease, 'cortical malformation' and unknown cause. Most reports used LF-rTMS, but alternate rTMS protocols were also used, including HF-rTMS to interrupt SE [12,13], HF-rTMS to interrupt SE followed by LF-rTMS for maintenance of seizure control [13], and 6 Hz priming stimulation prior to LF-rTMS [14]. Seizure reduction or control with rTMS occurred in 15 patients (71.4%), with 5 (23.8%) showing partial and 10 (47.6%) showing complete responses. Breaking down responders by seizure subtype, 8 of 10 (80%) with FSE were responders, as were 4 of 8 (50%) with FRSE, 2 of 2 (100%) with GRSE and 1 of 1 (100%) with unknown SE. The authors hypothesized that the 80% response in FSE versus 50% response in FRSE might suggest a benefit from earlier intervention with rTMS [11]. Given the low number of cases with GRSE, the review could not comment on the efficacy of rTMS in GRSE [11]. The conclusion of this systematic review was that there is an Oxford level 4 (case series and poor cohort studies) [15], GRADE D level of evidence (very low quality evidence based on either expert opinion or few studies with severe limitations) [16], suggesting a potential benefit of rTMS for FSE and FRSE. The authors acknowledged that publication bias likely exists within this literature [11]. Therefore, further prospective study is clearly needed. While the authors could not recommend routine use of rTMS for SE, the results pointed to potential for efficacy, especially in FSE.

Safety and Side Effects

The literature to date suggests that the use of LF-rTMS in individuals with epilepsy appears to be well tolerated with minimal risk. According to a 2007 review and analysis of the rTMS epilepsy literature [17], side effects attributed to rTMS were reported in 17% of 280 epilepsy patients. Side effects were mild, with headache being the most common, occurring in 9.6%. Dizziness and non-specific discomfort were other common side effects.

Perhaps the biggest concern when stimulating the brain of individuals with epilepsy is the risk of inducing a seizure. In the above-referenced 2007 review [17], seizures occurred in 4 of 280 epilepsy patients (1.4%), 2 during rTMS and 2 after a rTMS session. All subjects in whom seizures occurred had medically refractory seizures and were on seizure medication during rTMS. Three of the four patients had their typical seizure with regard to semiology and duration. One subject experienced an atypical seizure that arose from the region of stimulation during HF-rTMS, a type of TMS known to increase cortical excitability and induce seizures. The two patients who experienced seizures after LF-rTMS had frequent seizures at baseline (more than seven per week), and thus a causal relationship between the LF-rTMS session and their seizures was unclear. Since this 2007 review, a report of five patients who experienced in-session seizures provided additional insights into the risk [18]. All five patients experienced frequent seizures at baseline, ranging from 8 per week to 30 per day. All seizures were the same semiology as the baseline seizures and were of the same duration or shorter. Seizure risk did not increase with increasing TMS pulse accumulation, since the timing of seizures during the 30-minute session was evenly distributed across the session, ranging from 6–29 minutes into the session. Similarly, during their 10- to 15-day blocks of daily TMS sessions, seizures did not tend to cluster near the end of the block. Seizure frequency did not worsen after the in-session seizure, with no change in two patients and seizure reduction in three. In contrast to HF-rTMS that can provoke atypical seizures, the literature to date suggest that seizures that occur in epilepsy patients during LF-rTMS consist of the patients' typical baseline semiology, are of similar or shorter duration compared to baseline, tend to occur in patients with high baseline seizure frequency and result in no detriment to the patient.

Conclusion

Through a recent meta-analysis [3] and recent systematic reviews [1,10,11] of existing literature, evidence is mounting that LF-rTMS holds promise as a therapy for focal epilepsy and for focal status epilepticus, especially in individuals with a superficial epileptic focus and when LF-rTMS is administered with the coil positioned directly over the epileptic focus. While future research is needed to have higher level of evidence for efficacy, there is now direction for future research with regard to the type of patients that will most likely benefit from LF-rTMS and with regard to the likely benefit of more targeted LF-rTMS therapy. Importantly, evidence to date suggests LF-rTMS is safe and well-tolerated [17,18].

Key Points

- Due to heterogeneity and limitations of existing studies, recommendations for the use of LF-rTMS in epilepsy do not exceed Level C recommendations (possible efficacy) for 'focal LF-RMTS of the epileptic focus.' [1]
- Optimal candidates for LF-rTMS have an epileptic focus near the cerebral convexity, where it is more accessible to TMS delivered across the scalp and skull [10].
- The level of evidence of rTMS for focal status epilepticus or refractory focal status epilepticus is Oxford level 4 (case series and poor cohort studies) [15] and Grade D (very low quality evidence based on either expert opinion or few studies with severe limitations) [16], which allows for the suggestion of potential benefit [11].
- Evidence to date suggests the use of LF-rTMS in individuals with epilepsy is safe and well-tolerated [17,18].

References

1. Lefaucheur JP, André-Obadia N, Antal A, et al. Evidence-based guidelines on the therapeutic use of repetitive transcranial magnetic stimulation (rTMS). *Clin Neurophys* 2014;125:2150–206.

2. Tergau F, Naumann U, Paulus W, Steinhoff BJ. Low-frequency repetitive transcranial magnetic stimulation improves intractable epilepsy. *Lancet* 1999;353:2209.

3. Hsu WY, Cheng CH, Lin MW, et al. Antiepileptic effects of low frequency repetitive transcranial magnetic stimulation: a meta-analysis. *Epilepsy Res* 2011;96:231–40.

4. Theodore WH, Hunter K, Chen R, et al. Transcranial magnetic stimulation for the treatment of seizures: a controlled study. *Neurology* 2002;59:560–2.

5. Cantello R, Rossi S, Varrasi C, et al. Slow repetitive TMS for drug-resistant epilepsy: clinical and EEG findings of a placebo-controlled trial. *Epilepsia* 2007;48:366–74.

6. Fregni F, Otachi PT, Do Valle A, et al. A randomized clinical trial of repetitive transcranial magnetic stimulation in patients with refractory epilepsy. *Ann Neurol* 2006;60:447–55.

7. Sun W, Mao W, Meng X, et al. Low-frequency repetitive transcranial magnetic stimulation for the treatment of refractory partial epilepsy: a controlled clinical study. *Epilepsia* 2012;53:1782–9.

8. Tergau F, Neumann D, Rosenow F, et al. Can epilepsies be improved by repetitive transcranial magnetic sitmulation?–interim analysis of a controlled study. *Suppl Clin Neurophysiol* 2003;56:400–5.

9. Joo EY, Han SJ, Chung SH, et al. Antiepileptic effects of low-frequency repetitive transcranial magnetic stimulation by different stimulation durations and locations. *Clin Neurophysiol* 2007;118:702–8.

10. Bae EH, Theodore WH, Fregni F, et al. An estimate of placebo effect of repetitive transcranial magnetic stimulation in epilepsy. *Epilepsy Beh* 2011;20:355–9.

11. Zeiler FA, Matuszczak M, Teitelbaum J, Gillman LM, Kazina CJ. Transcranial magnetic stimulation for status epilepticus. *Epilepsy Res Treat* 2015;2015:678074:1–10.

12. Graff-Guerrero A, Gonzáles-Olvera J, Ruiz-García M, et al. rTMS reduces focal brain hyperperfusion in two patients with EPC. *Acta Neurol Scand* 2004;190:290–6.

13. Rotenberg A, Bae EH, Takeoka M, et al. Repetitive transcranial magnetic stimulation in the treatment of epilepsia partialis continua. *Epilepsy Behav* 2009;14:253–7.

14. Morales OG, Henry ME, Nobler MS, Wassermann EM, Lisanby SH. Electroconvulsive therapy and repetitive transcranial magnetic stimulation in children and adolescents: a review and report of two cases of epilepsia partialis continua. *Child Adolesc Psychiatr Clin N Am* 2005;14:193–210.

15. Phillips B, Ball C, Sackett D et al. Oxford Center for Evidence-Based Medicine Levels of Evidence. Version 2009. 2015;http://www.cebm.net/?o=1025.

16. Jaeschke R, Guyatt GH, Dellinger P, et al. Use of GRADE grid tor each decisions on clinical practice guidelines when consensus is elusive. *BMJ* 2008;337: a744.

17. Bae EH, Schrader LM, Machii K, et al. Safety and tolerability of repetitive transcranial magnetic stimulation in patients with epilepsy: a review of the literature. *Epilepsy Behav* 2007;10:521–8.

18. Rotenberg A, Bae EH, Muller PA, et al. In-session seizures during low-frequency repetitive transcranial magnetic stimulation in patients with epilepsy. *Epilepsy Behav* 2009;16:353–5.

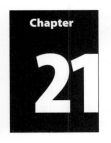

Diet Therapy for Medication-Resistant Epilepsy

Eric H. Kossoff and Daniel B. Lowenstein

Introduction

Although pharmacologic therapy remains the mainstay of treatment for most types of epilepsy, today the use of dietary therapy, most notably the ketogenic diet (KD), has become increasingly recognized as helpful, especially in those patients whose seizures are resistant to traditional anti-seizure medications. The history of using dietary manipulation for seizures dates back to the time of The Bible [1]. There are descriptions of Jesus curing 'possessed' patients with prayer and fasting [2,3].

The first modern use of fasting (a water diet) was by Marie and Guelpa, in 1911 [4], who reported improvement of seizures in 20 French children and adults. In the early part of the twentieth century, diet therapy was first introduced to the United States of America by Dr Hugh Conklin, an osteopathic physician [5]. In 1921, Dr Geyelin, an endocrinologist from New York City reported his research on fasting treatments at the convention of the American Medical Association [6]. His research was based on the previous work of Dr Conklin as well as Bernarr Macfadden, a physical fitness guru using a 'water diet' to help cure a 10-year-old boy with epilepsy.

During the 1920s, several other physicians began to first investigate the use of diets designed to mimic fasting, but for prolonged periods of time. Most notably, Dr Russell Wilder at the Mayo Clinic proposed using a high fat diet for an extended period of time as a treatment for seizures. The diet utilized fat for 90% of the caloric needs. Similar to today's use of the KD, a ratio of fats to carbohydrates plus protein of 3:1 to 4:1 was used to achieve ketosis. However, in the original version of the diet, calories and fluids were more restricted than in the more modern version.

Over the course of the twentieth century fasting diets went in and out of favour as new pharmacologic treatments were discovered. However, in 1993, at Johns Hopkins Hospital, the dramatic benefits seen using the ketogenic diet in the treatment of a two-year-old boy with intractable epilepsy named Charlie brought the KD back into the spotlight. Charlie had previously been treated with multiple anti-seizure medications. In addition, he had had a corpus callosotomy. Within weeks of starting the ketogenic diet his seizures had significantly improved. This triggered the creation of the Charlie Foundation, a great resource for families interested in the ketogenic diet [7].

The goal of this chapter is to provide information to epileptologists, neurologists and other healthcare providers who manage children and adults with epilepsy on the efficacy of the ketogenic diet, how to maintain the ketogenic diet, how the diet works, the side effects of the diet and diet alternatives, as well as specific indications for the diet.

Mechanisms of Action

Even though the ketogenic diet was first introduced into the modern era over a century ago we still only have a partial understanding of the exact mechanisms of action. It was initially thought that it was a combination of acidosis, hyperlipidaemia and dehydration that resulted in seizure reduction. However, this theory was replaced by the view that ketosis was the source of benefit [8]. There are three major types of ketone bodies, including acetoacetate, acetone and beta-hydroxybutyrate (BHB). Multiple animal studies have revealed that acetoacetate and acetone have anticonvulsant properties.

It is currently thought that there are multiple reasons for the diet's benefits [9]. Fasting in and of itself appears to have a benefit in seizure control. As previously mentioned, the ketones may have some benefit. However, it is not clear if is the ketones themselves are beneficial or if the ketones are simply a marker that the body has made the shift to using fat as its fuel source. Additionally, other mechanisms, including elevated plasma-free fatty acids, reduced glycolysis resulting in activation of ATP-sensitive potassium channels, elevated adenosine levels, caloric restriction and elevated amino acids may be beneficial in seizure control [10].

Diet Efficacy

Most people with epilepsy will respond to pharmacologic treatment. One study evaluated the natural history of childhood-onset epilepsy and followed 144 patients for an average of 37 years. They found that about 19% of patients had medication-resistant epilepsy [11]. For those individuals the ketogenic diet may be appropriate. It can be used in a large range of ages from infancy through to adulthood. A study in 2001 by Nordli proved that the ketogenic diet can be used in infants; 32 patients were enrolled and seizure freedom was achieved in 19.4% of patients, with an additional 35.5% who had greater than 50% reduction in seizure frequency [12].

Additionally, there was a more recent study in 2015 investigating the efficacy and safety of the KD in infants. In that study they compared 58 infants less than 1.5 years old (group A) to 57 infants greater than 1.5 years old (group B). There was no significant difference in responder rates between the two groups. They did find that more of the children in group A were seizure-free (34.5% vs. 19% at three months; 32.7% vs. 17.5% at 6 and 12 months, respectively). There were no significant differences between the two groups with regard to safety [13].

Typically, the ketogenic diet has been reserved as a treatment if medical intractability has been established. Medication-resistant epilepsy is traditionally defined as a failure of at least two adequately dosed anti-seizure medications. Two studies, published in 1998, supported the ketogenic diet as a helpful option for medication-resistant epilepsy in children [14,15]. The first was a multi-centre trial involving seven sites in the United States and enrolled 51 children. Of those who entered the study the frequency of seizures was reduced by greater than 50% in 54% at three months, 55% at six months and 40% at one year. Five patients (10%) were seizure-free at one year.

The second study, also completed in 1998, evaluated the efficacy of the KD in 150 children with medication-resistant epilepsy at Johns Hopkins Hospital. In this study, at three months after diet initiation, 34% had a >90% decrease in seizures. At six months, 32% had a >90% decrease in seizures. At one year, 27% had a >90% decrease in seizure frequency. By one year 45% of the children had discontinued the diet for various reasons. The most common reasons for discontinuing the diet were it being it being ineffective or too restrictive [15].

A meta-analysis was completed in 2006 by Henderson et al. at the University of Utah School of Medicine. They evaluated 19 studies, with a total sample size of 1084 patients. They found that the odds ratio of treatment success (>50% seizure reduction) among patients staying on the diet relative to those discontinuing the diet was 2.25. The reasons for diet discontinuation included <50% seizure reduction (47.0%), diet restrictiveness (16.4%) and intercurrent illness or diet side effects (13.2%)[16].

After the meta-analysis, other studies went on to confirm the efficacy of the ketogenic diet. The highest level of evidence came in the form of a randomized controlled trial at the Great Ormond Street Children's Hospital in London [17]

In 2008 a study examined when improvement typically occurs in those children who respond to the KD [18]. Of the 118 children started on the KD, 84% had documented seizure reduction. At three months on the diet 75% of children had a >50% seizure reduction and 48% had a >90% seizure reduction. At six months 71% had a >50% seizure reduction and 43% had a >90% seizure reduction.

In 2012 a Cochrane review was published, which included four new randomized studies. They were not able to perform a meta-analysis with their data due to the heterogeneity of the trials. However, they did find that at least 38% of the patients had a 50% reduction in their seizures compared to their comparative controls at three months and their response was maintained for up to a year [19].

It is important to note that they cited a study from 2001, which found that at three to six-year follow-up only 10% of patients remained on the KD. The reasons for discontinuation of the diet were mainly due to ineffectiveness or the restrictive nature of the diet [20].

Specific Indications and Contraindications for Diet Therapy

There are several epilepsy syndromes in which the use of dietary therapy has been well established, as well as several diseases in which the KD is contraindicated (Table 21.1)[1]. The most well-known indication for the ketogenic diet is GLUT-1 (glucose transporter-1) deficiency syndrome. This disease results from

Table 21.1 Indications and contraindications of the ketogenic diet

Indications
- Children with intractable epilepsy
- Epilepsy with intolerable anticonvulsant side effects
- Glucose transporter protein deficiency (GLUTI)
- Pyruvate decarboxylase deficiency

Suggested indications
- Infantile spams
- Myoclonic-astatic epilepsy (Doose syndrome)
- Tuberous sclerosis complex
- Rett syndrome
- Dravet syndrome
- Lennox–Gastaut syndrome
- Certain mitochondrial disorders

Contraindications
- Pyruvate carboxylase deficiency
- Porphyria
- Primary carnitine deficiency
- Fatty acid oxidation defects

mutation of the SLC2A1 gene, which encodes for the GLUT-1 receptor protein. The disease is characterized by a low glucose level in the CSF, thus leading to intractable epilepsy presenting in infancy. In addition, children with GLUT-1 deficiency classically have mild to severe developmental delay, acquired microcephaly, hypotonia, spasticity, ataxia and dystonia [21]. In 2010, one study looked at the efficacy of the KD in GLUT-1 deficiency. They found that of the 37 patients placed on the diet, 62% had complete seizure freedom, with an additional 24% with some seizure reduction [22].

The second major indication for the KD is pyruvate dehydrogenase (E_1) deficiency, in which the KD is first-line therapy. E_1 deficiency is an X-linked disorder with clinical heterogeneity among individuals even with the same mutation [22]. In these disorders there is impairment of conversion of pyruvate to acetate, leading to accumulation of pyruvate and lactate (lactic acidosis). Fatty acid oxidation furnishes acetate moieties for the Krebs cycle without resulting in pyruvate/lactate accumulation. In a study published in 1997, seven children with E_1 deficiency were enrolled and all received the ketogenic diet. They found that those who either had the diet initiated earlier in life or who were placed on greater carbohydrate restriction had increased longevity and improved development [23]. A recent report from Sweden that includes long-term follow-up of patients with this disorder confirms these findings [24].

Although not often used as a first-line therapy, the KD is often used today for refractory infantile spasms. In one study in 2002, a total of 23 children with difficult to treat infantile spasms were enrolled to investigate the efficacy of the ketogenic diet. Of all the children on the diet at 3, 6, 9 and 12 months, 38%, 39%, 53% and 46%, respectively, saw greater than 90% improvement in their seizure frequency (three were seizure-free at 12 months). In addition, 67%, 72%, 93% and 100% were >50% improved at 3, 6, 9 and 12 months, respectively [23]. However, evaluations did not involve the gold standard of video-EEGs consistently, and parental reports were used as a substitute.

In a separate study in 2008, the investigators examined the efficacy of the KD as first-line therapy for infantile spasms. This was a retrospective chart review comparing 13 children who were started on the KD as first-line therapy to 20 children who were started on ACTH. They found that 62% of the infants on the KD were spasm-free within one month of starting the diet as compared to 90% of those treated with ACTH. In the five children in whom the KD was unsuccessful, four became spasm-free subsequently with ACTH or topiramate. However, side effects were lower in the KD group, 31% as compared to 80% in the ACTH group (p = 0.006) [25]. Disappointingly, resolution of hypsarrhythmia and overall improvement in EEG was inconsistent in the group treated with the KD.

In another study, a total of 104 infants were enrolled. This is the largest study to date to investigate the efficacy of the KD in infantile spasms. There was a greater than 50% improvement in spasms in 64% of the patients at six months and 77% after one to two years. A total of 37% became spasm-free for at least a six-month period after starting the diet. Additionally, 62% reported improvement in development, 35% had EEG improvement and 29% were able to reduce concurrent anti-convulsants. Adverse effects were noted in 33% of the infants. Positive predictors for success of the KD included older age of onset of infantile spasms and fewer prior anticonvulsants [26].

Other suggested indications for the ketogenic diet include tuberous sclerosis complex, Lennox–Gastaut syndrome, Dravet's syndrome, mitochondrial disorders and myoclonic-astatic epilepsy (Doose syndrome) (listed in Table 21.1) [1]. There are also several diseases in which the KD is contraindicated, including pyruvate carboxylase deficiency, porphyria and primary carnitine deficiency as well as in fatty acid oxidation defects.

Implementation of the Classic Ketogenic Diet

The traditional ketogenic diet can be difficult to maintain at times. It requires a team approach, including the epileptologist, a trained dietician who is knowledgeable about the diet and the commitment of the patient and his/her family. In 2009, an international multi-centre consensus statement was published in the journal *Epilepsia*, which proposed guidelines for the use of the ketogenic diet [27].

The diet regimen has not changed much since its inception over 100 years ago. The regimen includes a ratio of grams of fat to carbohydrate of 4:1 as the most common starting ratio. However, starting ratios of 2:1 to 3:1 have been used. Calories and fluid amounts are typically not restricted any longer, but are still carefully measured and calculated using computer programs. The ketogenic diet protocol used at Johns Hopkins Hospital is outlined in Table 21.2 [1,10]. The KD is typically started in the inpatient hospital setting, but in select situations has been reported as feasible using an outpatient approach. Prior to the initiation of the diet, an extensive workup is recommended, as outlined in the 2009 consensus statement.

Often individuals will fast for 24 hours leading up to the hospital admission. However, many centres do not do this. While the patient remains in the hospital, he/she is monitored for vomiting, hypoglycemia and acidosis. Anti-convulsants are left unchanged during the admission. However, it is important to switch all medications to tablet form to minimize carbohydrates in the medication formulation.

A study done in 2005 compared the efficacy of rapid initiation of the diet vs. a gradual initiation [28]. A total of 48 children were enrolled in the study and were randomized into the two arms: FAST-KD and GRAD-KD. They found that there was no statistically significant difference in the efficacy of the two groups. However, they did find that those in the GRAD-KD group had fewer adverse events and better tolerance than those in the FAST-KD group.

Once the patient is discharged from the hospital they are closely monitored by the multi-disciplinary team every one to three months. Adjustment of the diet ratio may take place, depending on tolerability, side effects and seizure control.

Table 21.2 The ketogenic diet protocol at Johns Hopkins Hospital

Day 1 (Monday)
- Admitted to the hospital
- Blood glucose monitoring every six hours
- Use carbohydrate-free medications when possible
- Dinner given as one-half of calculated calories as eggnog or ketogenic formula
- Parents begin education programme

Day 2 (Tuesday)
- Breakfast and lunch given with one-half of calculated calories as eggnog or ketogenic formula
- Blood glucose checks discontinued after lunch, if lunch is tolerated
- Dinner given as full ketogenic diet
- Education continues

Day 3 (Wednesday)
- Full ketogenic diet breakfast and lunch given
- Education completed
- Prescriptions provided for carbohydrate-free anti-convulsants and supplements
- Child discharged to home

Three Variations on the Diet

In addition to the classic ketogenic diet there are three 'alternative' dietary therapies that have been developed. The Modified Atkins Diet (MAD) is one of these. It was developed at Johns Hopkins Hospital in 2003 as a less restrictive form of the ketogenic diet for use as treatment for epilepsy. It restricts adults and adolescent patients to 20 grams of carbohydrates per day and children to 10–15 grams per day [7]. This diet is somewhat easier to tolerate, especially in older children and adults who typically eat a normal diet. In the MAD there are no restrictions on protein and calories. Increased fat intake is encouraged to increase ketosis. See Table 21.3 for the MAD protocol currently used at Johns Hopkins Hospital.

In a recent review of studies of the MAD, there were 31 studies completed from multiple centres with a total of 423 children and adults enrolled across those studies. All together, 47% of patients had a >50% reduction in their seizures, which is comparable to the results found for the ketogenic diet. They noted that for children under the age of two years and those who receive formula-only nutrition the diet is preferable. For older adolescents and adults, the MAD is probably a better option due to increased tolerability [29].

Table 21.3 Modified Atkins Diet protocol

- Copy of a carbohydrate counting guide, recipes and web sites provided
- Complete blood count, liver and kidney functions, anti-convulsant levels and fasting lipid profile at baseline, three and six months
- Carbohydrates restricted to 10 g/day for the first month for children, 15 g/day for adolescents, 20 g/day for adults. Carbohydrates can be increased after two months in many patients
- Foods high in fat (e.g. oils, butter and mayonnaise) are strongly encouraged. KetoCal shake daily during the first month is advised
- Clear, carbohydrate-free fluids ad lib
- Daily low-carbohydrate multi-vitamin and calcium supplementation
- Urine ketones checked weekly for the first two months and weight checked weekly throughout dietary therapy
- Medications left unchanged for at least the initial month, but reformulated if necessary to tablet or sprinkle preparation
- Discontinue the diet if ineffective after two months

In the MCT diet, medium-chain triglycerides (MCT) oil is used to replace the long-chain fatty acids of the traditional ketogenic diet. As MCT oil is highly ketogenic, this allows for more carbohydrates. The MCT diet has been used since the 1970s. A randomized controlled prospective study from London in 2008 compared the MCT diet to the traditional KD. It found that although the traditional KD led to higher serum ketone levels, fatigue and mineral deficiencies, there was no difference in growth, efficacy and overall tolerability [10,30].

The third alternative version of ketogenic diet is the low glycaemic index treatment (LGIT), which was first studied for epilepsy at the Massachusetts General Hospital in 2005 by Thiele and colleagues. The LGIT uses a liberalized but still low carbohydrate intake, with carbohydrates supplied only in the form of low-glycaemic index foods (glycemic index of less than 50 relative to glucose) [31]. Of the 20 patients studied, 10 experienced a greater than 90% reduction in seizure frequency. The LGIT can be started as an outpatient without a fasting period. An updated study in 2009 also from the same group in Boston included 76 children, of which 50% of those remaining on the diet at three months had a >50% seizure reduction [10,32].

Side Effects of the Diet

Like the pharmacologic treatments for epilepsy, the ketogenic diet has side effects. Particularly during the initiation of the ketogenic diet, it is important to monitor for side effects closely. It is important to be mindful of the patient's underlying medical history, as children and adults with certain metabolic disorders can deteriorate quickly on the diet. The most common side effects include constipation, difficulty gaining weight and hypo-glycaemia. Other rarer side effects include pancreatitis, cardiomyopathy and prolonged QT syndrome, as well as vitamin or mineral deficiencies, most notably selenium and zinc. For this reason, it is important to supplement individuals on the ketogenic diet with a multi-vitamin.

Renal calculi have been reported to occur in 3–7% of children on the KD. Stone composition includes uric acid (50% of the stones), calcium oxalate, calcium phosphate and mixed calcium/uric acid stones. In general, they do not require diet discontinuation. Polycitra K appears to help prevent renal calculi from forming and has dropped the risk to <1% [28].

There has long been concern about the effects of the KD on linear growth of children. In a study by Vining in 2002 they enrolled 237 children who were all placed on the KD. There were 133 children who remained on it at one year and 76 at two years. Growth parameters were closely monitored. They found that the older children tended to have near normal growth, while the younger children had poor growth. However, they concluded that overall the KD does provide sufficient nutrition to allow for some growth [33].

The effects of the KD on vascular function was recently studied in an article published in 2014. In this study they enrolled 26 children who were followed for one year, 13 of which were followed for two years. They used high-resolution ultrasound-based assessment in order to evaluate carotid artery intima-media thickness (cIMT), carotid artery distensibility and carotid artery compliance. They also evaluated blood lipid, including high-density lipoprotein (HDL), low-density lipoprotein (LDL), total cholesterol (TC), apolipoprotein A (apoA), apolipoprotein B (apoB) and high-sensitivity C-reactive protein (hsCRP). They found a gradual decrease in carotid distensibility, as well as an increase in LDL, apoB, the ratios of TC to LDL and LDL to HDL at both three- and twelve-month evaluations. There were no statistical changes at the two-year follow-up [34]. See Table 21.4 for a more complete list of side effects [10].

Conclusion

Although we have made great advances in the pharmacologic and surgical management of epilepsy, the ketogenic diet represents a very helpful non-

Table 21.4 Side effects of the ketogenic diet

Common
- Lack of significant weight gain
- Constipation
- Hypoglycemia (typically with fasting)

Occasional
- Gastrointestinal upset or gastroesophageal reflux
- Dehydration or acidosis (more frequent with illness)
- Dyslipidemia
- Growth slowing (especially in younger children)
- Skeletal fractures (more common with long-term use)

Rare
- Renal calculi
- Pancreatitis
- Cardiomyopathy
- Bruising
- Prolonged QT syndrome
- Basal ganglia changes
- Selenium and zinc deficiencies (if not supplemented)
- Carnitine deficiency (symptomatic)

pharmacologic approach. It is particularly helpful for medication-resistant epilepsy due to GLUT1 deficiency, PDH deficiency, infantile spasms, Doose syndrome and Dravet syndrome. Many epilepsy centres have established ketogenic diet clinics to provide patients with a multi-disciplinary setting in order to evaluate if the ketogenic diet is an appropriate option for the individual and his/her family. However, the ketogenic diet has some adverse effects and should only be started after a proper evaluation has been completed and with appropriate supervision from an experienced medical team.

Key Points

- The ketogenic diet is a non-pharmacologic treatment used for children and adults with drug-resistant epilepsy.
- Side effects are mostly gastrointestinal and often preventable.
- It is helpful for all kinds of epilepsy, but the treatment of choice for GLUT1 deficiency disorder and pyruvate dehydrogenase deficiency.

References

1. Kossoff E, Haney C. Ketogenic diets. In: Shorvon S, Perucca E, Engel J Jr (eds.), The Treatment of Epilepsy, 4th ed. Oxford: Wiley 2016:288–297.
2. Wheless J. History of the ketogenic diet. *Epilepsia* 2008;**49**(Suppl 8):3–5
3. Huisjen D. Mark 9:14–29. *Today's Parallel Bible*. Grand Rapids, MI: Zondervan Corporation. 2000:2306–2308
4. Guelpa G, Marie A. La lutte contre l'e'pilepsie par la de' sintoxication et par la re'e'ducation alimentaire. *Rev Ther Medico-Chirurgicale* 1911;**78**:8–13
5. Conklin HW. Cause and treatment of epilepsy. *J Am Osteopathic Assoc* 1922;**26**:11–14
6. Geyelin HR. Fasting as a method for treating epilepsy. *Med Record* 1921;**99**:1037–1039
7. Abrahams J. *An Introduction to the Ketogenic Diet: A Treatment for Pediatric Epilepsy* (videotape). Santa Monica, CA: The Charlie Foundation, 1994.
8. Swink TD, Vining EPG, Freeman JM. The ketogenic diet: 1997 *Adv Pediatr* 1997;**44**:297–329
9. Rogawski MA, Löscher W, Rho JM. Mechanisms of action of antiseizure drugs and the ketogenic diet. *Cold Spring Harb Perspect Med* 2016;**6**(5):a022780
10. Hartman AL, Stafstrom CE. Harnessing the power of metabolism for seizure prevention: focus on dietary treatments. *Epilepsy Behav* 2013;**26**(3):173–178
11. Sillanpää M, Schmidt D. Natural history of treated childhood-onset epilepsy: prospective, long-term population-based study. *Brain* 2006;**129**:617–624
12. Nordli DR Jr, Kuroda MM, Carroll J, et al. Experience with the ketogenic diet in infants. *Pediatrics* 2001;**108**:129–133
13. Dressler A, Trimmel-Schwahofer P, Reithofer E, et al. The ketogenic diet in infants – Advantages in early use. *Epilepsy Res* 2015;**116**:53–58
14. Vining EPG, Freeman JM, Ballaban-Gil K, et al. A multicenter study of the efficacy of the ketogenic diet. *Arch Neurol* 1998;**55**:1433–1437
15. Freeman JM, Vining EPG, Pillas DJ, et al. The efficacy of the ketogenic diet – 1998: a prospective evaluation of intervention in 150 children. *Pediatrics* 1998;**102**:1358–1363
16. Henderson CB, Filloux FM, Alder SC, et al. Efficacy of the ketogenic diet as a treatment option for epilepsy: meta-analysis. *J Child Neurol* 2006;**21**:193–198
17. Neal EG, Chaffe H, Schwartz RH, et al. The ketogenic diet for the treatment of childhood epilepsy: a randomised controlled trial. *Lancet Neurol* 2008;**7**:500–506
18. Kossoff EH, Laux LC, Blackford R, et al. When do seizures improve with the ketogenic diet? *Epilepsia* 2008;**49**:329–333
19. Levy RG, Cooper PN, Giri P. Ketogenic diet and other dietary treatments for epilepsy. *Cochrane Database Syst Rev.* 2012;(3):CD001903

20. Hemingway C, Freeman JM, Pillas DJ, Pyzik PL. The ketogenic diet: a 3- to 6-year follow-up of 150 children enrolled prospectively. *Pediatrics* 2001;**108**:898–905

21. Leen WG, Klepper J, Verbeek MM, et al. Glucose transporter-1 deficiency syndrome: the expanding clinical and genetic spectrum of a treatable disorder. *Brain* 2010;**133**:655–670

22. Wexler ID, Hemalatha SG, McConnell J, et al. Outcome of pyruvate dehydrogenase deficiency treated with ketogenic diets: studies in patients with identical mutations. *Neurology* 1997;**49**:1655–1661

23. Kossoff EH, Pyzik PL, McGrogan JR, et al. Efficacy of the ketogenic diet for infantile spasms. *Pediatrics* 2002;**109**:780–783

24. Sofou K, Dahlin M, Hallböök T, et al. Ketogenic diet in pyruvate dehydrogenase complex deficiency: short- and long-term outcomes. *J Inherit Metab Dis* 2017;**40**:237–245

25. Kossoff EH, Hedderick EF, Turner Z, et al. A case–control evaluation of the ketogenic diet versus ACTH for new-onset infantile spasms. *Epilepsia* 2008;**49**:1504–1509

26. Hong AM, Turner Z, Hamdy RF, Kossoff EH. Infantile spasms treated with the ketogenic diet: Prospective single-center experience in 104 consecutive infants. *Epilepsia* 2010;**51**(8):1403–1407

27. Kossoff EH, Zupec-Kania BA, Amark PE, et al. Optimal clinical management of children receiving the ketogenic diet: recommendations of the international ketogenic diet study group. *Epilepsia* 2009;**50**:304–317

28. Bergqvist AGC, Schall JI, Gallagher PR, et al. Fasting versus gradual initiation of the ketogenic diet: a prospective, randomized clinical trial of efficacy. *Epilepsia* 2005;**46**(11):1810–1819

29. Kossoff EH, Cervenka MC, Henry BJ, Turner Z. A decade of the modified Atkins diet (2003–2013): results, insights, and future direction. *Epilepsy Behav* 2013;**29**(3):437–442

30. Neal EG, Chaffe H, Schwartz RH. A randomized trial of classical and medium-chain triglyceride ketogenic diets in the treatment of childhood epilepsy. *Epilepsia* 2009;**50**(5):1109–1117

31. Pfeifer HH, Thiele EA. Low-glycemic index treatment: a liberalized ketogenic diet for treatment of intractable epilepsy. *Neurology* 2005;**65**(11):1810–1812

32. Muzykewicz DA, Lyczkowski DA, Memon N, et al. Efficacy, safety, and tolerability of the low glycemic index treatment in pediatric epilepsy. *Epilepsia* 2009;**50**(5):1118–1126

33. Vining EPG, Pyzik P, McGrogan J, et al. Growth of children on the ketogenic diet. *Dev Med Child Neurol* 2002;**44**:796–802

34. Kapetanakis M, Liuba P, Odermarsky M, et al. Effects of ketogenic diet on vascular function. *Eur J Paediatr Neurol* 2014;**18**:489–494

Chapter 22

Botanical Treatments for Medication-Resistant Epilepsy

Steven C. Schachter

Introduction

Botanical treatments have been used by persons with epilepsy, especially for convulsive seizures, dating from 6000 BC in India [1], from 3000 BC in China and in Peru, and for centuries in Africa and South America. In traditional Western medicine, botanical treatments were widely used to treat seizures before the advent of compounds such as bromide and phenobarbital. For instance, Gowers documented his use of *Cannabis indica* (see also section on Cannabis and its Derivatives) and digitalis, the latter derived from the Foxglove plant (*Digitalis purpurea*) [2].

Currently, botanical treatments are widely used in regions where herbal medicines are an accepted part of the healthcare system (for example, Traditional Chinese Medicine (TCM) and Ayurveda). In general, these products are derived from plants, and in particular herbs and herbal materials, such as the roots, stems or leaves, and then extracted and taken in numerous formulations and routes of administration. Likewise, over-the-counter dietary supplements are often taken by patients in developed countries, usually without knowledge of their physicians, for control of seizures, to reduce side effects from anti-seizure medications (ASMs), for symptoms of one or more comorbidities of epilepsy, or for general health maintenance.

Published reports demonstrate that hundreds of plant-based products have anti-convulsant properties in animal models of epilepsy. For many of these, mechanisms of action have been identified related to actions of flavonoids, (furano) coumarins, phenylpropanoids and terpenoids on GABA receptors and voltage-gated ion channels [3]. Additionally, there is now evidence from randomized controlled trials of therapeutic benefit for the botanical treatment cannabidiol (CBD) for Dravet's syndrome and Lennox–Gastaut syndrome, as well as evidence suggesting the potential for some botanical products to worsen seizures or affect ASM metabolism [4].

Unfortunately, there are few published well-designed clinical trials of botanical treatments for medication-resistant epilepsy. Further, there is inadequate pre-clinical evaluation of most botanical treatments and their constituent compounds using validated scientific methods that would be needed to provide the scientific rationale to proceed to human studies.

This chapter reviews botanical therapies for the treatment of epilepsy, including medication-resistant seizures, provides an overview of historical use in TCM and Ayurveda, current use in developing and developed regions, regulatory aspects, safety issues and the example of cannabis, and concludes with an overview of an existing healthcare system that includes prescribing botanical treatments in a scientific medicine context.

Unmet Medical Need for Botanical Treatments

As documented throughout this book, a substantial proportion of patients with epilepsy who have access to and who adhere to ASMs continue to have seizures. Unfortunately, the extent of medication-resistant epilepsy has not substantially changed over time, in spite of the growing number of available approved ASMs. What is less often discussed but nonetheless critically important is that there are tens of millions of persons with epilepsy in the world, primarily in developing countries, who do not have access to, cannot pay for or do not take ASMs (comprising the global treatment gap), but for whom botanical treatments may be accessible, affordable and culturally acceptable [5,6].

Therefore, there is an opportunity to view botanical treatments as a potential source of new therapies for patients with medication-resistant seizures and, in addition, as a possible solution for bridging the global treatment gap. The basis for this statement derives from the centuries-old traditions of use for convulsions, contemporary anecdotal reports of efficacy and identification of relevant underlying mechanisms of action, all of which may be illustrated by the current interest in cannabis and its constituent compounds, including cannabidiol and other phytocannabinoids. As this chapter concludes, much more work is needed to advance botanical treatments to clinical use.

Extent and Pattern of Use of Botanical Treatments for Epilepsy

Historical Use in Traditional Chinese Medicine

The Chinese term for epilepsy, 'Dian Xian', suggests insanity and convulsion and reflects the traditional Chinese view of epilepsy as punishment from ghosts [7]. The use of botanical therapies in China dates back thousands of years. The Yellow Emperor's classic of internal medicine, *Huang Di Nei Ching*, written by a group of physicians between 770 and 221 BC, describes convulsive seizures [8]. Later publications expanded the description of epilepsy. For example, in 610 AD, Cao Yuan Fang noted five types of epilepsy: 'Yang Dian', 'Yin Dian', 'Feng (Wind) Dian', 'Shih (Wet) Dian', and 'Ma (Horse) Dian', though there is little correspondence of these categories to modern classifications of epilepsy. Conceptually, TCM attributes seizures to 'Liver Yang Rising', which generates Heat that disturbs the brain and Shen (Mind), producing Internal Wind (seizures) in any of five forms [8]. The causes of Liver Yang Rising in TCM, and therefore the targets of TCM therapies, include Liver Yin Deficiency, Liver Blood Deficiency, Phlegm, Blood Stagnation, Liver Fire and Liver Qi Stagnation.

Botanical therapies comprise an important component for TCM treatment, as based on the principles of 'Yin Yang Wu Xing', with other aspects including acupuncture, massage, food therapy and therapeutic exercise [7]. In TCM, multiple botanical therapies are typically selected for a particular patient for their purported synergistic actions against the presenting disease as well as their ability to counteract adverse effects of individual herbs and benefits for other constitutional symptoms that may be present; the combination is generally referred to as a formula.

Xiao et al. conducted extensive searches of Chinese online databases and PubMed and identified 23 botanical therapies that have been used in TCM to treat epilepsy for which potential mechanisms of action have been proposed, activity in animal models of epilepsy has been documented or results from clinical studies have been published [8].

Historical Use in Ayurveda

Ayurveda is both a functional science and system of medicine that emphasizes a holistic approach to the patient and that attributes bodily functions to three dynamic principles similar to humors (dosha) known as vata (responsible for movement), pitta (responsible for transformation) and kapha (responsible for anabolic activities) [9]. Disease states represent lack of harmony in bodily functions, as conceptualized by these principles, affecting the body's structural elements (dhatu) and the elimination of wastes (mala). Botanical therapies are the primary component of Ayurveda medicine.

A condition called Apasmara (apa, meaning negation or loss of; smara, meaning recollection or consciousness), similar to epilepsy, was described in Ayurveda literature including *Charaka Samhita*, *Sushruta Samhita* and *Ashtanga Hridaya* from approximately 800 BC–400 AD [9]. Apropos of current concepts of the psychiatric comorbidities of epilepsy, both physical and psychological manifestations were documented.

The selection of herbs for a patient with epilepsy in the Ayurveda system of medicine is based both on the manifestations of the disease and on host factors, resulting in herbal combinations or formulations administered in a variety of formulations, including freshly prepared juices of herbs (svarasa), pastes (kalka), lipid-based formulations (sneha – oil- or ghee-based preparations), decoctions (kashaya), powders (churna), fermented preparations (asava–arishta) and pills (vati) [9]. In addition to botanical therapies, other non-pharmacological treatments may be recommended such as oleation (snehana) and sudation (svedana), cleansing (shodhana), emesis (vamana) and purgation (virechana) [9].

Sriranjini et al. summarized the botanical formulations that have been widely prescribed for Apasmara, including Manasamitravatakam, Mritasanjeevani gutika, Apasmarahara rasa, Apasmarari rasayana, Bhootabhairava rasa, Smritisagara rasa, Chaturbhuja rasa, Chaturmukha rasa, Chintamani chaturmukha rasa, Tapyadi lauha, Vatakulantaka rasa and Yogendra rasa [9]. They further identified the specific herbs described in Ayurveda literature that have been individually tested for anti-convulsant activity.

Current Use in Developed Countries

The National Center for Complementary and Integrative Health (http://nccih.nih.gov) defines 'complementary health approaches' as 'practices and products that were developed outside of mainstream Western (conventional or scientific) medicine, and which include natural products, such as botanical therapies, that are widely available to consumers as dietary supplements, vitamins, minerals, and probiotics'.

In developed countries, botanical therapies are often used by the lay public for general health maintenance or for chronic conditions that respond poorly or incompletely to standard medical treatments [10]. Surveys in the United States or the United Kingdom suggest that up to one in three patients with epilepsy take botanical therapies and/or dietary supplements at some time, and that the majority do not inform their treating physicians [11]. One survey found that ginseng, St. John's wort, melatonin, gingko, garlic and black cohosh were most frequently used, while another study also identified soy and kava. People with epilepsy may take botanical therapies for ASM-related side effects or comorbid conditions, such as valerian for insomnia, St. John's wort for depression, or ginkgo for memory disturbance.

Current Use in Developing Countries

Botanical therapies for epilepsy in developing countries have evolved over time, often in conjunction with changing cultural beliefs, modifications in systems of healthcare and training of healthcare practitioners, and levels of public education [11]. A survey conducted in China in 1988 found that nearly 40% of people considered herbal medicine or acupuncture to be appropriate for treating epilepsy [12]. More recent studies found that less than 10% of patients with epilepsy in urban areas used TCM [13], while nearly one in four patients in rural west China took botanical therapies [14], generally because ASMs were unaffordable or for cultural reasons.

Botanical therapies in developing countries are generally available from traditional healers or practitioners, either instead of or in addition to medications prescribed by Western-trained physicians, and in some practice settings, healers and Western-style doctors work together in teams, so that botanical therapies may be taken together with ASMs [15].

Table 22.1 Dianxianning and Zhenxian pill TCM formulas for treatment of epilepsy

Name (Pinyin)	Generic name	Weight (g) for formula
Dianxianning		
Matixiang 马蹄香	Saruma henryi	5.0
Qianniuzi 牵牛子	Pharbitisnil choisy	2.0
Gouteng 钩藤	Uncaria rhynchophylla	2.0
Shichangpu	Acorus tatarinowii	5.0
Qianjinzi 千金子	Euphorbialathyris	1.5
Gansong 甘松	Nardostachys jatamansi	2.0
Bohe 薄荷	Mentha haplocalyx	0.3
Zhenxian pill		
Niuhuang 牛黄	Bos taurus domesticus	3.0
Guangyujin 广郁金	Curcuma longa	5.0
Tiannanxing 天南星	Arisaema erubescens	5.0
Fuling 茯苓	Poria cocos	7.0
Gancao 甘草	Glycyrrhiza uralensis	1.0
Shichangpu 石菖蒲	Acorus tatarinowii	5.0
Suanzaoren 酸枣仁	Ziziphus jujuba	10.0
Hongshen 红参	Radix ginseng rubra	5.0
Maidong 麦冬	Ophiopogon japonicus	7.0
Yuanzhi 远志	Polygala tenuifolia	5.0
Lianzixin 莲子心	Plumula nelambinis	5.0

Reprinted from [8] with permission.

In China, botanical therapies are covered under Chinese drug laws. *Monographs in the Pharmacopoeia of the People's Republic of China* (2010 edition) provides detailed information in the context of legally mandated standards [16]. As used in TCM, formulas of botanical therapies consist of fixed combinations of weighed herbs with no consideration of an individualized dose titration or dosing regimens [8]. The complexity of these formulas is exemplified by two of the most popular formulas (Dianxianning tablets and Zhenxian pills), as shown in Table 22.1.

Regulatory Aspects

Governmental regulations concerning the approval of botanical therapies for treatment of diseases vary around the world [16]. For example, in Germany, herbal medicinal products are integrated into primary healthcare, provided that they are produced according to good manufacturing practice (GMP) and that quality, safety and efficacy have been reviewed as part of a registration process and published in monographs [17,18]. Similarly, in Canada, a comprehensive draft guidance document, *Quality of Natural Health Products Guide*, specifies quality requirements for botanical therapies, including standards for characterization, identification and quantification [16].

In the USA, prescription drugs are regulated by the Federal Food, Drug and Cosmetic Act and available by prescription, whereas botanical therapies are regulated by the 1994 Dietary Supplement and Health Education Act (DSHEA) and available over-the-counter as dietary supplements, defined as products taken by mouth that contain dietary ingredients intended to supplement the diet, such as vitamins, minerals, herbs or other botanicals, amino acids, and substances such as enzymes, organ tissues, glandulars and metabolites (https://ods.od.nih.gov/About/dshea_wording.aspx). Under DSHEA, manufacturers of dietary supplements cannot claim effectiveness for a specific medical condition, such as epilepsy, but may claim an effect on a bodily part or function when accompanied by the sentences: 'This statement has not been evaluated by the FDA. This product is not intended to diagnose, treat, cure or prevent any disease'. Unlike for prescription drugs, no government agency was required by DSHEA to verify the labelling claims of dietary supplements or to independently assess their quality and safety. To address this problem, in June 2007, the FDA issued *Current Good Manufacturing Practice in Manufacturing, Packaging, Labeling or Holding Operations for Dietary Supplements* (www.fda.gov/regulatory-information/search-fda-guidance-documents/small-entity-compliance-guide-current-good-manufacturing-practice-manufacturing-packaging-labeling), which required new manufacturing standards for dietary supplements, though its impact on the quality of dietary supplements has not been systematically assessed in the literature.

Until relatively recently, botanical therapies in the USA were available only as dietary supplements and were marketed to consumers without the evidence base that physicians are accustomed to for prescription drugs. In 2004, the FDA issued a policy guidance for the evaluation of the safety and efficacy of botanical therapies (referred to as botanical drug products) in mitigating, treating, curing or diagnosing a disease, which provides the regulatory pathway for FDA approval of botanical therapies for specific medical indications, including, potentially, epilepsy. The guidance specifies rigorous requirements for pre-clinical studies, as well as for human safety and efficacy studies under an Investigational New Drug (IND) application. Botanical drug products were defined as products that contain ingredients of vegetable matter or its constituents as a finished product, including whole plants or plant parts, and also algae or macroscopic fungi and similar products, but not products of fermentation (yeast, bacteria), highly purified or chemically modified substances derived from botanical sources or homeopathic drugs [19]. Hoffman has reviewed the FDA regulations for botanical drug products in detail and highlighted features that differentiate botanical drug products from single compounds (Table 22.2) [19].

There are several unique challenges to conducting clinical trials of botanical drug products compared to trials of single active compounds or molecular entities. Published recommendations for conducting and reporting randomized clinical trials of botanical products emphasize the importance of completely describing the botanical product with regard to name, manufacturer, plant part used, type of preparation, source and authentication of the herbal material, pharmaceutical quality, dosage regimen and purity testing [20].

Safety Issues

While the public may generally regard over-the-counter botanical therapies as 'natural' and therefore safe, there is the potential nonetheless for serious or life-threatening side effects. Further, cannabidiol is the only botanical therapy widely taken by people with epilepsy that has been rigorously studied in this population for safety, the potential for interactions with ASMs or for worsening seizures [11].

Given the relatively lax manufacturing requirements for dietary supplements as compared to pharmaceuticals, dietary supplements could potentially be contaminated with, for example, microorganisms or pesticides, or admixed with potentially toxic levels of heavy metals, as has been documented for some Ayurveda products, or adulterated with other herbs or drugs [11].

Some botanical therapies have been anecdotally reported to cause seizures, including in patients with epilepsy, such as anisatin (a component of Japanese

Table 22.2 Characteristics of botanical and standard drugs

Characteristics	Botanical[a] drug	Standard[b] drug
Chemical composition	Complex heterogeneous polymolecular	'Simple' single molecule
Active(s)	Multiple active constituents; true active constituents may be unknown (entire drug substance is the 'active')	Single active ingredient
Characterization	High or low	High
Control	Process controlled	'Final vial' controlled
Source materials	'Dedicated' sourcing Good Agricultural and Cultivation Practices (GACPs) may apply	May or may not require dedicated sourcing
Dose/route/schedule	May already be known (prior human use)	Discovered through non-clinical and clinical testing
Predictors of efficacy	Clinical (prior human use)	Generally based on non-clinical testing
Mechanism of action known	Rarely	Often
Non-clinical toxicity testing	Scheduling may be negotiable (depends on prior human use)	Prior to starting clinical studies
Pharmacokinetics	Depends on product (may be infeasible)	Required
Clinical targets	Polymorphic	Single receptor
'Patent protected'	Sometimes, but not always	Generally
Expedited programmes apply	Yes	Yes
Generic equivalents	May be avoidable	Generally unavoidable

[a] Polymolecular drug substance, as defined by FDA Guidance for Industry on Botanical Drug Products
[b] Single molecular drug substance
Reprinted from [19] with permission.

star anise, which is used in Spain and other countries to treat infant colic), gingko nuts, essential oils, evening primrose, borage and ephedra (ma huang) [11,21].

The known interactions between botanical therapies and ASMs suggest that St. John's wort, garlic, echinacea, pine bark extract (also known as pycnogel, Pygenol, or Pychnogenol), milk thistle, American hellebore, ginkgo, mugwort and pipissewa have effects on cytochrome p450 and could therefore potentially alter serum concentrations of hepatically metabolized ASMs [11,22].

Status of Clinical Use of Botanical Therapies for Epilepsy

There is a surprising dearth of well-designed clinical trials to support the use of botanical therapies in patients, and specifically, there are no English-language full-length publications of randomized clinical trials of botanical therapies for the treatment of epilepsy other than cannabidiol [20]. A Cochrane review of TCM for epilepsy, published in 2009, reviewed seven Chinese clinical trials of herbal products given as monotherapy and compared with ASMs [23]. While epilepsy was diagnosed according to the International League Against Epilepsy (ILAE) classification, the review found substantial methodological problems, such as unclear study design, significantly unbalanced allocation of patients to intervention and control arms, poorly specified randomization procedures, and lack of blinding. Although the studies did report efficacy, the methodological flaws prevented firm conclusions of safety or efficacy.

A subsequent study from the Institute of Basic Research in Clinical Medicine, China Academy of Chinese Medical Sciences, Beijing, and published in English in abstract form, evaluated Dianxianning (Table 22.1) as add-on to ASMs in a three-month, multi-centre, prospective, randomized, placebo-controlled trial [24]. Nearly twice as many patients were randomized to the active intervention as to the control group. In the group receiving add-on Dianxianning, seizures were reduced by 37.84% compared to 13.18% reduction in the placebo group (p < 0.05).

Cannabis and its Derivatives

Fueled by widespread media reports about a young girl with epilepsy and her use of a cannabidiol-enriched strain of marijuana [25], as well as uncontrolled published surveys [26,27], there has been a resurgence of interest in cannabis for epilepsy, and in particular cannabinoids such as cannabidiol (CBD) that are either extracted from cannabis or chemically synthesized. Several recent reviews outline the pharmacological basis for developing cannabis for medication-resistant epilepsy [28–30].

A Cochrane review of CBD clinical studies published between 1979 and 1990, including 48 patients with epilepsy, concluded that 200–300 mg/day CBD in adults was generally well tolerated, but drew no conclusions about long-term safety, and evidence for efficacy was absent, given the low number of enrolled patients [31]. Another review evaluated eight studies with a total of 105 children and adults with epilepsy treated with placebo or cannabis compounds, including CBD, tetrahydrocannabinol (THC), and CBD/THC combinations with less than 10% THC and found that 61% of patients receiving cannabinoids had improved seizure control with no reported serious adverse events [32].

More recently, three double-blind, placebo-controlled trials of CBD have identified efficacy for two forms of epilepsy. The trials had the standard efficacy trial rigor, and the results were the basis for an FDA approval of the investigated CBD formulation in 2018. Two of the trials investigated efficacy for reducing drop seizures due to Lennox–Gastaut syndrome and together included 396 patients [33,34]. The other trial investigated efficacy for convulsive seizures due to Dravet's syndrome and included 120 patients [35]. As such, the FDA's CBD approval is for seizures associated with these specific forms of epilepsy. Determination of the efficacy of CBD for other forms of epilepsy and seizure types is ongoing along with investigations of other phytocannabinoids, such as cannabidivarin [20].

Therapeutic Use of Botanicals in a Western-Style Clinical Healthcare System and Public Dissemination of Botanical Knowledge

The significant challenge of obtaining reliable information on the medical use of botanicals, especially in regard to their relative effectiveness [36], and particularly in the context of principles of Western medicine, has spawned the scientific field of ethnobotany. This field is the basis for a present-day model of clinical practice known as anthroposophic medicine, in which detailed information on medical uses of botanicals is systematically collected from experienced practitioners and put into a compendium called the *Vademecum of Anthroposophic Medicines* [37]. Anthroposophic medicine is a comprehensive system of integrative medicine, including the use of botanical therapies, that was founded in the 1920s in Switzerland and Germany, and which is practiced worldwide as well as in specifically dedicated, acute care hospitals in Germany, Switzerland and Sweden in conjunction with conventional Western medicine [37].

To further facilitate research and development efforts in botanical therapies, a publically available wiki called Epilepsy Naturapedia (www.epilepsynaturapedia.com/index.php/Main_Page) launched under the auspices of the ILAE. It constitutes the most comprehensive repository available of current scientific and medical knowledge regarding botanical therapies in epilepsy, written and updated by credentialled experts who have published relevant research in peer-reviewed journals.

Conclusion

Despite the significant and centuries-long use of botanicals by people with epilepsy around the world, as well as the growing literature of laboratory studies demonstrating the anti-convulsant properties of botanical products, there is a striking lack of controlled evidence to support their use for patients with medication-resistant epilepsy, and some anecdotal reports suggest that certain botanical therapies may pose a safety risk to this population. Absence of proof of efficacy and safety, however, is not necessarily proof of absence, and the centuries-old traditions of use of botanical therapies for epilepsy provide a rational foundation for systematic pre-clinical studies using widely accepted, modern scientific methods to identify promising botanical therapies for further clinical study under appropriate regulatory guidelines [8,38].

As illustrated by the ongoing work on cannabis and its derivatives, some botanical therapies may eventually emerge as new treatment options for patients with medication-resistant epilepsy and in addition may represent culturally acceptable treatments for the millions of people around the world who live with untreated epilepsy.

Key Points

- Botanical treatments are widely used in regions where herbal medicines are an accepted part of the healthcare system.
- Except for cannabidiol, controlled evidence does not support the use of botanical treatments for patients with medication-resistant epilepsy.
- Anecdotal reports suggest that certain botanical therapies may pose a safety risk.

References

1. Jain S. Ayurveda: the ancient Indian system of medicine. In: Devinsky O, Schachter S, Pacia S (eds.), *Complementary and Alternative Therapies for Epilepsy.* New York: Demos Medical Publishing, 2005:123–128

2. Gowers WR. *Epilepsy and Other Chronic Convulsive Diseases: Their Causes, Symptoms, & Treatment.* London: Churchill, 1881:264–268, 271

3. Sucher NJ, Carles MC. A pharmacological basis of herbal medicines for epilepsy. *Epilepsy Behav* 2015;**52**(Part B):308–318

4. Samuels N, Finkelstein Y, Singer SR, Oberbaum M. Herbal medicine and epilepsy: proconvulsive effects and interactions with antiepileptic drugs. *Epilepsia* 2008;**49**:373–380

5. Mbuba CK, Ngugi AK, Newton CR, Carter JA. The epilepsy treatment gap in developing countries: a systematic review of the magnitude, causes, and intervention strategies. *Epilepsia* 2008;**49**:1491–1503

6. Ngugi AK, Bottomley C, Kleinschmidt I, Sander JW, Newton CR. Estimation of the burden of active and life-time epilepsy: a meta-analytic approach. *Epilepsia* 2010;**51**:883–890

7. Lai CW, Lai YH. History of epilepsy in Chinese traditional medicine. *Epilepsia* 1991;**32**:299–302

8. Xiao F, Yan B, Chen L, Zhou D. Review of the use of botanicals for epilepsy in complementary medical systems: traditional Chinese medicine. *Epilepsy Behav.* 2015;**52**(Part B):281–289

9. Sriranjini SJ, Sandhya K, Mamta VS. Ayurveda and botanical drugs for epilepsy: current evidence and future prospects. *Epilepsy Behav.* 2015;**52**(Part B):290–296

10. Wahner-Roedler DL, Elkin PL, Vincent A, et al. Use of complementary and alternative medical therapies by patients referred to a fibromyalgia treatment program at a tertiary care center. *Mayo Clin Proc* 2005;**80**:55–60

11. Schachter SC Herbs and botanicals. In: Rho JM, Sankar R, Strafstrom CE (eds.) *Epilepsy: Mechanisms, Models, and Translational Perspectives.* Boca Raton, FL: CRC Press. 2010:403–411

12. Lai CW, Huang X, Lai, YHC, et al. A survey of public awareness, understanding and attitudes toward epilepsy in Henan Province, China. *Epilepsia* 1990;**31**:182–187

13. Hong Z, Qu B, Wu X-T, et al. Economic burden of epilepsy in a developing country: a retrospective cost analysis in China. *Epilepsia* 2009;**50**:2192–2198

14. Hu J, Si Y, Zhou D, et al. Prevalence and treatment gap of active convulsive epilepsy: a large community-based survey in rural West China. *Seizure* 2014;**23**:333–337

15. Danesi MA, Adetunji JB. Use of alternative medicine by patients with epilepsy: a survey of 265 epileptic patients in a developing country. *Epilepsia* 1994;**35**:344–351

16. Govindaraghavan S, Sucher NJ. Quality assessment of medicinal herbs and their extracts: criteria and prerequisites for consistent safety and efficacy of herbal medicines. *Epilepsy Behav* 2015;**52**(Part B):363–371

17. Liu FX, Salmon JW. Herbal medicine regulation in China, Germany and the United States. *Integr Med* 2010;**9**:54–61

18. Blumenthal M, Busse WR. *The Complete German Commission E Monographs: Therapeutic Guide to Herbal Medicines: Developed by a Special Expert Committee of the German Federal Institute for Drugs and Medical Devices.* Austin, TX: American Botanical Council.1998.

19. Hoffman FA. Botanicals as 'new' drugs: US development. *Epilepsy Behav* 2015;**52**(Part B):338–343

20. Ekstein D. Issues and promise in clinical studies of botanicals with anticonvulsant potential. *Epilepsy Behav* 2015;**52**(Part B):329–332

21. Luciano DJ, Spinella M. Herbal treatment of epilepsy: phytotherapy. In: Devinsky O, Schachter S, Pacia S (eds.) *Complementary and Alternative Therapies for Epilepsy,* New York: Demos Medical Publishing. 2005:143–155

22. Delgoda R, Westlake AC. Herbal interactions involving cytochrome p450 enzymes: a mini review. *Toxicol Rev* 2004;**23**:239–249

23. Li Q, Chen X, He L, Zhou D. Traditional Chinese medicine for epilepsy. *Cochrane Database Syst Rev* 2009;(3):CD006454

24. He L, Wen T, Yan S, et al. Reevaluation of the effect of Dianxianning on seizure rate of refractory epilepsy as additive treatment in clinical practice. *Front Med* 2011;**5**:229–234

25. Maa E, Figi P. The case for medical marijuana in epilepsy. *Epilepsia* 2014;**55**:783–786

26. Porter BE, Jacobson C. Report of a parent survey of cannabidiol-enriched cannabis use in pediatric treatment-resistant epilepsy. *Epilepsy Behav* 2013;**29**:574–577

27. Hussain SA, Zhou R, Jacobson C, et al. Perceived efficacy of cannabidiol-enriched cannabis extracts for treatment of pediatric epilepsy: a potential role for infantile spasms and Lennox–Gastaut syndrome. *Epilepsy Behav* 2015;**47**:138–141

28. Reddy DS, Golub V. The pharmacological basis of cannabis therapy for epilepsy. *J Pharmacol Exp Ther* 2016;**357**(1):45–55

29. Rosenberg EC, Tsien RW, Whalley BJ, Devinsky O. Cannabinoids and epilepsy. *Neurotherapeutics* 2015;**12**:747–768

30. Devinsky O, Cilio MR, Cross H, et al. Cannabidiol: pharmacology and potential role in epilepsy and other neuropsychiatric disorders. *Epilepsia* 2014;**55**:791–802

31. Gloss D, Vickrey B. Cannabinoids for epilepsy. *Cochrane Database Syst Rev* 2014;(3):CD009270

32. Szaflarski JP, Bebin EM. Cannabis, cannabidiol, and epilepsy: from receptors to clinical response. *Epilepsy Behav* 2014;**41**:277–282

33. Thiele EA, Marsh E, French JA, et al. Cannabidiol in patients with seizures associated with Lennox-Gastaut syndrome (GWPCARE4): a randomized, double-blind, placebo-controlled phase 3 trial. *Lancet* 2018;**391**:1085–1096

34. Devinsky O, Patel AD, Cross JH, et al. Effect of cannabidiol on drop seizures in the Lennox–Gastaut syndrome. *N Engl J Med* 2018;**378**:1888–1897

35. Devinsky O, Cross JH, Laux L, et al. Trial of cannabidiol for drug-resistant seizures in the Dravet syndrome. *N Engl J Med* 2017;**376**:2011–2020

36. Schachter SC. Botanicals and herbs: a traditional approach to treating epilepsy. *Neurotherapeutics* 2009;**6**:415–420

37. Elsas SM. A model on how to obtain data from botanical practitioners. *Epilepsy Behav* 2015;**52**(Part B):333–337

38. Schachter SC. Herbal therapies for epilepsy. In: Schwartzkroin PA (ed.) *Encyclopedia of Basic Epilepsy Research*. Oxford: Academic Press.2009:1450–1454

Psychiatric Comorbidities in Medication-Resistant Epilepsy

Andres M. Kanner

Introduction

The clinical manifestations of epilepsy are not restricted to epileptic seizures. They often include psychiatric and cognitive comorbidities, which need to be identified and treated as part of the comprehensive management of any patient with epilepsy (PWE). This is particularly relevant in patients with treatment-resistant epilepsy in whom the prevalence of these comorbidities is significantly higher.

Psychiatric disorders can be identified in 25% to 70% of PWE and include depression, anxiety, psychotic and attention deficit disorders as well as personality disorders; while they may be clinically identical to primary psychiatric disorders, they often display atypical clinical manifestations, which, as discussed below, is not unusual in medication-resistant epilepsy (MRE) [1–3]. While psychiatric comorbidities are often considered to reflect a complication of the seizure disorder, this may not always be the case, as their onset may often precede the first epileptic seizure [4, 5].

In patients with MRE, psychiatric symptomatology can be divided according to its temporal relation to the epileptic seizure and thus, can be the expression of an *interictal* psychiatric disorder, or can represent *peri-ictal* phenomena, which include *pre-ictal* symptomatology (when it precedes the seizure), *ictal*, when it is the expression of seizure activity and *postictal*, when the symptoms occur following seizures, typically after a symptom-free period that can range between a few hours to up to seven days [6]. In addition, psychiatric symptomatology can be the expression of a *para-ictal* phenomenon, that is, when their onset and remission are associated with the onset and/or remission of the seizure disorder [7]. Finally, psychiatric symptomatology can be the expression of an *iatrogenic* process associated with pharmacologic and/or surgical treatments of the seizure disorder.

The pathogenic mechanisms operant in psychiatric disorders of patients with MRE are multifactorial and their severity may be accentuated by the underlying seizure and neurologic disorders as well as by iatrogenic complications and /or psychosocial consequences of a 'chronic life with epilepsy'. For example, in a population-based study carried out in the Isle of White in Great Britain, Rutter and collaborators found behavioural disorders in 28.6% of children with uncomplicated seizures, and 58.3% of children with both seizures and additional central nervous system pathology (e.g. cerebral palsy and intellectual disabilities) [8]. Yet, in certain types of epileptic syndromes in which seizures are responsive to pharmacotherapy with anti-seizure drugs (ASMs), psychiatric disturbances may be the more serious problem. This phenomenon is illustrated by behavioural and cognitive disturbances in childhood absence epilepsy, benign focal epilepsy of childhood and juvenile myoclonic epilepsy (JME). For example, in a study of 100 patients with JME, psychiatric diagnoses were found in 49 patients. Anxiety and mood disorders were diagnosed in 23 and 19 patients, respectively, while a personality disorder was identified in 20 patients [9].

A comprehensive review of the psychiatric comorbidities in all forms of MRE would require a separate textbook and cannot be done justice in one chapter. Therefore, the aim of this chapter was restricted to provide a pragmatic review of the more common psychiatric comorbidities in adults with MRE, which includes an analysis of the available epidemiologic data of mood, anxiety, psychotic and personality disorders, a review of psychiatric symptomatology that is mainly identified in MRE, a summary of treatment strategies of common psychiatric comorbidities and their impact on the pharmacologic and surgical management of the seizure disorder. ADHD will not be included in this review, as its data in adults with MRE are very limited.

Epidemiologic Considerations

As stated above, patients with MRE have been found to be at higher risk of suffering from mood, anxiety, psychotic and personality disorders [1–3, 10–14]. Unfortunately, the epidemiologic data of psychiatric comorbidities in MRE has several limitations: 1) The reported prevalence rates vary widely among studies, based on the methodology used to identify the psychiatric phenomena. Some studies used screening instruments designed to identify "psychiatric symptoms", while others have relied on structured and semi-structured interviews aimed at identifying categorical psychiatric disorders based on the Diagnostic and Statistical Manual of Mental Disorders (DSM) classifications. 2) Psychiatric disorders often present with atypical clinical manifestations and do not always meet diagnostic criteria suggested in one of the DSM editions. 3) Most of the available studies have investigated mood, anxiety and psychotic disorders, while little data exist on personality disorders. 4) Very few studies that have investigated peri-ictal psychiatric symptomatology and those available have limited their investigation to postictal psychotic episodes, while very little data are available on peri-ictal depression and anxiety episodes despite the fact that they occur with a relatively high frequency in MRE [6]. Taking into consideration these limiting factors, a review of published case series of patients with MRE suggests that the prevalence-rates of psychiatric comorbidities range from 30% to 70%.

Depression has been reported to be the most frequent psychiatric comorbidity in PWE and three separate community-based studies found higher prevalence rates (21% and 33%) among those with persistent seizures than seizure-free patients (4 to 6%) [1–3]. Yet, high lifetime prevalence rates have been identified in a population-based study carried-out in Canada, in which a 30 to 35% lifetime history of depression and anxiety disorder was found in PWE [1]. Since this study was not limited to people with MRE, the question of whether a higher prevalence is more likely to occur in treatment-resistant epilepsy has to be re-evaluated. This point is supported by a study which consisted of a meta-analysis of 27 studies which investigated the pooled prevalence rates of mood and anxiety disorders encompassing more than 3000 patients [15]. The authors found prevalence rates of 22% and 23%, respectively and no difference between seizure-free patients and patients with MRE. Depression has been more frequently associated with focal epilepsy of temporal or frontal lobe origin, which is not surprising, given the involvement of limbic structures [16, 17].

Anxiety is the second most common psychiatric comorbidity in PWE, with an estimated prevalence between 15 and 25% [1, 2, 3, 4, 12, 15]. For example, in 174 consecutive patients with epilepsy from five epilepsy centers, half of whom had treatment-resistant epilepsy a current DSM-IV diagnosis of anxiety disorder was found in 30% of patients [18].

Psychotic disorders in PWE include interictal psychotic episodes, which can be identical to the primary schizophreniform disorder, schizophrenia-like psychosis of epilepsy (SLPE), postictal psychotic (PIP) episodes and para-ictal psychotic episodes that result from the phenomenon of alternative psychosis or 'forced normalization'. The prevalence of interictal psychotic disorders in epilepsy has been found to range from 7% to 10%, compared to rates of 0.4% and 1%, in the general population [19]. The prevalence rates of SLPE have ranged between 3% and 7%, corresponding to six to twelve times higher in epilepsy than in the general population [20]. The prevalence of postictal psychotic episodes is yet to be established but has been estimated to range between 6% and 10%, while recurrent postictal psychotic symptoms have been found in 7% of 100 consecutive patients with refractory partial epilepsy [21]. Finally, alternative psychosis (also known as forced normalization) have been estimated to occur in approximately 1% of patients with MRE [14, 20].

The association between MRE and an increased risk of schizophrenia was illustrated by a population-based study conducted in Israel. The authors found that among 861 062 17-year-old male adolescents consecutively screened by the Israeli Draft Board and found to be free of major mental illness, MRE was identified in 0.06%, while 0.25% had epilepsy which was in remission and an additional 0.16% had a history of seizures which had abated 5 or more years prior to screening [22]. Subjects were followed for an average follow-up of 9.6 ± 1.0 years (range: 1.0–10.0 years). Compared to the general population, adolescents with MRE had a significantly increased risk for hospitalization for schizophrenia (HR = 3.89, 95% CI = 1.75–89.67), while this was not seen for male seizure-free adolescents.

Personality disorders are a group of psychiatric comorbidities that result from individual endogenous and/or genetically facilitated disturbances and/or environmental maladaptive developmental conditions that yield behavioural traits that are deviant from sociocultural norms. These disorders interfere with the individual's capacity to cope with potential stressors and facilitate a psychiatric decompensation. Despite the significant negative impact that personality disorders have in PWE, there are very little data available. In a review of the literature, Devinsky et al. identified nine studies, two of which were large series of patients with MRE [10, 23], while the other were small series comparing personality disorders in PWE and psychogenic non-epileptic seizures [24]. In the two large case series, prevalence rates were 18% [10] and 61% in the other [23]. The higher prevalence in the latter study may be accounted for by the inclusion of a population of patients with a more chronic and severe epilepsy, associated with more psychiatric and psychosocial disabilities.

A Bidirectional Relation Between Psychiatric Disorders and Epilepsy and Its Impact in MRE

As stated above, psychiatric comorbidities may precede or follow the onset of the seizure disorder. Furthermore, epidemiologic studies have suggested that not only do PWE have a higher risk of developing a psychiatric disorder, but patients with primary psychiatry disorders have a higher risk of developing epilepsy. For example, Hesdorffer et al (2012) conducted a longitudinal cohort study using the United Kingdom's General Practice Research Data Base to investigate the temporal relation between the onset of psychiatric disorders and epilepsy in individuals 10 to 60 years old [4]. A total of 3 773 subjects that wenton to develop epilepsy were compared to 14 025 controls who went on to develop eczema; they were matched by year of birth, gender, general practice and years of medical records before the index date. The incidence rate ratios of psychosis, anxiety and depression were significantly higher during the three years preceding and during the three years that followed the diagnosis of epilepsy, while for suicidality there was a higher incidence rate ratio during the three years before the onset and one year after the diagnosis of epilepsy. In a Swedish population-based study, investigators compared the risk of developing unprovoked seizures or epilepsy among patients who had been hospitalized for a primary psychiatric disorder (n = 1 885) to a group of controls, matched for gender and year of diagnosis selected randomly from the register of the Stockholm County population [25]. The age-adjusted OR (95% confidence interval) for

unprovoked seizures was 2.5 (1.7–3.7) after a hospital discharge diagnosis for depression, 2.7 (1.4–5.3) for bipolar disorder, 2.3 (1.5–3.5) for psychosis, 2.7 (1.6–4.8) for anxiety disorders, and 2.6 (1.7–4.1) for suicide attempts. In a separate population-based study in Taiwan, patients with primary schizophreniform disorder had a 5.9-fold higher risk of developing epilepsy than controls (HR: 5.88; CI: 4.71–7.36), while patients with newly diagnosed epilepsy had a sevenfold higher risk of developing a schizophrenic disorder (HR: 7.65; CI: 6.04–9.69) [34].

It appears that this bidirectional relation may have an impact on the risk to develop MRE. For example, in a study of 780 patients with new onset epilepsy, individuals with a history of psychiatric disorders, and particularly depression, were two-fold less likely to be seizure-free with ASMs after a median follow-up period of 79 months compared to patients without a psychiatric history [26]. Likewise, in a prospective study of 138 patients with new onset epilepsy, those with symptoms of depression and anxiety at the time of diagnosis of epilepsy and before the start of pharmacotherapy with ASM were significantly less likely to be seizure-free at 12 months of follow-up [27]. Furthermore, several studies have found a worse post-surgical seizure outcome in patients with a lifetime history of psychiatric disorders, including depression, anxiety, psychosis and a personality disorder [28–31]. For example, in a study of 100 consecutive patients with treatment resistant TLE who had an anterotemporal lobe resection, those with a lifetime history of depression were significantly less likely to achieve complete freedom from auras and disabling seizures [28]. The largest case study, which included 434 patients whose psychiatric diagnosis was established with a formal psychiatric evaluation by an expert neuropsychiatrist, revealed that a prior history of personality disorder without and with another psychiatric disorders, were the worse predictors of post-surgical seizure outcome after temporal lobectomy [31]. These findings, however, have been refuted by other studies which have only focused on the impact of presurgical depression on post-surgical seizure outcomes [32, 33].

Psychiatric Phenomena That is Particular to MRE

As stated above, psychiatric comorbidities in PWE are often identical to primary psychiatric disorders and have been described in several publications by this and other authors and do not need to be reviewed again here. Instead, this section will focus on clinical expressions of psychiatric disorders that are identified mainly in MRE. These include: 1) postictal psychiatric symptoms and episodes; 2) para-ictal psychiatric episodes; 3) among interictal psychiatric disorders, the Interictal Dysphoric Disorder [17] and SLDE [20].

Postictal Psychiatric Phenomena

While cognitive, motor and sensory deficits typically occur during the immediate postictal phase (e.g., the period that follows a seizure and which typically has a duration of a few minutes to two hours but may occasionally last for up to 48 hours) postictal psychiatric symptoms (PPS) occur characteristically during a 'delayed' postictal phase, which follows a symptom-free period of 12 hours to up to seven-days duration. Postictal psychiatric phenomena may be the expression of de-novo isolated symptoms and/or clusters of PPS mimicking a depressive, anxiety or psychotic episode, but can also include postictal exacerbation in severity of interictal psychiatric symptoms. With the exception of PIP, PPS and non-psychotic postictal psychiatric episodes remain unrecognized by clinicians and have been investigated by very few authors.

Postictal Psychiatric Symptoms

The largest and most comprehensive study included 100 patients with MRE [6]. The PPS were identified with a 42-item questionnaire (The Rush Postictal Psychiatric Questionnaire) designed to identify 30 PPS and five cognitive symptoms. The PPS included symptoms of mood disorders (e.g. depression and mania), anxiety disorders (i.e. general anxiety, panic attacks, agoraphobia), obsessions and compulsions, psychotic symptoms, and neurovegetative symptoms. Each question inquired about the frequency of each symptom during the postictal and interictal periods in the course of the last 3 months. The postictal period was defined as the 72 hours that followed a seizure. Only symptoms that patients reported to occur after more than 50% of seizures were coded as PPS, so as to reflect a "habitual" phenomenon. For each symptom, patients were asked to estimate the average duration. For symptoms identified during both interictal and postictal periods, only symptoms reported to be significantly more severe during the postictal period were recorded and coded as postictal exacerbation of interictal symptoms. Seventy-nine patients had seizures of temporal and 21 of extratemporal lobe origin. Focal

seizures with loss of consciousness and secondarily GTC seizures were identified in about 50% of patients, while 78% of patients had more than one seizure per month. Fifty-four patients had a past psychiatric history and 11 had one or more psychiatric hospitalizations. A mean of 8.9 postictal symptoms (range 0 to 25; median 8.5) were identified among the 100 patients, including a mean of 2.8 postictal cognitive symptoms (PCS) (range 0 to 5; median 3) and a mean of 5.95 PPS (range 0 to 22; median 5). Seventy-four patients experienced at least one type of PPS; 68 reported PPS and PCS and 6 only PPS, while 14 patients experienced only PCS. Postictal symptoms of depression were identified in 43 patients, which included 13 patients with habitual postictal suicidal symptoms and 22 patients reported hypomanic symptoms; 45 patients endorsed postictal symptoms of anxiety, seven psychotic symptoms and 62 experienced postictal neurovegetative symptoms (e.g. change in appetite, sleep patterns, sexual drive). Of note, there was a high correlation in the occurrence of mood, anxiety, psychotic and neurovegetative symptoms. The median duration of these symptoms was 24 hours with ranges between 1 and 208 hours.

Postictal Psychiatric Episodes

Postictal psychiatric episodes are defined as clusters of PPS that mimic a psychiatric disorder with a minimal duration of 24 hours.

Postictal Depressive Episodes

The prevalence of postictal depressive episodes has yet to be established. In Kanner's study cited above [6], 18 patients experienced a minimum of six postictal symptoms of depression for a period of at least 24 hours; the semiology mimicked a typical major depressive episode, with the exception that the duration of the event was significantly shorter than the required 2 weeks of such episodes. Yet, patients may at times experience PDE of 1–3 weeks' duration.

Postictal Psychotic Episodes

In contrast to non-psychotic postictal psychiatric episodes, PIP have been recognized for the last 50 years, and in particular, since the advent of video-EEG monitoring studies, during which a drop in ASM doses and/or their discontinuation facilitate the occurrence of secondarily GTC seizures in clusters. PIP occur in patients who have suffered from a MRE for more than 10 years. As in the case of PPS, there is a symptoms-free period between the onset of psychotic symptoms and the last seizure. A period of agitation and/or insomnia often heralds the PIP by 12 hours. In patients with recurrent postictal psychotic episodes, families need to learn to recognize these symptoms so that a timely administration of a low dose neuroleptic drug (e.g. 1 to 2 mg of risperidone) can avert their evolution into a full psychotic episode. PIP are relatively short in duration (from hours up to a few weeks long) and include affect-laden delusional thinking with religious and/or grandiose contents, auditory and visual hallucinations, which tend to respond readily to low dose neuroleptic medication or even benzodiazepines [21, 34, 35]. A significant number of PIP follow the occurrence of clusters of secondarily generalized tonic–clonic seizures.

The presence of PIP should alert for the presence of bilateral independent *interictal* and *ictal foci* [35–37]. For example, in a study of 16 consecutive patients with MRE, a history of PIP was associated with bilateral independent *ictal* foci in close to 90% of patients [36]. Accordingly, patients with a prior history of PIP, or those who developed a PIP in the course of the presurgical evaluation may require longer video EEG monitoring studies with the aim of recording a larger number of seizures but avoiding their occurrence in clusters. Often, these patients may need a repeat video-EEG study with intracranial electrodes, in which case prophylactic treatment with low dose neuroleptic drugs (e.g. risperidone, quetiapine, apiprazole) can avert the occurrence of such episodes during the invasive video-EEG monitoring studies.

Patients who experience PIP are at increased risk of developing *interictal* psychotic episodes (IPE) [38, 39]. For example, Tarulli et al. found that 6 of 43 patients with an initial history of PIP went on to have episodes that met all the criteria for both PIP and IPE [39]. Five of the six patients had multiple documented PIP before they became chronically psychotic. The time period of 7 to 96 months separated the first PIP and the first IPE. Kanner and Ostrovskaya found that 7 of 18 patients with PIP went on to develop IPE, compared to 1 of 18 controls [38]. Other investigators have reported PIP preceding and/or following the occurrence of IPE [20].

Alternative Psychosis or "Forced Normalization"

The concept of alternative psychosis was derived from the initial observations by Landoldt in 1953, who reported the development of a *de-novo* psychotic episode associated with total remission of epileptic seizures in patients with MRE [40]. He described a 'normalization' of the EEG recordings (e.g. disappearance of the epileptiform activity) with the appearance of the psychiatric symptoms and coined the term 'forced normalization'. Forced normalization is a rare phenomenon which has been reported in patients with MRE and generalized epilepsies, with estimated prevalence rates of 1% [41]. As with other forms of psychosis of epilepsy, the psychotic manifestations were identified after a 15.2-year history of epilepsy in 23 patients reported by Wolf [14]. Both Landoldt and Wolf reported a pleomorphic clinical presentation with a paranoid psychosis without clouding of consciousness being the most frequent manifestation. A premonitory phase involving insomnia, anxiety, a feeling of oppression, and social withdrawal may occur in a prodromal phase. The clinical expression of the forced normalization phenomenon is not limited to psychotic episodes, but can also manifest as conversion symptoms, hypochondriasis, depression or mania.

Interictal Psychiatric Episodes

In patients with MRE, interictal mood and psychotic disorders may have atypical clinical manifestations. These include interictal dysphoric disorder and the SLPE.

Interictal Dysphoric Disorder

Interictal Dysphoric Disorder was initially described by Kraepelin in the beginning of the 20th century [42] and 20 and 30 years later by Bleuler [43] and Gastaut [44], respectively, but it was Blumer, in the second half of the 20th century, who brought it to the attention of the epilepsy community. It is estimated that 20 to 50% of the depressed PWE present this atypical type of depressive episode. It has a chronic course and includes a pleomorphic cluster of symptoms of depression, hypomania, anxiety, irritability and pain that waxes and wanes in severity and which are interrupted by symptom-free periods ranging from days to weeks. Yet, the belief that this form of depression is specific to epilepsy was disproven by Mula et al., who identified this type of depressive episode in patients with migraine [45].

Interictal Psychotic Episodes

As stated before, primary schizophreniform disorders may precede the onset of epilepsy and even increase the risk of developing epilepsy. On the other hand, patients with a chronic MRE can develop a psychotic disorder that differs clinically from a primary schizophreniform disorder and for which Slater coined the term SLPE, which is characterized by *the absence* of negative symptoms, better premorbid history, and less common deterioration of the patient's personality than those seen in primary schizophreniform disorder. In addition, this SLPE is less severe and more responsive to therapy [46].

Impact of Psychiatric Comorbidities on The Life of Patients with MRE

Psychiatric comorbidities impact the life of patients with MRE at several levels, which include: (a) worse quality of life; (b) worse tolerance of ASMs; (c) increased risk of iatrogenic psychiatric adverse events of ASMs and psychiatric complications of epilepsy surgery; (d) interference with the presurgical evaluation and ability to make a decision to proceed with surgery; (e) interference with postsurgical achievement with gainful employment and independent living; (f) worsening of cognitive functions; (g) increase suicidality risk. All of these result in-turn in an increased economic burden on the patient, the family and society as a whole. We will briefly review these issues below.

(a) Worse Quality of Life

Multiple studies have demonstrated a worse quality of life of PWE than in control subjects [47]. Furthermore, in patients with MRE, the presence of psychiatric comorbidities, particularly depression and anxiety have been found to account for worse health-related quality of life measures than the actual seizure frequency and type of seizures. For example, in a study of patients with MRE of temporal lobe origin, Gilliam et al. found that high ratings of depression and neurotoxicity from ASMs were the only independent variables significantly associated with poor quality of life scores on the QOLIE-89 summary score [48]. The authors *did not* find any correlation between the type and/or the frequency of seizures. These data were supported by a study by Lehrner et al. who found that depression was the single strongest predictor for each domain of health-related quality of life which persisted after controlling for seizure frequency, seizure severity, and other psychosocial variables [49]. Perrine et al., found that mood had the highest correlations with scales of the Quality of Life in Epilepsy Inventory-89 (QOLIE-89) and was the strongest

predictor of poor quality of life in regression analyses [50], while Kanner et al. found that the negative impact on QOL was not restricted to major depressive episodes or established anxiety disorders but was also associated with sub-syndromic forms of depression that had as negative an impact on quality of life as major depressive episodes and anxiety disorders [18]. Of note, reduction in seizure frequency has not been associated with a significant improvement in QOL measures, until a seizure-free state was reached.

The level of education and employment play a paramount role in the QOL of PWE. Unemployment and underemployment are significantly higher among PWE with some studies citing >50% of patients unemployed. These data are driven in particular by patients with MRE. Comorbid psychiatric disorders play a significant obstacle in patients attempting to seek vocational evaluations and gainful employment and the unemployment, inturn, worsens an underlying poor self-image and mood disorder. This vicious circle is also fed by the negative impact of comorbid mood disorder on cognitive functions, which interferes with the patient's educational needs to achieve employment.

Clearly, these data highlight the need to recognize at an early stage of the patient's seizure disorder and at every outpatient visit, the presence of comorbid psychiatric disorders and to incorporate their treatment into their comprehensive management. Sadly, implementation of these strategies remain an exception, rather than the rule, including in major epilepsy centers.

(b) Worse Tolerance of ASMs

The presence of comorbid mood and anxiety disorders has been associated with a worse tolerance of ASMs [51, 52]. For example, using the Adverse Event Profile to quantify the prevalence and severity of ASM-related adverse events, Kanner et al. demonstrated that compared to asymptomatic patients, patients with SSDE, MDE, anxiety disorders only or mixed MDE/anxiety disorders had significantly higher scores indicating, more severe AEs to ASMs [51]. These findings persisted even after deletion of mood and anxiety symptoms included in the AEP. Of note, these studies did not investigate the impact of psychotic attention-deficit and personality disorders, which are likely to yield a similar, if not greater impact.

Given the relatively high prevalence of psychiatric comorbidities in patients with MRE, these data bear significant implications in the analysis of tolerability of any ASM being tested for its safety and efficacy, which is first studied in this patient population. Thus, it is essential that the psychiatric profile of all subjects enrolled in these trials be accounted not only to assess if such therapies have an impact on the psychiatric disorder, but also to establish whether the psychiatric disorders may significantly modify their tolerability.

(c) Increased Risk of Iatrogenic Psychiatric Adverse Events of ASMs

A personal and/or a family psychiatric history have been identified in several studies as a risk factor for the development of psychiatric adverse events to ASMs including perampanel [53], topiramate [54], and levetiracetam [55, 56]. The development of iatrogenic psychiatric adverse events is mediated through three mechanisms: 1) The introduction of ASMs with negative psychotropic properties (barbiturates, benzodiazepines, topiramate, levetiracetam, zonisamide, vigabatrin, perampanel and brivaracetam). 2) The discontinuation of ASMs with mood stabilizing properties (e.g., carbamazepine, oxcarbazepine, valproic acid, lamotrigine) and/or anxiolytic properties (e.g. benzodiazepines, tiagabine, gabapentin, pregabalin) in patients whose mood and /or anxiety disorders had remitted and/or was kept in remission with one of these ASMs. 3) The introduction of ASMs with enzyme-inducing properties (e.g., carbamazepine, phenytoin, barbiturates) in PWE taking psychotropic drugs, whose clearance may be accelerated by these ASMs.

Patients with MRE, particularly those who are not candidates for epilepsy surgery are likely to be considered for trials with ASMs that may also have negative psychotropic properties. It is of the essence, therefore, that clinicians be aware of their personal and family psychiatric history when recommending these ASMs. While a psychiatric history is not a contraindication to start these ASMs, patients and family members need to be educated on the type of psychiatric adverse events they are at risk of developing so that they may be recognized in case and as soon as they occur. Conversely, the same considerations must be entertained before discontinuing an ASM with positive psychotropic properties.

(d) Impact on Epilepsy Surgery

The option of epilepsy surgery is the first treatment modality that is considered when a patient is diagnosed with MRE. As stated above, psychiatric comorbidities are relatively frequent in this patient population, with prevalence rates ranging between 40 and 70%. Current and/or past comorbid psychiatric histories can have an impact on the surgical treatment of epilepsy at several levels:

1) On the patient's ability to consider the surgical option and/or collaborate with the various studies involved in the presurgical evaluation and on their ability to make an informed consent. Indeed, depressed patients are more likely to be pessimistic about the potential benefits of any treatment option, and hence to reject outright the possibility of a possible cure of their seizure disorder with respective surgery or other treatment modalities. Furthermore, rapid discontinuation of ASMs with mood stabilizing properties during the video-EEG monitoring study in patients with a prior mood anxiety disorder may trigger panic attacks and resurgence of anxiety symptoms, which would derail the study. In addition, epileptologists in many epilepsy centers may disqualify patients from consideration for epilepsy surgery solely based on a prior psychiatric history, in particular psychotic disorders, even if they could be good surgical candidates from a neurophysiologic and a neuroimaging perspective.

2) On the development of psychiatric complications of epilepsy surgery. A presurgical psychiatric history has been associated with an increased risk of postsurgical psychiatric disturbances in patients undergoing a temporal lobectomy. Indeed, two reviews of the literature revealed that approximately 30% of patients undergoing epilepsy surgery are expected to develop a worsening and/or recurrence of a presurgical depressive and/or anxiety disorder during the first three to six months after surgery and approximately 10 to 15% of these may fail to remit after several pharmacologic interventions [58, 59]. For example, in a study of 60 patients undergoing a temporal lobe resection, a lifetime history of depression was identified in 43% of patients [60]. In the 12 months after surgery, 20 patients (33%) experienced a major depressive episode, identified in 70% in the first 3 months and persisting for at least 6 months in 65% of patients. A preoperative history of depression and poor postoperative family dynamics

were predictive of depression after surgery. The association of a presurgical history of depression with postsurgical recurrence has been replicated in several studies [60–62]. In one study, patients with a preoperative psychiatric history had more than six times the odds of developing a postoperative psychiatric disorder [62]. Furthermore, presurgical history of depression has been associated with post-surgical memory deficits in patients undergoing a left temporal lobectomy [63].

Completed suicide is the most serious post-surgical complication of temporal lobe resections. In one multicenter study that included 396 patients, 27 deaths were reported after surgery, four of which were attributed to suicide [64]. The standardized mortality ratio, compared with suicides in the U.S. population and adjusted for age and gender was 13.3 (95% CI = 3.6–34.0).

A history of personality disorders remains largely unexplored. Yet, one of the few studies that have investigated the impact of this psychiatric comorbidity on epilepsy surgery revealed an increased risk for the development of de-novo post-surgical psychotic episodes in these patients [23].

Conversely, remission of presurgical psychiatric disturbances after surgery is an under-recognized benefit of epilepsy surgery, affecting between 30 and 50% of patients [59]. In one study, post-surgical remission of depression was associated with good seizure control [65].

3) Interfering with a favourable post-surgical psychosocial outcome. It is assumed that patients with MRE who become seizure-free are likely to seek full employment and an independent living. While these goals are achieved by a significant percentage of seizure-free patients, this may not be the case in patients with presurgical history of anxiety disorders, associated with poor social interactions [66].

Clearly, these data call for the inclusion of a thorough psychiatric evaluation as part of the presurgical evaluation in every patient. Based on this evaluation, patients and family members need to be advised of the increased risk of psychiatric complications post-surgically.

(e) Impact on Suicidal Risk

Patients with epilepsy are at increased risk of suicide. In fact, suicide was found to account for an average of 11.5% of all deaths of PWE in a review of 21 studies that investigated suicide as the cause of death in this patient population [67]. A past psychiatric history increases significantly the risk. For example, in a Danish population-based study, PWE had a two-fold higher risk of completed suicide in the absence of any psychosocial problem. This risk increased by 32-fold in the presence of a mood disorder and 12-fold in the presence of an anxiety or schizophreniform disorders [68]. In a population-based study conducted in Sweden, mood disorders and substance/alcohol abuse were associated with an increased risk of premature death due to non-epilepsy related causes [69]. Finally, PIP have been also associated with an increased suicide risk [34].

(f) On Cognitive Functions

In patients with MRE, cognitive functions are very frequently affected. These may be further compromised by comorbid psychiatric disorders. For example, Hermann and collaborators identified three cognitive profiles in patients with focal epilepsy of temporal lobe origin [70]: Cluster 1, termed minimally impaired and which comprised almost 50% of the subjects studied identified lower scores in tests assessing immediate and delayed memory functions, language and psychomotor speed than those of controls, but had minimal clinical implications. Cluster 2 involved one fourth of the patients, whose neuropsychological profile displayed greater and significant involvement of immediate and delayed memory functions, with lesser involvement in the other cognitive domains, while Cluster 3 included the remaining patients with significant impairment across all cognitive domains. Patients in Cluster 2 were those with a chronic epilepsy in whom decrease in grey matter volumes extended beyond mesial temporal structures to temporal lateral neocortex and minimal involvement in frontal and parietal regions, while those in Cluster 3 had multilobar grey matter and diffuse white matter involvement and most likely corresponding to patients with MRE. Depression is known to have a negative impact on cognitive functions mediated by frontal lobes and, in fact, Hermann's team was also the first to point out that neuropsychological testing in TLE patients with a comorbid depressive disorder may present dysfunction of frontally mediated cognitive functions. There is agreement that mood disorders have a negative impact on the subjective perception of memory processing, while their impact on neuropsychological memory tests is still a source of discussion.

Treatment of Psychiatric Comorbidities in MRE: Practical Considerations

Given the data discussed above, any reasonable reader of this chapter would expect to see a plethora of data available on the management of psychiatric comorbidities in MRE. Sadly, nothing is further from the truth. In fact, there is only one controlled trial which has compared the efficacy of sertraline to cognitive behaviour therapy in the treatment of major depression in PWE [71]. This study demonstrated remission of symptoms of depression in 60% of patients treated with either therapy. No other controlled trials exist on the pharmacologic management of anxiety and psychotic disorder in PWE, despite their frequent atypical manifestations. Accordingly, clinicians must use the therapeutic strategies followed in the management of primary psychiatric disorders with the assumption that they apply as well to patients with MRE [72].

A long-held concern that psychotropic drugs are associated with a proconvulsant effect has been an obstacle in the pharmacologic treatment of PWE, and even more in patients with MRE, for fear that these drugs would further worsen the seizure disorder. Yet, a review of the available data on the proconvulsant properties of psychotropic drugs suggest the following facts: With respect to antidepressant drugs, an association between seizure occurrence and exposure to these agents was established when these drugs are used at toxic doses, particularly in the case of overdoses. In fact, in one study conducted in patients with primary psychiatric disorders who were participating in phase II and III multicenter, randomized, placebo-controlled trials between 1985 and 2004, the investigators compared the incidence of seizures between those randomized to a psychotropic drug and those given placebo [73]. The trials included antidepressants of the tricyclic (TCA), selective serotonin-reuptake inhibitor (SSRI) and serotonin-norepinephrine reuptake inhibitor (SNRI) families as well as bupropion, anxiolytic drugs and atypical antipsychotic drugs. Subjects suffering from mood and anxiety disorders randomized to antidepressants were 52% less likely (69% less likely when excluding bupropion immediate release formulation) to develop seizures compared to those randomized to placebo. In

addition, patients randomized to placebo were 19 times more likely to experience a seizure compared to the expected incidence in the general population. The investigators found an increased seizure incidence in patients randomized to clomipramine (indicated for the treatment of obsessive compulsive disorder) and bupropion in its immediate release form. With respect to antipsychotic medications, an increase seizure incidence was found among subjects randomized to the antipsychotics clozapine and olanzapine and to a lesser degree quetiapine, than those given placebo. Among the first- and second-generation antipsychotic chlorpromazine at doses >1000 mg/day and loxapine are the drugs with proconvulsant properties, while those with a lower seizure risk include haloperidol, molindone, fluphenazine, perphenazine and trifluoperazine [85]. The risk of seizure occurrence or worsening of seizures with psychotropic drugs in PWE has not been well studied. Pacia and Devinsky reviewed the incidence of seizures among 5629 patients treated with clozapine [74]. Sixteen of these patients had epilepsy before the start of this APD and all patients experienced worsening of seizures while on the drug: eight patients at doses lower than 300 mg/day, three patients at doses between 300 and 600 mg/day, and five at doses higher than 600 mgs/day. Higher doses of clozapine were associated with greater risk of seizures than lower dose therapy. It goes without saying that clozapine should be avoided or used in exceptional circumstances with extreme caution in patients with epilepsy.

Most antipsychotic drugs can cause EEG changes consisting of slowing of the background activity particularly when used at high doses, while epileptiform discharges have been reported with the use of clozapine, although they are not predictive of seizure occurrence. Data from studies by Tiihonen et al. suggest that a severe disorganization of the EEG recordings is a better predictor of seizure occurrence [75].

Clinicians must also consider the pharmacokinetic and pharmacodynamic interactions between psychotropic drugs and ASMs. Induction of hepatic enzymes following the introduction of enzyme inducing ASMs may result in an increase of the clearance of most antipsychotic and antidepressant drugs including TCAs, SSRIs, mirtazapine, trazadone, first generation antipsychotic (including chlorpromazine, fluphenazine and haloperidol) and atypical antipsychotics (including clozapine, olanzapine, risperidone [with the exception of phenytoin which inhibits its clearance], quetiapine, aripiprazole and ziprazidone). By the same token, discontinuation of an ASM with enzyme inducing properties may result in a decrease in their clearance, which in turn can lead to extrapyramidal side effects caused by an increase of the serum concentrations of certain antipsychotic drugs.

Finally, certain antiepileptic drugs, like valproic acid, can decrease the clearance of certain TCAs (amitriptyline, nortriptyline) and antipsychotic drugs (clozapine, olanzapine, quetiapine). Given that the second and third-generation ASMs are in general less reliant upon the CYP isoenzyme system for their disposition, it is likely that there will be fewer opportunities for pharmacokinetic interactions with other ASMs, psychotropic drugs and other concomitant medications.

Conversely, several psychotropic drugs can inhibit the clearance of some enzyme-inducing ASMs, in particular phenytoin and carbamazepine. The psychotropic drugs include the antidepressants of the SSRI family fluoxetine, fluvoxamine and paroxetine, some of the first-(haloperidol and loxapine) and second-generation antipsychotic drugs (risperidone, quetiapine). Citalopram and escitalopram do not have an inhibitory effect on other drugs, while the inhibitory effect of sertraline is minimal. Although definitive studies are lacking, it has also been suggested that venlafaxine and duloxetine are unlikely to cause significant interactions with currently available ASMs. Accordingly, clinicians must remember to adjust the dose of psychotropic drugs and ASMs to achieve optimal serum concentrations.

The following pharmacodynamic interactions between psychotropic drugs and ASMs need to be considered when prescribing the former:

(a) All antipsychotic drugs can potentially increase the QT interval; among the first-generation antipsychotic drugs, haloperidol, fluphenazine and trifluoperazine are the ones with the higher risk, while ziprasidone is the second-generation antipsychotic drug with the greater risk. Accordingly, EKG studies should be performed before starting these drugs and once a target dose is reached, given that PWE are at increased risk of sudden death where prolonged QT has been one of the possible pathogenic mechanisms.

(b) Antidepressant drugs of the SSRI and SNRI families can increase the risk of bleeding. Thus, they should be used in a cautious manner in PWE on anticoagulants and NSAIDs.

(c) Antidepressant drugs of the SSRI family can facilitate the development of hyponatraemia by causing a syndrome of inappropriate antidiuretic hormone. Thus, serum electrolytes must be monitored in patients taking these drugs and in particular if they are on the ASMs carbamazepine, oxcarbazepine and eslicarbazepine.

(d) Drugs of the SSRI family have been associated with the development of osteopaenia and osteoporosis in population-based studies [76]. Thus, in addition to the supplementation of vitamin D3 and calcium, bone mineral density studies should be performed, particularly in PWE who are taking enzyme-inducing ASMs.

Obstacles to Treatment of Psychiatric Comorbidities in Patients with MRE

While there is a universal acceptance of the need to identify and treat psychiatric comorbidities in patients with MRE, it has yet to translate into the implementation of treatment strategies. Several reasons account for this contradiction: 1) Most epilepsy centers (including in the United States National Association of Epilepsy Centers (NAEC) level-4) do not have psychiatrists as part of the epilepsy team and very few centers include a psychiatric evaluation as part of the presurgical work-up. 2) In a majority of centers, psychiatric evaluations are replaced by neuropsychological evaluations, which are complementary but different from psychiatric evaluation. 3) In most centers, psychiatric evaluations are conducted by psychiatrists from the Liaison and Consultation team, who often lack the knowledge and expertise of psychiatric aspects of epilepsy. 4) All of these problems may be probably self-inflicted by neurologists who have failed to recognize the need to have a psychiatrist as part of the epilepsy team. Indeed, while the NAEC guidelines recognize the need to identify and treat psychiatric comorbidities, they do not list psychiatrists as essential personnel of an epilepsy center. Clearly, this bizarre phenomenon is symptomatic of a more serious problem of the lack of meaningful communication and interaction between psychiatrists and neurologists, the cause of which are multiple, but most importantly, the lack of education by neurologists on psychiatric comorbidities of neurologic disorders and vice-versa the poor training by psychiatrists of the neurologic and psychiatric aspects of psychiatric comorbidities of neurologic disorders. Until both disciplines start to recognize and act on this fundamental problem and try to find objective solutions, psychiatric comorbidities of PWE will continue to go under-treated. After all, Goethe summarized this problem in 'Faust' when he wrote: 'We see what we know'.

Key Points

- Psychiatric comorbidity is frequent in treatment-resistant epilepsy.
- It accounts, to a greater degree than seizures, for the poor quality of life of these patients.
- Postictal and para-ictal psychiatric episodes are identified primarily in treatment-resistant epilepsy.
- Psychiatric disorders preceding the onset of epilepsy appear to be a risk factor for treatment-resistant epilepsy.
- Treatment of psychiatric comorbidities must be part of the comprehensive management of the treatment-resistant epilepsy.
- Psychotropic drugs do not worsen seizures when used at therapeutic doses in patients with treatment-resistant epilepsy.

References

1. Tellez-Zenteno JF, Patten SB, Jetté N, Williams J, Wiebe S. Psychiatric Comorbidity in Epilepsy: A Population-Based Analysis. *Epilepsia*, 2007; **48**:2336–2344

2. Jones JE, Herman BP, Berry JJ, Gilliam F, Kanner AM, Meador KJ. Clinical assessment of Axis I psychiatric morbidity in chronic epilepsy: a multicenter investigation. *J Neuropsychiatry Clin Neurosci* 2005 Spring;**17**(2):172–179

3. O'Donoghue MF, Goodridge DM, Redhead K, Sander JW, Duncan JS. Assessing the psychosocial consequences of epilepsy: a community-based study. *Br J Gen Pract* 1999;**49**(440):211–214

4. Hesdorffer DC, Ishihara L, Mynepalli L, Webb DJ, Weil J, Hauser WA. Epilepsy, suicidality, and psychiatric disorders: a bidirectional association. *Ann Neurol* 2012;**72**:184–191

5. Hesdorffer DC, Ludvigsson P, Olafsson E, Gudmundsson G, Kjartansson O, Hauser WA. ADHD as a risk factor for incident unprovoked seizures and epilepsy in children. *Arch Gen Psychiatry.* 2004;**61**:731–736

6. Kanner AM, Soto A, Gross-Kanner H. Prevalence and clinical characteristics of postictal psychiatric symptoms in partial epilepsy. *Neurology* 2004; 62:708–713

7. Robertson, M. Forced normalization and the etiology of depression in epilepsy. In: M.R. Trimble, B. Schmitz (Eds.) *Forced Normalization and Alternative Psychosis of Epilepsy.* Wrightson Biomedical, Petersfield, UK; 1998:143–168.

8. Rutter M, Graham P, Yule W.A. *Neuropsychiatric Study in Childhood.* Philadelphia: JB Lippincott, 1970.

9. Filho G, Rosa V, Lin K, Caboclo L, Sakamoto A, Yacubian EMT. Psychiatric comorbidity in epilepsy: a study comparing patients with mesial temporal sclerosis and juvenile myoclonic epilepsy. *Epilepsy Behav* 2008;**13**:196–201

10. Manchanda R, Schaefer B, McLachlan RS, et al. Psychiatric disorders in candidates for surgery for epilepsy. *J Neurol Neurosurg Psychiatry* 1996;**61**:82–89

11. Sanchez-Gistau V, Pintor L, Sugranyes G, et al. Prevalence of interictal psychiatric disorders in patients with refractory temporal and extratemporal lobe epilepsy in Spain. A comparative study. *Epilepsia* 2010;**51**:1309–1313

12. Brandt C, Schoendienst M, Trentowska M, et al. Prevalence of anxiety disorders in patients with refractory focal epilepsy-a prospective clinic based survey. *Epilepsy Behav* 2010;**17**:259–263

13. Jones JE, Hermann BP, Barry JJ, Gilliam FG, Kanner AM, Meador KJ. Rates and risk factors for suicide, suicidal ideation, and suicide attempts in chronic epilepsy. *Epilepsy Behav* 2003;**4**(Suppl 3):S31–38

14. Wolf P., Trimble M. R. (1985). Biological antagonism and epileptic psychosis. *Br J Psychiatry*, 146;272–276

15. Scott AJ, Sharpe L, Hunt C, and Gandy M. Anxiety and depressive disorders in people with epilepsy: A meta-analysis. *Epilepsia*, **58**(6):973–982, 2017

16. Kanner AM, Ettinger A. Anxiety disorders in epilepsy. In: J Engel and T Pedley, eds. *Epilepsy: A Comprehensive Textbook.* Lippincott, Williams and Wilkins: Baltimore, 2008.

17. Kanner AM and Blumer D. Affective disorders in epilepsy. In: J Engel and T Pedley, eds. Epilepsy: A Comprehensive Textbook. Lippincott, Williams and Wilkins: Baltimore, 2008.

18. Kanner AM, Barry JJ, Gilliam F, Hermann B, Meador KJ. Anxiety Disorders, Sub-Syndromic Depressive Episodes and Major Depressive Episodes: Do they Differ on their Impact on the Quality of Life of Patients with Epilepsy? *Epilepsia*, 2010; **51**:1152–1158.

19. Toone BK, Garralda ME, Ron MA. The psychosis of epilepsy and the functional psychosis: a clinical and phenomenological comparison. *Br J Psychiat*, 1982;**141**:256–261

20. Kanner AM, Rivas-Grajales AM. Psychosis of epilepsy: a multifaceted neuropsychiatric disorder. *CNS Spectr*, 2016 Jun;**21**(3):247–257

21. Kanner AM, Stagno S, Kotagal P, Morris HH: The incidence of postictal psychiatric events in prolonged video-EEG monitoring studies. *Archives of Neurology*, 1996, **53**:258–263

22. Fruchter E, Kapara O, Reichenberg A, Yoffe R, Fono-Yativ O, Kreiss Y, Davidson M, Weiser M. Longitudinal association between epilepsy and schizophrenia: a population-based study. *Epilepsy Behav* 2014 Feb;**31**:291–294

23. Koch-Stoecker S. Personality disorders as predictors of severe post-surgical psychiatric complications in epilepsy patients undergoing temporal lobe resections. *Epilepsy Behav* 2002;526–531

24. Devinsky O, Vorkas C, Barr W, Hermann B. Personality Disorders in Epilepsy. In: J Engel Jr and TA Pedley, Eds. *Epilepsy:A Comprehensive Textbook.* Second Edition. Lippincott, Williams & Wilkins: New York, pp 2105–2112.

25. Adelow C, Anderson T, Ahlbom A, Tomson T. Hospitalization for psychiatric disorders before and after onset of unprovoked seizures/epilepsy. *Neurology* 2012;**78**:396–401.

26. Hitiris N, Mohanraj R, Norrie J, et al. Predictors of pharmacoresistant epilepsy. *Epilepsy Res* 2007;**75**:192–196

27. Petrovski S, Szoeke CEI, Jones NC, Salzberg MR, Sheffield LJ, Huggins RM, et al.Neuropsychiatric symptomatology predicts seizure recurrence in newly treated patients. *Neurology* 2010;**75**:1015–1021

28. Kanner AM, Byrne R, Chicharro A, et al. A lifetime psychiatric history predicts a worse seizure outcome following temporal lobectomy. *Neurology* 2009;**72**:793–739

29. Cleary RA, Thompson PJ, Fox Z, Foong J. Predictors of psychiatric and seizure outcome following temporal lobe epilepsy surgery. *Epilepsia* 2012;**53**(10):1705–1712

30. de Araújo Filho GM, Gomes FL, Mazetto L, Marinho MM, Tavares IM, Caboclo LO, et al. Major depressive disorder as a predictor of a worse seizure outcome one year after surgery in patients with temporal lobe epilepsy and mesial temporal sclerosis. *Seizure* 2012;**8**:619–623

31. Koch-Stoecker SC, Bien CG, Schulz R, May TW. Psychiatric lifetime diagnoses are associated with a reduced chance of seizure freedom after temporal lobe surgery. *Epilepsia* 2017 Jun;**58**(6):983–993

32. Lackmayer K, Lehner-Baumgartner E, Pirker S, et al. Preoperative depressive symptoms are not predictors of postoperative seizure control in patients with mesial temporal lobe epilepsy and hippocampal sclerosis. *Epilepsy Behav* 2013; **26**:81–86

33. Adams SJ, Velakoulis D, Kaye AH, et al. Psychiatric history does not predict seizure outcome following temporal lobectomy for mesial temporal sclerosis. *Epilepsia* 2012; **53**:1700–1704

34. Kanemoto K, Kawasaki J, Kawai I. Postictal psychosis: a comparison with acute interictal and chronic psychoses. *Epilepsia* 1996;**37**:551–556

35. Logsdail SJ, Toone BK. Post-ictal psychoses. A clinical and phenomenological description. *Br J Psychiatry* 1998;**152**:246–252

36. Kanner AM and Ostrovskaya A. Long-term significance of postictal psychotic episodes II. Are they predictive of interictal psychotic episodes? *Epilepsy Behav* 2008 Jan;**12**(1):154–156

37. Umbricht D, Degreef G, Barr WB, Lieberman JA, Pollack S, Schaul N. Postictal and chronic psychoses in patients with temporal lobe epilepsy. *Am J Psychiatry* 1995;**152**:224–231

38. Kanner AM and Ostrovskaya A. Long-term significance of postictal psychotic episodes I. Are they predictive of bilateral ictal foci? *Epilepsy Behav* 2008 Jan;**12**(1):150–153

39. Tarulli, A., Devinsky, O., & Alper, K. (2001). Progression of postictal to interictal psychosis. [Case Reports]. *Epilepsia* **42**(11),1468–1471

40. Landoldt, H. (1953). Some clinical electroencephalographical correlations in epileptic psychosis (twilight states). *Electroencephalogr Clin Neurophysiol 5*, 121 (abstract)

41. Schmitz B, Trimble MR: Epilogue. In: Trimble MR, Schmitz B, ed. *Forced Normalization and Alternative Psychoses of Epilepsy*. Petersfield: Wrightson Biomedical Publishing, 1998:221–227

42. Kraepelin E. *Psychiatrie*, vol **3**. Leipzig: Johann Ambrosius Barth, 1923.

43. Bleuler E. *Lehrbuch der Psychiatrie*, 8th ed. Berlin: Springer, 1949.

44. Gastaut H, Roger J, Lesèvre N. Différenciation psychologique des épileptiques en fonction des formes électrocliniques de leur maladie. *Rev Psychol Appl* 1953;**3**:237–249

45. Mula M, Jauch R, Cavanna A, Collimedaglia L, Barbagli D, Gaus V, Kretz R, Viana M, Tota G, Israel H, Reuter U, Martus P, Cantello R, Monaco F, Schmitz B. Clinical and psychopathological definition of the interictal dysphoric disorder of epilepsy. *Epilepsia* 2008 Apr;**49**(4):650–656

46. Slater E, Beard A W, Glithero E. The schizophrenialike psychoses of epilepsy. *Br J Psychiatry* 1963 **109**:95–150

47. Gilliam, F. (2002). Optimizing health outcomes in active epilepsy. *Neurology, 58*(8 Suppl 5)S9–20

48. Gilliam F, Kuzniecky R, Faught E, Black L, Carpenter G, Schrodt R. Patient-validated content of

epilepsy-specific quality-of-life measurement. *Epilepsia* 1997, **38**(2)233–236

49. Lehrner J, Kalchmayr R, Serles W, Olbrich A, Pataraia E, Aull S, Baumgartner C. Health-related quality of life (HRQOL), activity of daily living (ADL) and depressive mood disorder in temporal lobe epilepsy patients. *Seizure* 1999, **8**(2)88–92

50. Perrine K, Hermann B P, Meador K J, Vickrey B G, Cramer J A, Hays R D, Devinsky O. The relationship of neuropsychological functioning to quality of life in epilepsy. *Arch Neurol* 1995, **52**(10)997–1003

51. Kanner AM, Barry JJ, Gilliam F, Hermann B, Meador KJ. Depressive and anxiety disorders in epilepsy: Do they differ in their potential to worsen common antiepileptic drug-related adverse events? *Epilepsia* 2012. 53(6):1104–1108

52. Perucca P, Jacoby A, Marson AG, Baker GA, Lane S, Benn EK, Thurman DJ, Hauser WA, Gilliam FG, Hesdorffer DC. Adverse antiepileptic drug effects in new-onset seizures: a case-control study. *Neurology* 2011 Jan 18;**76**(3):273–279

53. Kanner AM, perampanel

54. Mula M, Trimble MR, Lhatoo SD, Sander JW. Topiramate and psychiatric adverse events in patients with epilepsy. *Epilepsia* 2003 May;**44** (5):659–663

55. Josephson CB, Engbers JDT, Jette N, Patten SB, Singh S, et al.Prediction Tools for Psychiatric Adverse Effects After Levetiracetam Prescription. *JAMA Neurol* 2019 Apr 1;**76**(4):440–446

56. Mula M, Trimble MR, Yuen A, Liu RS, Sander JW. Psychiatric adverse events during levetiracetam therapy. *Neurology* 2003;**61**(5):704–706

57. Kanner AM. Management of psychiatric and neurological comorbidities in epilepsy. *Nat Rev Neurol* 2016 Feb;**12**(2):106–116

58. Fasano RE, Kanner AM. Psychiatric complications after epilepsy surgery… but where are the psychiatrists? *Epilepsy Behav* 2019; **98**, Part B:318–321

59. Wrench JM, Rayner G, Wilson SJ. Profiling the evolution of depression after epilepsy surgery. *Epilepsia* 2011;**52**:900–908

60. Ring HA, Moriarty J, Trimble MR. A prospective study of the early postsurgical psychiatric associations of epilepsy surgery. *J Neurol Neurosurg Psychiatry* 1998 May;**64**(5):601–604

61. Wrench J, Wilson SJ, Bladin PF. Mood disturbance before and after seizure surgery: A comparison of temporal and extratemporal resections. *Epilepsia* 2004;**45**:534–543

62. Barbieri V, Cardinale F, Luoni A, et al. Risk factors for postoperative depression in 150 subjects treated for drug-resistant focal epilepsy. *Epidemiol Psychiatr Sci* 2011;20:99–105

63. Sawrie SM, Martin RC, Kuzniecky R, et al. Subjective versus objective memory change after temporal lobe epilepsy surgery. *Neurology* 1999; 53:1511–1517

64. Hamid H, Devinsky O, Vickrey BG, et al. Suicide outcomes after resective epilepsy surgery. *Epilepsy Behav* 2011;20:462–464

65. Devinsky O, Barr WB, Vickrey BG, et al. Changes in depression and anxiety after resective surgery for epilepsy. *Neurology* 2005; 65:1744–1942

66. Ferguson SM, Rayport M. The adjustment to living without epilepsy. *J Nerv Ment Dis* 1965; 140:26–37

67. Jones JE, Hermann BP, Barry JJ, Gilliam FG, Kanner AM, Meador KJ. Rates and risk factors for suicide, suicidal ideation, and suicide attempts in chronic epilepsy. *Epilepsy Behav* 2003 4 (Suppl 3): S31–S38

68. Christensen J, Vestergaard M, Mortensen PB, Sidenius P, Agerbo E. Epilepsy and risk of suicide: a population-based case–control study. *Lancet Neurol* 2007;6:693–698

69. Fazel S, Wolf A, Långström N, Newton CR, Lichtenstein P. Premature mortality in epilepsy and the role of psychiatric comorbidity: a total population study. *Lancet* 2013 Nov 16;**382**(9905):1646–1654

70. Hermann B, Jones J, Sheth R, Dow C, Koehn M, Seidenberg M. Children with new-onset epilepsy: neuropsychological status and brain structure. *Brain* 2006 Oct;**129**(Pt 10):2609–2619

71. Gilliam FG, Black KJ, Carter J, Freedland KE, Sheline YI, Tsai WY, Lustman PJ. A Trial of Sertraline or Cognitive Behavior Therapy for Depression in Epilepsy. *Ann Neurol* 2019 Oct;**86**(4):552–560

72. Kerr MP, Mensah S, Besag F, et al. International consensus clinical practice statements for the treatment of neuropsychiatric conditions associated with epilepsy. *Epilepsia* 2011;52:2133–2138

73. Alper K, Schwartz K A, Kolts R L, Khan A. Seizure incidence in psychopharmacological clinical trials: an analysis of Food and Drug Administration (FDA) summary basis of approval reports. *Biol Psychiatry* 2007 **62**(4), 345–354

74. Pacia SV, Devinsky O. Clozapine-related seizures: experience with 5,629 patients. *Neurology* 1994 Dec;**44** (12):2247–2249

75. Tiihonen J, Nousiainen U, Hakola P, Leinonen E, Tuunainen A, Mervaala E, Paanila J. EEG abnormalities associated with clozapine treatment. *Am J Psychiatry* 1991 Oct;**148**(10):1406

76. Wang CY, Fu SH, Wang CL, Chen PJ, Wu FL, Hsiao FY. Serotonergic antidepressant use and the risk of fracture: a population-based nested case-control study. *Osteoporos Int* 2016 Jan;**27**(1):57–63

Index